PLACENTA

A NEGLECTED EXPERIMENTAL ANIMAL

PLACENTA
A NEGLECTED EXPERIMENTAL ANIMAL

Proceedings of a Round Table Discussion held at Bedford College, University of London, October 1978, under the auspices of the Special Commission on Internal Pollution

Editors

PETER BEACONSFIELD

Bedford College, University of London

CLAUDE VILLEE

Harvard Medical School, Boston, USA

Technical Editors

Rebecca Beaconsfield and George Birdwood

PERGAMON PRESS

OXFORD · NEW YORK · TORONTO · SYDNEY · PARIS · FRANKFURT

U.K. — Pergamon Press Ltd., Headington Hill Hall, Oxford OX3 0BW, England

U.S.A. — Pergamon Press Inc., Maxwell House, Fairview Park, Elmsford, New York 10523, U.S.A.

CANADA — Pergamon of Canada, Suite 104, 150 Consumers Road, Willowdale, Ontario M2J 1P9, Canada

AUSTRALIA — Pergamon Press (Aust.) Pty. Ltd., P.O. Box 544, Potts Point, N.S.W. 2011, Australia

FRANCE — Pergamon Press SARL, 24 rue des Ecoles, 75240 Paris, Cedex 05, France

FEDERAL REPUBLIC OF GERMANY — Pergamon Press GmbH, 6242 Kronberg-Taunus, Pferdstrasse 1, Federal Republic of Germany

First edition 1979

British Library Cataloguing in Publication Data

Placenta.
1. Placenta - Congresses
2. Medicine, Experimental - Congresses
I. Beaconsfield, Peter II. Villee, Claude
III. Special Commission on Internal Pollution
619 QP281 79-40046

ISBN 0-08-024430-0 Hard cover
ISBN 0-08-024435-1 Flexi cover

In order to make this volume available as economically and as rapidly as possible the authors' typescripts have been reproduced in their original forms. This method unfortunately has its typographical limitations but it is hoped that they in no way distract the reader.

Printed and bound at William Clowes & Sons Limited Beccles and London

CONTENTS

Section II. Cell replication

Section III. Immunology

Section IV. Ageing

CONTRIBUTORS AND INVITED PARTICIPANTS

R.J. AITKEN

M.R.C. Reproductive Biology Unit,
Edinburgh.

E.C. AMOROSO

A.R.C. Institute of Animal Physiology,
Cambridge.

J. MAXWELL ANDERSON

Department of Surgery,
Royal Infirmary, Glasgow.

PETER BEACONSFIELD

SCIP Research Unit,
Bedford College, University of London.

REBECCA BEACONSFIELD

SCIP Research Unit,
Bedford College,
University of London.

J.N. BLACK

Principal, Bedford College,
University of London.

W.D. BILLINGTON

Department of Pathology,
Medical School, University of Bristol

L. BRENT

Department of Immunology,
St. Mary's Hospital Medical School,
London

A.D.H. BROWNE

Department of Obstetrics & Gynaecology,
Royal College of Surgeons in Ireland,
Dublin.

B. CRABTREE

Animal Physiology & Nutrition,
University of Leeds.

D.G. CRAMP

Department of Chemical Pathology,
Royal Free Hospital, London.

P.P. DENDY

Biomedial Physics & Bioengineering,
University of Aberdeen.

M.U. DIANZANI

Institute of General Pathology,
University of Turin.

G.C. EASTY

Ludwig Institute,
Royal Marsden Hospital, Sutton, Surrey.

C.W. ELSTON

Department of Pathology,
City Hospital, Nottingham.

W.P. FAULK

McIndoe Laboratories,
Queen Victoria Hospital,
E. Grinstead, Sussex.

H. FOX

Department of Pathology,
University of Manchester.

R.L. GARDNER

Department of Zoology,
University of Oxford.

OLGA GENBACEV

Department of Physiology & Radiobiology
INEP, Zemun,
Yugoslavia

JEAN GINSBURG

Department of Medicine,
Royal Free Hospital,
London.

R.J.C. HARRIS

Microbiological Research Establishment,
Porton Down, Wilts.

SIR WILLIAM HENDERSON

Genetic Manipulation Advisory Group,
Medical Research Council, London.

W. HIJMANS

Institute for Experimental Gerontology,
Rijswijk, The Netherlands

R. HOLLIDAY

National Institute of Medical Research,
Mill Hill, London.

P.M. JOHNSON

Department of Immunology,
University of Liverpool.

EVA KLEIN

Department of Tumour Biology,
Karolinska Institutet, Stockholm.

J.A. McINTYRE

Department of Pathology,
Medical University of S.Carolina,
Charleston, U.S.A.

ROSALIND MELDRUM

Biomedical Physics & Bioengineering,
University of Aberdeen.

H.MUNRO

Department of Nutrition & Food Science,
M.I.T., Cambridge, Mass., U.S.A.

A. NEUBERGER

Lister Institute of Preventive Medicine,
London.

E.A. NEWSHOLME

Department of Biochemistry,
University of Oxford.

F. POCCHIARI

Istituto Superiore di Sanità, Rome.

J. PONTÉN

Wallenburg Laboratory,
University of Uppsala

H. THEORELL

Nobel Medical Institute,
Stockholm.

CLAUDE VILLEE

Laboratory of Human Reproduction,
Harvard Medical School, Boston.

DOROTHY VILLEE

Department of Pediatrics,
Harvard Medical School, Boston.

G. VOISIN

Centre d'Immuno-Pathologie,
INSERM, Hôpital St. Antoine,
Paris

A.E. WILD

Department of Biology,
University of Southampton.

ELUNED WOODFORD-WILLIAMS

Department of Geriatric Medicine,
University of Manchester.

MAUREEN YOUNG

Department of Gynaecology,
St. Thomas's Hospital, London

D.L. YUDILEVICH

Department of Physiology,
Queen Elizabeth College,
University of London.

Technical Editors

REBECCA BEACONSFIELD and GEORGE BIRDWOOD

FOREWORD

The quest for a suitable model on which to base human medical research is as long as the history of medicine itself. Only time will show how important a milestone on this journey the placenta may prove to be. As yet, it has been neglected, as the title of this book suggests, and somewhat surprisingly, when we consider how much effort has been applied to seemingly less satisfactory and less freely available alternatives.

The placenta's remarkably complete spectrum of cellular and biochemical activity, as well as its hormonal and endocrinological roles and its short life-cycle, adds to its suitability for studying the processes of cell replication, immune mechanisms - notably graft acceptance and rejection - and perhaps ageing.

Both the meeting itself and this account of it make two breaks with tradition. The small number of participants were invited as experts in their fields in the hope they would tackle one another's concepts and plant seeds for further research in each other's minds. In short, the whole emphasis was on future progress rather than past accomplishments. This spirit is extended into the book, which differs from the usual proceedings in that it consists of broad-ranging reviews instead of accounts of personal research. But more important still is the fact that the discussion has been written up in narrative form - so as to present information and ideas as challenges for the future. More questions are posed than answered. But that, after all, is the proper basis for scientific progress. A reasonably attentive reader of this book could find a dozen ideas for research projects to engage his attention at first glance - and many more on careful reading. The one proposed for cancer studies interests me particularly.

The imprint of the book's senior editor, Peter Beaconsfield, who originally proposed an interdisciplinary get-together to discuss the placenta as an experimental model, was also clearly in evidence at the meeting itself. He succeeded in producing an exchange of ideas between experts in many fields, which must have sent participants home with thoughts stimulated by round-table discussion, enlivened by an unusually wide yet highly pertinent range of scientific view-points.

It was roughly ten years ago that Peter consulted me about launching a programme to study the effect of various pollutants and chemicals and non-disease related drugs on biological systems - which he has since called more simply 'internal pollution'. That evocative term has of course now become a household word outside the scientific milieu. I told him I thought it was a very important project, but also a very difficult and ambitious one. This book marks the beginning of another of his interesting ambitious endeavours, and I have no hesitation in repeating the comment I made on that earlier occasion:

'All new ideas are difficult to launch, but we have to start somewhere - so why don't we begin now?'

Hugo Theorell

Nobel Medical Institute
Karolinska Insitutet
Stockholm

PLACENTAL PREVIEW

Rebecca Beaconsfield

Tradition makes conformists of us all. A conventional speech of welcome, appearing as 'introductory remarks' in the proceedings, was something we originally felt to be superfluous at an informal gathering like this one. Straight to work - on the interdisciplinary lines already agreed - was to have been the order of the day. Yet, after last night's get-together, my husband expressed doubts whether everybody had really understood the aims set out in our invitations or the pattern of work by which we hope to accomplish them. Hence this reminder - which he kindly 'offered' me the task of presenting to you!

The room is deliberately arranged for round-table discussion. The formal review papers, to be published in full in the proceedings, will each be given - by way of groundwork to facilitate and stimulate discussion between experts working in different fields. We believe this cross-fertilisation of ideas to be vital if the placenta is to be fully utilised as a research tool in the fields with which this meeting is principally concerned: biochemistry, metabolism, cell replication and growth, cancer, immunology and ageing. Perhaps, after all, tradition is right to demand that professional meetings should begin with a more or less formal reminder of this kind. But we do still hope to avoid being conformist in other ways. For example, you have been asked to show few if any slides, because the success of the meeting will largely depend on discussion of ideas for future research, rather than the more conventional presentation of detailed data on work already done. In short, we see this more as a forum for asking - and refining - new questions than for answering old ones. That means breaking with another altogether too well-established tradition: that speakers from different disciplines hesitate to venture into one another's fields. To fulfill its potential this gathering needs to be not merely multidisciplinary - it is already that thanks to your presence here - but truly interdisciplinary. In addition, the clinicians among you must get together with the basic scientists if we are to see the fruits of placental research applied in practice. And that is, of course, our ultimate aim.

Although only one of many possible research models, the human placenta offers many advantages. It consists of human tissue. It is readily available. And it possesses the unique properties of differentiating and growing from embryonal tissue to maturity and what many clinicians consider to be senescence in only nine months. During that conveniently short period, it passes through the stages of graft acceptance, differentiation, invasive growth, cessation of both growth and invasiveness, and finally 'rejection' - while sustaining and protecting fetal development by a multitude of metabolic and immunological processes. All are accessible for study, together with their control mechanisms.

It would be unduly pretentious to compare this meeting with the Solvay conferences of the first 30 years of this century where the birth and flowering of modern nuclear physics took place. Yet there is currently potential for such a great leap forward in biology, and - in however small a contribution to that end - we might profitably emulate their approach. We believe that the Solvay conferences owed their success to something more than assembly of the right experts at the right stage in the growth of knowledge. Those who attended them were more interested in conceptual ideas than technical innovation, and more concerned with broad-ranging intellectual curiosity - or honest enquiry, if you like - than with being right or (in the modern idiom) confirming their findings. Our approach should be no less broad. The necessary range of biological knowledge is assembled here and, if only we can bring it to bear effectively, your combined experience should be sufficient to influence future progress.

Most meetings, as we all know for our sins, are very different. Attendance may be motivated by the opportunity to visit an unknown place at somebody else's expense. After the second world war - well over 30 years ago now, so its's high time for a change - there was an understandable desire to move freely round the world again, to exchange ideas with colleagues we had long missed or never met. Since then, aided and abetted by air travel, attending the 'congress circuit' has become as much part of a scientist's seasonal rhythm as balls and parties were to a pre-war socialite's. Yet, like the social season before them, international congresses have now largely outlived their usefulness. No great advances are ever announced at their sessions, and few if any original ideas are ever exchanged in the midst of a crowd - there or elsewhere. The size of a meeting seems to be in inverse proportion to its usefulness, with the most useful work being done outside the conference sessions, often over a drink. Yet we all go on attending mammoth congresses, uneasily aware that their great expense cannot be justified (except perhaps as a means of keeping conference hotels and airlines in business - so that the circus can go on). So it is that we continue to earn Arthur Koestler's apt soubriquet of 'call girls' - for those who come when money beckons.

A fresh start is badly needed. Here we hope to recreate, with minimal funding, the sort of informal small-scale discussion that normally takes place outside the conference room - albeit without alcoholic facilitation. We should all be able to learn something from each other's experience and stimulate each other's ideas on promising lines of future enquiry. Suppose you were 30 years younger, yet possessed of your present knowledge and experience, what avenues would you want to explore in your own - or other - fields? The courage to speculate along those lines should certainly ensure a stimulating meeting. Assessment of its ultimate usefulness we must leave to the future ...

SECTION I

PLACENTAL METABOLIC PROCESSES

A NEGLECTED EXPERIMENTAL ANIMAL

Editors' Note: In obstetrics the placenta tends to be taken for granted, except in the rare instances where it appears to fail. As an experimental model it is seldom even considered. Hence the deliberately provocative heading (which also subtitles the proceedings) to this first editorial note. Others introduce each of the later sections and a final one concludes the whole book. Their purpose is simply to guide and inform the reader.

Placental studies are so patently of importance in obstetrics and antenatal care - especially for research into threatened and spontaneous abortion, fetal anomalies, concealed haemorrhage, rhesus incompatibility and other disorders of pregnancy and parturition - that their neglect is hard to explain. Those are not, however, the subject of the placental studies reported here. The meeting on which these proceedings are based was devoted almost exclusively to consideration of the placenta as a research model in five main fields: biochemistry, cell replication, cancer, immunology and ageing. That these types of placental research, more or less remote from obstetric problems, should have been neglected is somewhat easier to understand. Perhaps because there is no obvious connection with childbirth, few have been suggested and fewer still done. But the matter seems to go deeper than that. Animal instincts dictate that the afterbirth should be promptly abandoned or tidied away, often by the mother eating it, while man disposes of the placenta almost ritually by burial or burning. The realistic conclusion that it has no further use seems to be reinforced by a deep but seldom voiced conviction that the placenta should not be exploited for other purposes. Absurd though they seem, such superstitious beliefs may still need to be overcome if the human placenta is to be widely accepted as an experimental model.

Other hinderances also need to be overcome - as indicated in Rebecca Beaconsfield's opening remarks - if cross-fertilisation by exchange of ideas and information is to take place between different research disciplines and between them and clinical medicine. Such difficulties of communication are not of course peculiar to the placenta. But they also raise primaeval echoes, of tribal identity and territoriality, and they were compounded at this meeting by their technological successor - the complexity of much of the specialised subject-matter. As the edited discussions show, so it may as well be frankly admitted here, few of the assembled experts ventured into each other's fields ...

But then, consider Peter Beaconsfield's statement that at least a million different biochemical processes are taking place in a typical mammalian cell each second. How many of those do we really know much about? How much less can we hope to understand all the processes of metabolism, growth, immunology and ageing - to name only the fields discussed here - that underlie them? Rash indeed the biochemist who laid claim to such omniscience. Rasher still the specialist in one of these other fields who rushed in with ill-founded comments or suggestions. And yet much progress has come from initially improbable ideas. Indeed, this meeting was planned in part as a forum for generating and refining them - with the first session devoted to the basic biochemical background.

It will be apparent from Eric Newsholme's opening review that much is now becoming known about the control of biochemical processes. Research is moving on from elucidation of reactions to the mechanisms which determine when, how, why and to what extent they are brought into play. In other words, biochemistry is beginning to be integrated with biological function. Few would question the interdisciplinary value of that development, which is also reflected in the following paper - in which Peter Beaconsfield and Jean Ginsburg discuss placental metabolism, with special reference to carbohydrates, fats and protein.

In the third paper, Hamish Munro turns to higher levels of control - describing what is known about the ways in which nucleic acids direct placental development. Chemical mediators obviously play a major part in transmitting those directions, though little is yet known of their details. But much has recently been learned about a subsequent stage in biochemical control of development, as shown by Dorothy Villee's review of the endocrine functions of the placenta. The theme of biochemical control is also taken up by Olga Genbačev discussing prostaglandins in the regulation of placental function.

Towards the end of this first section, Maureen Young describes techniques for studying placental metabolism and transfer, to which David Yudilevich adds a note (in discussion) on a promising new method of investigation.

Finally, drug metabolism: Peter Beaconsfield contributes a personal view of the need for work in this important and neglected field. It is a curious fact that, despite the stimulus the thalidomide disaster gave to drug safety testing in general, relatively little attention has been paid to placental drug metabolism. Yet the placenta does not merely pass most drugs to the fetus. It has the power to modify some and may expose the fetus to higher concentrations of drug or metabolite than are present in the mother. The dearth of work in this field emphasises the need for basic studies - whose practical importance is beyond question.

Much the same can be said of the later sections - on cell replication, immunology and ageing. They make the need for more interdisciplinary meetings unmistakeably clear - and by no means only on the subject of the placenta. The proceedings of this one make no claim to be a definitive review. At best, they make an early staging post on what promises to be a productive way forward.

SECTION I

PLACENTAL METABOLIC PROCESSES

Chairman: Claude Villee

The placenta used to be regarded simply as a barrier between mother and fetus that allowed good things through and kept bad things from reaching the fetus or the mother. But, about 25 years ago, biochemists began to become interested in the placenta, and it was discovered that things went back and forth from mother and fetus, not simply by physical diffusion but by a variety of active transport systems. We now know that the placenta has a full range of metabolic capabilities, and their rate compares favourably with the liver or kidney.

More recently, there has been interest in the synthetic abilities of the placenta, and the studies of its rapid development and ageing provide means of learning about those processes in other tissues. The first papers in this section are concerned with the biochemical background, as most people here are not biochemists. Since we take it for granted that the placenta has all the metabolic capabilities of any other tissue, one of the first questions to be answered is how these various metabolic pathways are regulated.

THE PRINCIPLES OF METABOLIC REGULATION WITH SPECIAL REFERENCE TO DEVELOPMENT AND AGEING

Eric A. Newsholme (Speaker) and Bernard Crabtree

During the earlier part of this century, biochemical research revealed the various sequences of reactions by which complex substances are degraded to simpler compounds in order to produce biological energy. When it became clear that a specific series of reactions was responsible for the metabolism of each complex substance, these sequences were called metabolic pathways (e.g. glycolysis for converting glucose to pyruvate or lactate, and the citric acid cycle for oxidising acetate to carbon dioxide and water. Elucidation of their biochemical details showed each individual reaction in these metabolic pathways to be catalysed by a specific enzyme. In the last 25 years, detailed biochemical research into the molecular details of the individual reactions has been particularly directed to clarifying the catalytic mechanism mediated by each of these enzymes. Another line of investigation, during the same period, has been devoted to the mechanisms which control the rate of the individual reactions in a pathway and hence the flux through the pathway as a whole.

This paper is primarily concerned with regulation, concentrating on general principles rather than the details of individual reactions and pathways. By way of example, reference will be made to glycolysis and glycogenolysis (glycogen degradation) in muscle, since a wealth of knowledge is available on these pathways. In addition to describing the principles of control, the reasons why different mechanisms are necessary will be discussed, noting the possible advantages and disadvantages of each. This will enable the control of other systems to be considered, concluding with an outline of how these principles of metabolic regulation may be applied to the control of the complex processes of development and ageing.

First, it is necessary to consider the basic concept of metabolic pathways since some knowledge is essential to an understanding of their regulation. The processes needed for the metabolic degradation of complex substances proceed via a series of enzyme-catalysed reactions, because the amount of chemical change that any one enzyme can produce is limited. A large chemical change requires a series of different enzymes. This is true not only of metabolic degradation: it applies equally to complex biosynthetic processes (e.g. protein synthesis, RNA and DNA synthesis) and also to processes not normally associated with metabolic pathways, such as mechanisms of regulation. (Examples are control of glycogen degradation via the enzyme cascade,[1] and the control of cyclic-AMP levels[2] described later. It is likely that a series of related reactions also plays a part in the regulation of cell division and in antibody production. Since application of the term metabolic pathway to a control system is an extension of its usual meaning, and may be unfamiliar, the next section sets out the basic properties of such pathways.

STRUCTURES OF METABOLIC PATHWAYS

1. Closed and open systems

All chemical (and hence enzymatic) reactions are reversible, but some are more reversible than others. With metabolic pathways, particularly *in vivo*, the rate of the forward component of a reaction can be much greater than that of the reverse component - to the extent that the reaction is regarded as irreversible. Consider the following hypothetical enzyme-catalysed reaction:

$$x \underset{v_2}{\overset{v_1}{\rightleftharpoons}} y$$

The reactants are x and y, and $v_1$and v_2 represent the rates of the forward and reverse components. If such a reaction is isolated from its surroundings, so that there is no production or removal of x or y from the system, the concentrations of these substances will approach values that equate v_1 and v_2. Such a state, in which the rates of the forward and reverse reactions are equal, is referred to as *equilibrium*. For an isolated (i.e. *closed*) system, equilibrium is the only state in which the concentrations of x and y do not vary with time. However, at equilibrium there is no *net* interconversion of the reactants (since $v_1 = v_2$) and, as classical thermodynamics shows, such a system can do no useful work. A closed system does not therefore provide a valid model of the metabolism in living cells, which interconvert substances at constant (through variable) rates and are capable of doing work on their surroundings. Nonetheless, some *individual* cell reactions may be at equilibrium under certain conditions, and some reactions in metabolic pathways may be very close to equilibrium.

Metabolic systems are examples of *open* thermodynamic reactions, characterised by continuous interchange of matter and energy with their surroundings. Such an open system can be illustrated as follows:

$$\xrightarrow{A} x \underset{v_2}{\overset{v_1}{\rightleftharpoons}} y \xrightarrow{B}$$

This system contains the same hypothetical reaction as the closed system described above. But, in this case, the preliminary reaction A continuously supplies x from the surroundings,while the subsequent reaction B continuously removes y from the system; reactions behaving in this way have been designated *non-equilibrium*. An important property of an open system is that the concentrations of x and y can be independent of time, even if the reaction $x \rightleftharpoons y$ is displaced from equilibrium (e.g. when v_1 is greater than v_2). In the above example, such a situation would arise if the rate of reaction A were constant and the rate of reaction B was a function of the concentration of y. The rate of conversion of one substance into the other would then be constant, and the system in *steady-state*, the rate of overall throughput being referred to as the *flux*.

Although the steady-state serves as a model for the operation of metabolic pathways, open systems can take other forms. Those in which the concentrations of substrate (or metabolic intermediates) are continuous functions of time include both transient (exponential) states, when the flux through a steady-state system changes, and oscillatory states.

2. Generation of flux in steady-state systems

The main characteristics of a system in steady-state are the time-independence of the concentrations of the intermediates and the presence of a constant flux; indeed, constancy of flux is the main factor determining steady-state. A steady-state system therefore consists of two types of reaction:

> One which provides (or generates) the constant flux, and
>
> Other reactions which adjust to the flux, by responding to changes in substrate concentration.

For example, in a steady-state system such as the following:

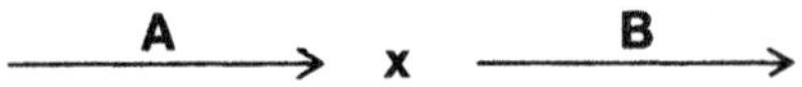

a constant flux is generated at reaction A. The rate of reaction B is determined by the concentration (which is constant) of its substrate x. The flux through reaction B is therefore equal to the rate of reaction A. For steady-state to be maintained, reaction A could not be isolated and substrate-dependent, because the concentration of the substrate, and hence the flux, would decline as the reaction progressed. In short, reaction A must be substrate-saturated if it is to generate a flux for the other reactions in the pathway to transmit. While such *flux-generating reactions* need to be substrate-saturated for a system to reach steady-state, other reactions which follow later in the pathway are substrate-dependent.

The term substrate needs to be used with care, as illustrated by the following hypothetical example:

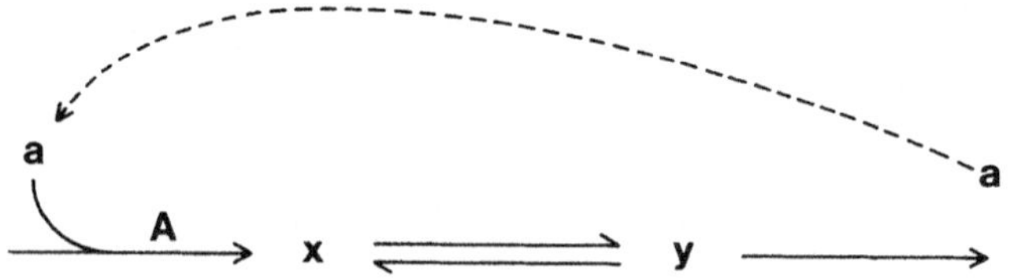

A cofactor (a) is involved in the flux-generating reaction (A), and this cofactor is regenerated at some subsequent reaction in the pathway. In this example reaction A must be saturated with the *pathway-substrate*, which provides the flow of matter through such an open system, but it need not necessarily be saturated with co-factor a. Since the latter is continuously regenerated, it can be considered to belong to a 'conserved system of metabolites', whereas the pathway-substrate has to be made constantly available from an outside source - in the same or another tissue.

The reactions that make up a metabolic system need not necessarily be confined to just one cell or tissue; a pathway can span several tissues linked by the circulation. For example, the flux-generating reaction may be located in one tissue while many of the subsequent reactions take place elsewhere:

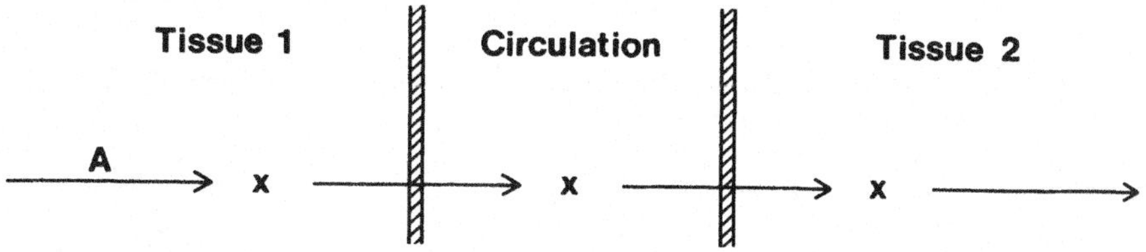

The flux here is generated by reaction A in tissue 1, and the rate of utilisation of x by tissue 2 will be a function of its concentration in the circulating fluid.

A flux-generating reaction can be identified by the following criteria:

The reaction is non-equilibrium in type

The substrate concentration _in vivo_ is considerably higher than the Michaelis constant (K_m)* of the enzyme catalysing the reaction, and

Changes in the substrate concentration cause no change in the flux through the pathway.

The early non-equilibrium reactions of glycolysis are given in Table I. Comparison of the _in vivo_ concentrations of pathway-substrates with the K_m values of the relevant enzyme reactions shows that glycolysis-from-glucose does not have a flux-generating step within the muscle. It follows that the flux-generating step for glycolysis from glucose must take place elsewhere, most probably in the liver. Hepatic phosphorylase, which catalyses the degradation of liver glycogen to glucose 1-phosphate, is thought to be flux-generating for subsequent glycolysis in muscle. The glucose 1-phosphate is then converted to glucose 6-phosphate, and that is hydrolysed by glucose 6-phosphatase to form glucose, which is released by the liver. The glucose is then transported to muscle via the circulation. These reactions are outlined in Fig. 1, which may be compared with the hypothetical example given above, reaction A representing the action of hepatic phosphorylase on liver glycogen, while x corresponds to glucose, which is present in the liver, bloodstream and muscle.

The concept of the flux-generating step is fundamentally important in understanding the regulation of metabolic pathways, and also assists in their definition.

* The substrate concentration at which the velocity of an enzyme reaction is _half_ the maximum (at infinite substrate concentration).

TABLE 1.

Glycolysis in muscle: K_m values and *in vivo* substrate concentrations for non-equilibrium reactions.

Enzyme or process	K_m for enzyme or process (mM)	Substrate concentrations *in vivo* (mM)
Phosphorylase	1.0	20-30
Glucose transport	10.0	5.0
Hexokinase	0.1	<0.1
Phosphofructokinase	c.0.1*	<0.1

* The enzyme kinetics are such that if it is inhibited by ATP, the concentration of fructose 6-phosphate cannot be saturating.[1]

It generally seems to have been tacitly assumed, in the absence of a proper definition, that a metabolic pathway existed by virtue of its presence in a given textbook or wall-chart - where it most probably gained its place because the particular series of reactions involved was amenable to biochemical study. Glycolysis-from-glucose, for example, is usually accepted as a pathway because it is possible to measure both glucose uptake by a muscle and the appearance of pyruvate or lactate. The accessibility of this process, together with the obvious biochemical linkage between the reactions led to acceptance of glycolysis as a metabolic pathway in muscle and other tissues. However, this has been questioned recently because it does not include the initial flux-generating step now considered an essential feature of such pathways. Glycolysis in muscle should therefore be reguarded as part of a pathway that begins with phosphorylation of liver glycogen.

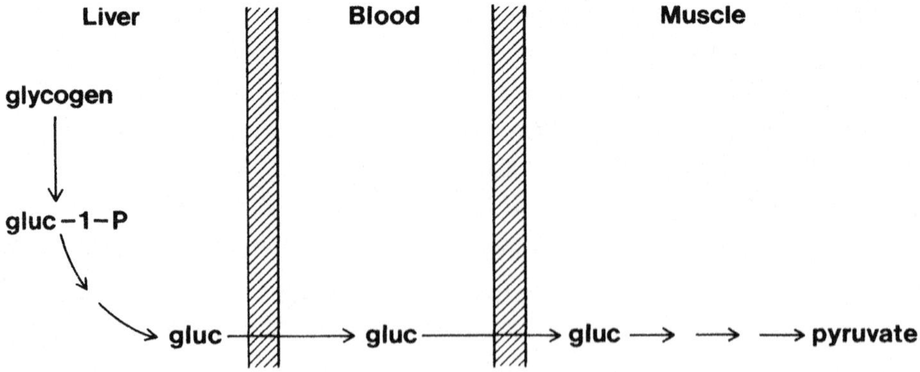

Fig. 1. Flux-generating step for muscle glycolysis.

In general, a metabolic pathway can be defined as a long or short series of reactions that are initiated by a flux-generating step and terminate in a reaction preceding another flux-generating step or in loss of the end-product to the enviornment.

This definition allows for metabolic pathways to span several tissues, another example being the metabolism of fatty acids which are made available from triglyceride in adipose tissue and transported via the circulatory system for utilisation in muscle (Fig.2). But it also raises an important question. What regulates the overall flux through a metabolic pathway, especially one that spans several tissues?

Consider hepatic phosphorylation, the flux-generating step for glucose utilisation in muscle: phosphorylase activity must be increased by a mechanism related

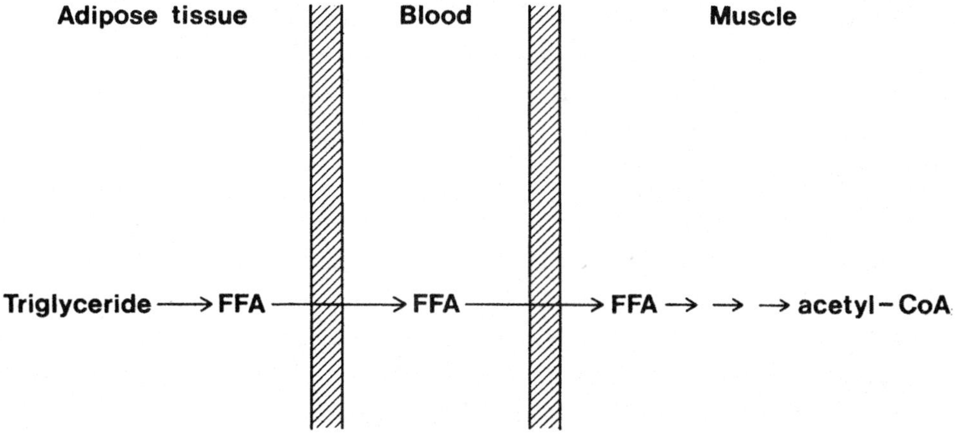

Fig. 2. Flux-generating step for beta-oxidation of fatty acids in muscle.

to the rate of energy utilisation by the muscles. And it is known that the activity of hepatic phosphorylase is modified by the hormones adrenaline, glucagon and insulin, whose concentrations during sustained exercise show appropriate changes (i.e. higher concentrations of adrenaline and glucagon, which increase phosphorylation, and lower concentration of insulin which decreases it). But can changes in the concentrations of these hormones regulate hepatic phosphorylase with sufficient precision to meet the energy demands of muscle during mechanical activity? The authors consider that hormonal regulation alone cannot produce sufficient precision and postulate an additional feedback mechanism for regulating the flux generating-step in the liver in accordance with energy demand by muscle. However, no such feedback mechanism has yet been identified.

3. Regulation of flux in steady-state systems

The general factors which determine the magnitude of the flux through a metabolic system (i.e. those factors which ultimately regulate the rate of operation of metabolic pathways) must now be considered. A simple hypothetical pathway shows the various possibilities:

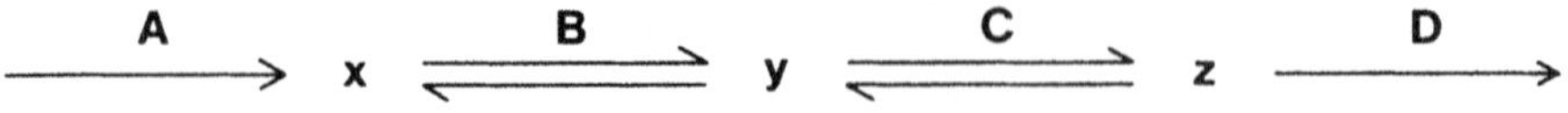

The magnitude of the flux is determined by reaction A and can only be modified by a change in the activity of its catalytic enzyme. The activity of this enzyme, and hence the rate of reaction A, could be modified either directly (e.g. via inhibition or activation by a regulatory metabolite) or indirectly (e.g. via modifications of the activity of the enzyme which catalyses reaction B). Influences acting on reaction B could modify the flux-generating reaction A by changes in the concentrations of x. However, for this to be the case, the enzyme that catalyses reaction A would have to be inhibited allosterically by its product x (since product x can have no mass-action effect on reaction A because this is a non-equilibrium reaction). An increase in the concentration of x would then lead to a reduction in the flux through the system.

It is therefore possible to regulate the flux through a system by modifying the activity of a reaction other than the flux-generating step. But can the concentration of the product x change sufficiently to provide satisfactory control of reaction A? If x is an allosteric inhibitor of reaction A, its concentration must fall to stimulate the rate of the flux-generating reaction and hence increase the flux through the overall pathway. However, if the concentration of x has to fall very low in order to increase the rate of reaction A, this could reduce the rate of reaction B for which x is the substrate. For this mechanism to operate effectively, small changes in the concentration of x must produce large changes in the rate of reaction A. In other words, the control mechanism would have to be very sensitive. Means for increasing sensitivity in metabolic control are outlined in the next main section.

How does the reversibility of reactions influence their control? It is known that non-equilibrium (irreversible) reactions provide more favourable conditions for allosteric regulation than near-equilibrium (reversible) reactions - a conclusion based on their different sensitivity to changes in the concentration of potential regulatory metabolites.[4] However, it would certainly be incorrect to regard non-equilibrium reactions as the only possible sites for regulation.

4. Non-equilibrium and near-equilibrium reactions - their significance in metabolic control.

Three types of reaction occur in metabolic pathways, namely:

Near-equilibrium

Non-equilibrium, not saturated with substrate, and

Non-equilibrium, saturated with substrate (i.e. the flux-generating step).

A reaction in a metabolic system kept in non-equilibrium because the concentration of the product(s) of the reaction and the catalytic activity of the enzyme are maintained low, so that the rate for the reverse component of the reaction is very much less than the rate of the forward component.

Conversely, a reaction is in near-equilibrium if the concentration of the product(s) and the catalytic activity of the enzyme are high enough to produce a rate for the reverse component (90 in the following example) which approaches that of the forward component (100) and therefore far exceeds the overall flux (10 in this case):

$$\longrightarrow x \underset{v_2 = 90}{\overset{v_1 = 100}{\rightleftharpoons}} y \longrightarrow$$

Probably the most important control function of a near-equilibrium reaction is to increase sensitivity to changes in the concentrations of the substrate and/or products of the reaction, as described in the next section. These are therefore ideal reactions to transmit the flux initiated by the flux-generating reaction. However, their increased sensitivity means that near-equilibrium reactions are much less sensitive to the effects of allosteric regulators; they do not therefore provide sites for feedback control or for hormonal control via secondary messengers.

Non-equilibrium reactions not saturated with substrate have an important role in providing directionality in a pathway, particularly towards its end or in the middle of a long pathway. Furthermore, the sensitivity of near-equilibrium reactions earlier in the pathway is dependent upon the properties and control of the subsequent non-equilibrium reactions.[5] The major advantage of non-equilibrium reactions in metabolic control is that they can be controlled by allosteric factors, and are thus open to feedback inhibition and hormonal control via secondary messengers. Their disadvantage is lack of sensitivity both to changes in substrate concentration and to allosteric effectors. Means for increasing sensitivity in such reactions are discussed below.

The importance of non-equilibrium reactions saturated with substrate, i.e. the flux-generating step, has already been discussed. These reactions also provide directionality at the beginning of the pathway and lack sensitivity to changes in the concentrations of allosteric effectors and other regulators.

SENSITIVITY IN METABOLIC CONTROL

The number of individual control mechanisms is probably at least as large as the number of processes to be regulated. It is possible to classify some of the many hundreds of such mechanisms into groups, illustrating different principles of metabolic regulation, which are thought to have developed primarily to improve the sensitivity of control.

Sensitivity can be defined as a measure of the magnitude of the response to a given stimulus, e.g. the change in flux through a metabolic pathway in response to a change in substrate concentration. This is expressed as the ratio between the relative percentage change in response and the relative change in stimulus.[6] The net sensitivity can therefore be calculated, using the power equation[5] given below, from measurements of stimulus and response, provided the relationship between them remains constant during the reaction (despite changes in their actual values):

$$J = \lambda(S)^{s_S^J}$$

where S = stimulus, J = response, s = sensitivity, and λ is an integration constant. A useful approximation can also be obtained when the relationship between stimulus and response does vary during the reaction, so long as the changes in their values do not exceed about 10%. For larger changes, the response must be calculated indirectly by numerical approximation. Despite this limitation, the equation provides a useful means for comparing the effectiveness of various mechanisms that increase the sensitivity of metabolic control.

Non-equilibrium reactions and sensitivity in control

We must consider how changes in substrate concentration affect enzyme activity and thus the flux through a non-equilibrium reaction. Similar effects can be produced by changes in the concentration of an allosteric effector, which could either increase or decrease enzyme activity. Since the reverse component exerts an insignificant effect on the overall flux through a non-equilibrium reaction, only the forward process need be considered in relation to flux changes. This means that *in vitro* measurements of the effects of concentration changes of substrate and/or allosteric effectors on enzyme activity may be relevant to changes in enzyme activity (and hence to flux changes) *in vivo*.

If an enzyme's activity responds in a hyperbolic manner to changes in substrate concentration, the power equation noted above will give sensitivity values between 1 and 0. The response to changes in substrate concentration well below the Michaelis constant (K_m) for the reaction is approximately unity; it approaches zero as the concentration rises towards saturation (see Table II). This appears to be the usual response between an enzyme and its regulator, whether substrate or allosteric effectors. It may be considered a basic response, with which any mechanism for improving a sensitivity can be compared. Obviously, if a change in substrate

TABLE II

The sensitivity provided by biochemical mechanisms involved in non-equilibrium reactions.

Mechanism for increasing sensitivity	Intrinsic sensitivity (s)
Hyperbolic response linear if s << K_m [1]	1.0
Positive cooperativity: sigmoid response of activity to change in substrate concentration [10]	1 - 2
Substrate cycle [6]	$1 + \frac{\text{cycling rate}}{\text{flux}}$
Interconversion cycle [10]	> 1

concentration within the cell lies below the K_m value, the enzyme activity will respond linearly. If, however, the total change in enzyme activity is larger (e.g. from 10% to 90% of maximal activity), which is not unusual for certain enzymes, the change in regulator concentration required will be considerably greater than the change in enzyme activity it produces. A nine-fold change in enzyme activity (e.g. from 10% to 90%) may require an 81-fold change in regulator concentration.[1]

Where much greater changes in enzyme activity are required, this relationship may be reversed. It can be shown, for instance, that the rate of glycolysis must increase 2000-fold to produce the increase in energy demanded by a man sprinting compared with that required when his muscles are at rest. If the response of the non-equilibrium reactions of glycolysis to the regulator were one-to-one (i.e. linear), a 2000-fold increase in regulator concentration would be needed. But the concentrations of the metabolites considered to regulate glycolysis (and glycogenolysis) in muscle in relation to the energy demand[1,7] change remarkably little, perhaps three- to four- fold for each regulator (see Table III).

TABLE III

Effects of exercise on metabolite concentrations in human skeletal muscle, rat heart and skeletal muscle, and locust flight muscle.

Metabolite concentration (μmol/g of fresh muscle)

Metabolite	Human quadriceps femoris		Rat heart isolated and perfused		Rat calf muscle isolated and perfused		Locust flight muscle whole insect	
	Rest	Exercise	Low Work	High Work	Rest	Exercise	Rest	Exercise
ATP	4.63	2.98	5.3	4.5	6.09	3.39	5.06	4.32
ADP	0.95	0.88	1.1	1.3	0.69	0.74	0.43	1.10
AMP	0.10	0.09	0.09	0.17	0.04	0.09	0.06	0.12
IMP					0.10	2.13		
Ammonia			0.27	0.51			0.77	1.21
P_i			3.9	5.9			9.3	11.9
Phosphocreatine	17.0	3.2	8.6	5.0	20.8	5.9		
Creatine								
Glucose 6-phosphate	0.35	2.25	0.14	0.10	0.17	0.47	0.10	0.22
Fructose bisphosphate			0.03	0.02			0.05	0.12
Phosphoenolpyruvate								
Pyruvate	0.14	0.14					0.06	0.24
Lactate	1.1	26.7			1.4	16.5		
Oxaloacetate			0.0008	0.0016			0.0020	0.0038
Acetyl-CoA							0.06	0.03
Citrate	0.067	0.054	0.14	0.11	0.11	0.13	0.79	0.16
2-Oxoglutarate			0.08	0.18			0.10	0.07

Human muscle obtained by biopsy 10-15 s after end of exercise.[26] Perfused heart and perfused hind-limb muscles of rat freeze-clamped during the period of increased work or exercise.[27,28] Whole locusts freeze-clamped and muscle obtained by dissection of frozen insect.[29]

The concentrations of these regulators cannot change by large amounts because one of their two roles in the cell requires a reasonable degree of constancy in concentration. The metabolites in question (e.g. ATP, AMP, NH_4^+, IMP, creatine phosphate, glucose 6-phosphate, fructose diphosphate, P_i, citrate) have roles both as metabolic regulators and as metabolic intermediates. Since these metabolites arise at important positions in the course of metabolism, they provide informational links between the metabolic process and the key regulatory enzymes. This is their regulatory role, for which metabolite concentrations must change to provide information about changes in metabolism. But since these metabolites also form part of a metabolic pathway or pathways, their concentration cannot change too severely or the structure of the metabolic pathway would break down. A change of ten- or 100-fold in the concentration of the product of a non-equilibrium reaction might, for instance be sufficient to convert a non-equilibrium reaction into a near-equilibrium one. This would change dramatically the organised kinetic 'structure' of the pathway.

It is well established that large changes do not occur in the relative concentrations of ATP/ADP which act as an energy source in many metabolic reactions. The importance of maintaining this value reasonably constant in relation to kinetic efficiency has been established in detail.[8,9]

The concentration of some important regulators of glycolysis and glycogenolysis that take place in human muscle after exhaustive exercise are given in Table III. These changes are considered to produce an increase in the rate of certain glycolysis reactions by approximately 2000-fold. This appears to be true of the near-equilibrium reactions, mediated by phosphoglucose isomerase, phosphoglucomutase, and glyceraldehyde 3-phosphate dehydrogenase in response to concentration changes of their substrates and/or products. It is,however, very unlikely to be the case for non-equilibrium reactions mediated by phosphorylase and phosphofructokinase unless the sensitivity of the non-equilibrium reaction is increased.

MECHANISMS FOR INCREASING SENSITIVITY OF METABOLIC CONTROL

1. Sigmoid response of enzyme activity to substrate concentration.

If an enzyme which catalyses a non-equilibrium reaction responds in a sigmoid manner to a change in substrate concentration over a certain range of activity, the sensitivity (s) will be greater than unity, its actual value depending upon the portion of curve considered. For simple globular enzymes, assuming that a reasonable portion of the response curve is considered (e.g. between 20 and 80% of maximal activity), it is likely that the sigmoidicity will produce s-values of up to 2 (see Table II). Some factors that limit the degree of sigmodicity in enzyme response have been discussed elsewhere.[10]

2. Substrate cycles

It is possible for a reaction which is non-equilibrium in the forward direction of a pathway (x$\longrightarrow$y, in the diagram below) to be opposed by a chemically distinct reaction that is non-equilibrium in the reverse direction of the pathway (x$\longleftarrow$y). These two separate reactions would be catalysed by different enzymes (E_2 and E_3). If the two enzymes act simultaneously, a substrate cycle will be established.

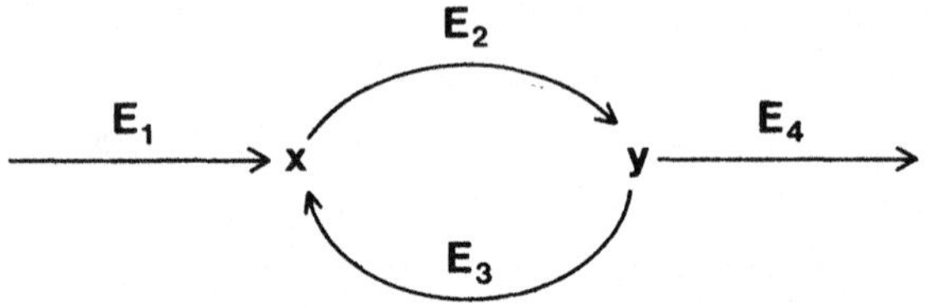

The precise quantitative role of substrate cycles in improving sensitivity has been developed in the course of our work,[6] the intrinsic sensitivity being given by: $1+\frac{\text{cycling rate}}{\text{flux}}$ (see Table II). This sensitivity factor has several important facets.

First, it is assumed that the response between substrate concentration and enzyme activity is first order. If a change in regulator concentration produces less than a linear response in enzyme activity (e.g. when the substrate concentration is above the K_m of the enzyme) the intrinsic sensitivity of the cycle will be less than : $1 + \frac{\text{cycling rate}}{\text{flux}}$; if the change in substrate concentration produces a greater than linear response (i.e. the response of enzyme activity to substrate concentration in sigmoid) the sensitivity will be greater than: $1 + \frac{\text{cycling rate}}{\text{flux}}$. In this latter case, the improvements in sensitivity from both cooperativity and cycling should be multiplied to give the overall improvement.

Second, it has been emphasised[6] that the sensitivity factor, $1 + \frac{\text{cycling rate}}{\text{flux}}$, represents <u>intrinsic</u> sensitivity - on the assumption that other factors which could modify sensitivity remain constant. For example, in the hypothetical cycle given above, if the concentration of the product (y) of the 'forward' enzyme (E_2) were increased by a similar extent to that of the substrate (x), the overall sensitivity of the cycle would be unaffected since the activity of E_3 could be increased to match that of E_2 . There are, however, various ways in which the effect of a change in product concentration (y) could be reduced or negated.[11] If the reverse enzyme (E_3) were saturated with its substrate (y) concentration changes above the saturation level could not affect the rate of cycling. Or the activity of the reverse enzyme (E_3) could be inhibited either by a changed concentration of an allosteric effector or by decreased concentration of a co-substrate. By inhibiting reverse enzyme activity, such changes could nullify the effect of an increased concentration of the product (y) which forms the substrate of the reverse reaction.

Comparison of cycling with the other mechanisms for increasing sensitivity shown in Table II reveals the quantitative importance of the relationship between cycling rate and overall flux. This will obviously be most sensitive to substrate or other regulator changes under 'basal' or 'resting' conditions, i.e. when the flux is low. Consequently, substrate cycling can be regarded as a metabolic control mechanism that is 'kinetically primed' to respond to a change in regulator signal (whereas the cooperative mechanism can be considered 'structurally primed'). The rate of energy utilisation that maintains the cycle in this 'primed' condition was at one time thought too large for the organism to 'permit' cycling.[8] However, the rise in body temperature resulting from conversion of chemical energy into heat may be the major limitation to the cycling rate.[6,12]

3. Interconvertible forms of enzymes

The regulation mechanism mediated by conversion of an enzyme from an inactive to an active form, and vice versa, has similarities to a substrate cycle, of which this 'interconversion cycle' represents a logical extension.[10] However, as noted above the substrate cycle mechanism may produce heat too rapidly to provide satisfactory control. That problem may be overcome by cycling between active and inactive forms of an enzyme (e.g. between phosphorylase a and phosphorylase b, or pyruvate dehydrogenase a and pyruvate dehydrogenase b). Interconversion cycling of this kind provides a control mechanism somewhat similar to the substrate cycle - but at a lower rate and, consequently, with less heat generation. The precise quantitative role of interconversion cycles in increasing sensitivity has not yet been defined, but qualitative general descriptions of their sensitivity are available.[10,13]

4. Near-equilibrium reactions

Many reactions in metabolic pathways are close to equilibrium, which confers biochemical advantage in conservation of energy.[1] But the major advantage of near-equilibrium reactions may lie in high sensitivity of enzyme activity to concentration changes of substrates and/or products. The power equation given earlier cannot be applied here because it applies only to non-equilibrium reactions. The intrinsic sensitivity of a near-equilibrium reaction to a change in substrate concentration is directly proportional to the reversibility of the reaction (R) - defined as the ratio between the rate of the forward reaction and the overall flux.[4,5,6]

The nearer a reaction is to equilibrium the greater is the value of R and the greater its sensitivity to concentration changes of substrates and/or products. Since such reactions are very sensitive to changes in product concentration (proportional to R-1), the change in product concentration should be small,[5] in order to retain some of the advantages of sensitivity to changes in substrate concentration.

The high level of sensitivity explains why a cell produces far more enzyme-protein for a near-equilibrium reaction than is necessary to accommodate the flux through the reaction.

THE FRUCTOSE 6-PHOSPHATE/FRUCTOSE BISPHOSPHATE CYCLE AND CONTROL OF GLYCOLYSIS IN MUSCLE.

Since the concept of substrate cycles in metabolic control is somewhat novel, an example may help to clarify their significance as control mechanisms and the means by which their sensitivity may be varied. Both features are exemplified by the fructose 6-phosphate/fructose bisphosphate cycle which regulates one step of glycolysis in muscle.

A major problem in providing adequate energy for muscle during exercise is that the rate of glycolysis must increase from a very low level in resting muscle to a high level during exercise. This is particularly a problem for human sprinting and for speed of escape in many animals. Most of the energy for such activities is obtained from the conversion of glycogen to lactate (anaerobic glycolysis) and the degradation of creatine phosphate. Compared with complete oxidation of glucose, this is a very inefficient means of energy production. Only 3 ATP molecules are produced for each glucose residue of glycogen metabolised, whereas complete oxidation would produce 36-38 ATP molecules. Since the power output of sprinting (or escape activity) is very high, the flux through this comparatively inefficient glycolytic process must be equally high. Since the energy demand of muscle at rest is very low, the transition from rest to maximal demand requires an enormous increase in the glycolysis rate - of approximately 2000-fold.[12]

The two non-equilibrium reactions involved in the control of glycolysis, both in the early portion of the pathway from glycogen, are catalysed by phosphorylase and phosphofructokinase. The control of phosphorylase activity is complicated by the existence of both an interconversion cycle, between phosphorylase _a_ and phosphorylase _b_, and a substrate cycle between glycogen and glucose 1-phosphate. Furthermore, phosphorylase _b_ may be controlled in a cooperative manner via changes in AMP concentration.[1] Consequently, this control mechanism may be very sensitive to changes in the concentrations of metabolic regulators. On the other hand, the activity of phosphofructokinase appears to be regulated by changes in the concentrations of ATP, creatine phosphate, AMP, P_i, fructose bisphosphate and NH_4^+ which have direct effects on the enzyme (via mechanisms discussed in detail elsewhere.[1,7])

The large increase (ca. 2000-fold) in the activity of phosphofructokinase necessary to provide the energy for muscular activity that depends on anaerobic glycolysis cannot, in our view, be obtained from the sensitivity afforded even by a sigmoid response to some or all of the above regulators. It could, however, be argued that high sensitivity is not required, since the concentration changes of the metabolic regulators might be very large during exercise. But this is not the case. Measurement of the total concentrations of these regulators in muscle at rest and during activity indicates that the changes are not very large (Table III).

Changes in the concentration of all these regulators depend upon the concentration ratio, ATP/ADP, in the muscle. A large change in the ratio would be necessary to produce comparably large changes in the concentrations of these regulators, despite the amplification provided via the adenylate kinase and possibly the AMP-deaminase reactions.[7,14] Moreover, both the concentrations of creatine phosphate, ATP and ADP and the ATP/ADP concentration ratio change very little in muscle, even in response to severe energy stress.[8,9]

The distribution of fructose bisphosphatase in a wide variety of muscles from many different types of animals led us to postulate that this enzyme played a role in the regulation of glycolysis via the operation of a substrate cycle between fructose 6-phosphate and fructose bisphosphate.[15] In recent years, the existence of such a cycle in skeletal muscle and liver has been directly demonstrated by specific isotope methods.[16,17] Its role in muscle could be to increase the sensitivity of metabolic control, at the level of fructose 6-phosphate phosphorylation, to changes in the concentrations of the phosphofructokinase regulators (e.g. creatine phosphate, ATP, AMP, P_i, NH_4^+).

The sensitivity of this fructose 6-phosphate/fructose bisphosphate cycle would be greatest when the ratio between cycling rate and flux was maximal - as in the cases already noted. But too high rates of cycling could lead to undue heat production and possible hyperthermia.[6,12] This problem may be overcome by variation of cycling rates, controlled by hormones or nervous activity.[6,12]

According to this hypothesis, the cycling rate would be very low when the subject is resting in the basal metabolic state. When exercise is anticipated, the rate of cycling would be raised, to increase the sensitivity of the metabolic control system. Hormones that might be involved in controlling rates of cycling in this way are adrenaline, noradrenaline, glucagon and glucocorticoids. There are at least two advantages in this form of control:

> First, high rates of cycling are only required for short periods, the rate being reduced to lower levels if the stress is withdrawn or if the exercise prepared for actually takes place and the glycolytic flux increases. Limiting the duration of high cycling

rates would minimise the amount of heat produced.

Secondly, the effect of the hormones (or nervous activity) would be confined to increasing the sensitivity of the metabolic control process to changes in the concentrations of endogenous regulators. The hormones (or nervous activity) would exert no direct effect on the rate of glycolysis or the basic cellular control mechanism.

In the case of the fructose 6-phosphate phosphorylation step in muscle, the basic cellular control mechanism is based on changes in the ATP/ADP concentration ratio. Since these are caused in active muscle by the activity of the myofibrillar ATPase (i.e. the activity of the contractile process per se), the regulatory mechanism for modulating the rate of fructose 6-phosphate phosphorylation (via changes in the concentrations of ATP, creatine phosphate, AMP, NH_4^+ and P_i) provides feedback control between energy utilisation and energy production. Consequently, the hormones do not interfere in this feedback link; they only improve the sensitivity of the control mechanism to changes in the concentrations of regulatory metabolites.

We believe that some hormones have an important effect in increasing the cycling rate in certain substrate cycles, to produce a marked rise in the sensitivity of the system to changes in metabolic (or other) regulators. Which hormones affect what cycles remains to be discovered.

HORMONE ACTION ON METABOLIC PROCESSES

Most current work on hormones influencing metabolic processes is directed towards understanding the mechanism of interaction between hormone and receptor and the identification and role of the secondary messenger in hormone action. Such detailed studies have diverted attention from the general principles of hormone action on metabolism. In the following paragraphs, recent findings are therefore discussed in relation to some of the principles of metabolic control already described.

1. The secondary messenger concept

The concept of the secondary messenger was proposed by Sutherland and colleagues in 1965 to account for the role of cyclic-AMP in mediating the intracellular response to a hormone.[18] In their elegant scheme, the hormone is seen as a primary messenger which, after release from the endocrine gland and transport via the blood stream, modifies metabolism within the target tissue(s) by changing the concentration of a secondary messenger.

Since 1965, a considerable amount of work has been directed towards understanding both the molecular events by which a hormone acts extracellularly, to influence the intracellular concentration of cyclic-AMP, and how the latter produces the physiological response in the target tissue. It is known that some hormones bind to a specific receptor on the cell surface, and that this binding enhances the activity of adenylate cyclase, which leads to an increase in the steady-state concentration of cyclic-AMP in the tissue. However, until recently, the precise quantitative roles played by adenylate cyclase and the phosphodiesterases (the enzymes that produce and utilise cyclic-AMP) in the maintenance of that steady-state concentration had not been considered. A number of models have now been proposed to account for the maintenance of steady-state cyclic-AMP concentrations and for changes in them.[2,19]

A simple model for the control of the concentration of a hypothetical secondary messenger is described below. The secondary messenger (X) is produced from compound A, via enzyme E_1, and X is utilised* by conversion to B via enzyme E_2.

$$A \xrightarrow{E_1} X \xrightarrow{E_2} B$$

The concentration of A must be provided from somewhere (i.e. a 'source' reaction is required to produce it), while B must be converted to another compound so that it does not accumulate (i.e. a 'sink' reaction is required for its removal). The reactions catalysed by the enzymes, E_1 and E_2, are non-equilibrium in type. In this model, enzyme E_1, is saturated with its substrate, A, this reaction being the flux-generating step, whereas the concentration of X is below the K_m of enzyme E_2 for this substrate in the second reaction. The system can be described mathematically, enabling the concentration of X to be calculated from the properties of the enzymes E_1 and E_2.

The most important points about control of the cyclic-AMP concentration in this model are that there is *always* a steady-state flux through the cyclic-AMP system, and that this flux is modified by the action of hormones - to produce changes in the steady-state concentration of cyclic-AMP. The usefulness of the model is that a knowledge of the *quantitative* effect(s) of the hormone on enzymes E_1 and/or E_2 can be used to predict the *precise* change in the concentration of the secondary messenger. Such effects of hormones on enzymes can be investigated *in vitro* with partially-purified enzymes,[2] as outlined below.

Although this simple model provides a useful introduction to the principles of hormone action, it is an oversimplification. The utilisation process actually

* The term 'utilised' is employed in the context of secondary or local messengers to mean conversion of such a messenger into a less active or non-active metabolite.

comprises at least two reactions, which may be entirely different or the same but have different functions. This complication must be included in the model. In the cyclic-AMP system, for example, the V_{max} and K_m values of the two phosphodiesterases are different. This can be illustrated by modifying the second stage of the hypothetical model as follows:

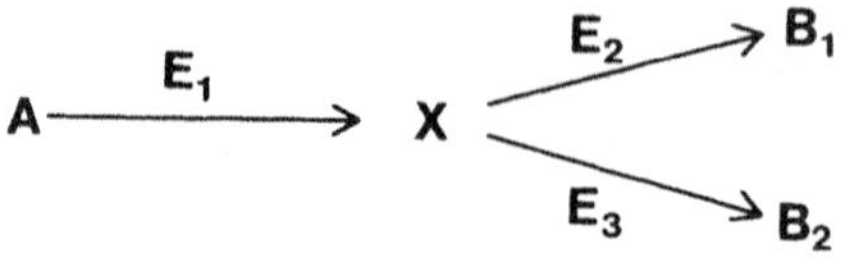

The actual sequence by which ATP is first transformed to cyclic-AMP, and then to AMP by two parallel reactions, takes the following form:

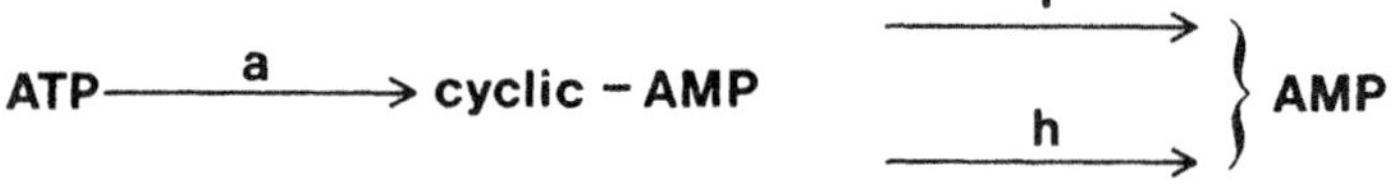

The activities of adenylate cyclase in the first stage, and of high- and low-K_m phosphodiesterases in the second are represented by a, l and h, respectively. The following assumptions are implicit in the model:

Adenylate cyclase is saturated with substrate (i.e.it is a flux-generating step)

All three enzymes catalyse non-equilibrium reactions

Both phosphodiesterases obey Michaelis-Menten kinetics.

The basal concentration of cyclic-AMP in a tissue can be calculated from in vitro measurements of V_{max} values for all three enzymes and of K_m values for the two phosphodiesterases. The increase in cyclic-AMP concentration produced by the action of hormones can also be calculated if the hormone effect on the activity of the cyclase and/or phosphodiesterase enzymes is known. If a hormone only affects adenylate cyclase activity, its maximum effect on cyclic-AMP concentrations can be obtained from knowledge of adenylate cyclase stimulation by fluoride in vitro, since this is considered to represent maximal hormonal stimulation of the enzyme.[20] The V_{max} value for fluoride-stimulated adenylate cyclase thus measured in vitro enables the stimulated (or maximal) concentration of cyclic-AMP in a tissue to be calculated.

Since the basal and fluoride-stimulated activities of adenylate cyclase and the activities and K_m values of the two phosphodiesterases have been measured in many different tissues,[2] the relevant concentrations of cyclic-AMP can be calculated according to the model. Where possible, such calculated tissue concentrations of cyclic-AMP have been compared with the measured concentrations reported in the literature[2] (Table IV). In general, calculated and reported concentrations are in reasonable agreement, but there are marked differences for both basal and hormone-stimulated concentrations in certain tissues (gastrocnemius muscle of mouse and rat and heart ventricle of frog). In these cases, calculation gives concentrations almost an order of magnitude lower than measurement. However, if the effect of hormone stimulation in raising the basal concentration is expressed as a ratio, i.e. stimulated concentration/basal concentration, there is remarkable agreement (except in the action of glucagon on rat liver). As shown in Table IV, the calculated ratios range from 1.7 to 7.4, and the measured ones from 1.7 to 4.0. This suggests that the model has some validity in assessing hormone-induced changes in concentration.

2. Hormone action and the flux-generating step

When a hormone modifies the flux through a metabolic pathway, its effect is generally mediated through the action of an intracellular secondary messenger such as cyclic-AMP. We have already seen how hormone action changes the concentration of the secondary messenger and how the amplification that might be necessary for this to produce the desired change in enzyme activity could be brought about. But one major question remains: which reactions in the pathway should (must) the hormone affect? To influence flux, it must plainly change the activity of the flux-generating step, directly or indirectly. In other words the secondary messenger may exert a direct effect on the activity of the enzyme that catalyses the flux-generating step, or it may act via another reaction whose product exerts such an effect. The cyclic-AMP secondary messenger system is a good example of this, since it modulates the activity of protein kinase which then modulates the activity of 'flux-generating' enzyme.

Once the activity of the flux-generating step has been increased by external control, via the action of the secondary messenger, the remainder of the reactions in the pathway could simply respond to the increases in the concentrations of pathway substrates produced by increased flux (internal control). However, the change in pathway-substrate concentration may not provide sufficient stimulus, particularly at non-equilibrium reactions, because of their innate insensitivity. It is therefore possible that the secondary messenger may also need to modulate the activity of 'non-equilibrium' enzymes that catalyse reactions following the flux-generating step. It should be emphasised that a hormone or secondary messenger acting solely upon a reaction (or reactions) other than the flux-generating step would not change the overall flux through the pathway. It could only lower substrate concentration at the reaction in question. The purpose of modifying the activity of later non-equilibrium reactions in addition to the flux-generating step

TABLE IV

Reported and calculated cyclic-AMP concentrations in different tissues

			Content of cyclic AMP (nmol/g of fresh tissue)[2]					
			Basal conditions		Stimulated conditions		Stimulated content / Basal content	
Animal	Tissue Preparation	Hormone addition	Measured	Calculated	Measured	Calculated	Measured	Calculated
Frog (*Rana pipiens*)	Heart ventricle strip during diastole	Adrenaline (10μM)	0.55	0.05	0.92	0.10	1.7	2.0
(*Rana catesbeiana*)	Muscle *in situ*	Adrenaline (50 nmol/kg body wt. injected into heart)	0.59	0.21	1.59	0.40	2.7	1.9
Mouse	Whole brain		1.1-1.3	1.7				
	Liver		0.95	0.15				
	Gastrocnemius muscle *in situ*	Adrenaline (25 nmol/kg body wt. injected intravenously)	1.95	0.16	4.8	0.46	2.5	2.9
Rat	Whole brain *in situ*	Adenosine (o.5μmol injected into cerebral ventricle)	1.9	2.2	5.0	3.7	2.6	1.7
	Perfused liver	Adrenaline (0.3μM)	0.5	0.28	2.0	2.1	4.0	7.4
		Glucagon (20 nM)	0.5	0.28	38.0	2.1	76.0	7.4
	Heart *in situ*	Adrenaline (10 nmol/kg body wt. per min)	0.5	0.74	1.8	3.0	3.6	3.0
	Gastrocnemius muscle *in situ*	Adrenaline (50 nmol/kg body wt. injected into heart)	0.68	0.09	1.82	0.30	2.7	3.3

is to prevent the concentration of metabolic intermediates in the pathway (i.e. pathway substrates) from changing markedly. Increased flux-generation alone could otherwise lead to bottle-necks at later reactions unable to cope with substrate build-up. The overall kinetic structure of the pathway has to be maintained.

METABOLIC REGULATION IN DEVELOPMENT AND AGEING

The processes that underlie the phenomena of development and ageing are of course much more complex than the process of glycolysis. It is nevertheless possible, at least in broad outline, to consider how the principles of metabolic control may be applied to these systems.

Development

The process of development involves control of transcription[21] - the means by which genetic information is transferred from DNA to the more mobile form of RNA molecules. In addition, there is some evidence that regulation of metabolic processes by general mechanisms, such as allosteric regulation and interconvertible forms of enzymes,[22] may be concerned in control of development. These general mechanisms are, however, assumed to be totally different from the specific mechanism that regulates the transcription process. This is usually known as repression, i.e. inhibition of the activity of DNA-dependent RNA polymerase towards part of the genome.

Repression is considered to involve physical restriction preventing the polymerase enzyme from transcribing specific parts of the genome. Non-histone proteins or special RNA molecules (or a combination of both) which may be involved in this physical restriction are known as repressor molecules. The presence of the repressor prevents the formation of messenger-RNA and thus the synthesis of specific proteins, which are therefore lacking in cells when this repressor is active. Removal of the repressor permits that portion of the genome to be transcribed, so that new specific proteins, which have important structural and catalytic properties in the cell, will be produced. This is, of course, what happens in development.

Let us assume that the repressor is a protein molecule that binds to a particular regulatory (or operator) site on the genome and prevents binding of the polymerase enzyme, so that transcription of that portion of the genome cannot take place. And suppose that the process of development requires that this portion of genome should be totally occluded, to prevent messenger-RNA synthesis of the corresponding protein molecules because they are not wanted in the cell. To achieve this, the repressor protein would have to bind so tightly to the genome that all available sites were fully occupied. One means would be covalent attachment. Removal of the repressor action could then be achieved only by specific cleavage of the covalent bond, for which a separate enzymatic reaction would be required. That enzyme would need to be totally (or almost totally) inactive in the repressed state yet highly active in the de-repressed state. Such large changes in activity could only be achieved by an interconversion cycle, or possibly by a substrate cycle combined with an interconversion cycle.

Alternatively, the repressor molecule could bind reversibly to the DNA, but the concentration of repressor would have to be very high to achieve total occupancy of all sites. De-repression would then present a problem: in order to facilitate dissociation from the DNA, the concentration of the repressor molecule would have to fall to extremely low levels. Such large changes in concentration could probably be achieved only via a substrate cycle, in which the concentration of the repressor (X) would be controlled by both 'information' and 'utilisation' reactions:

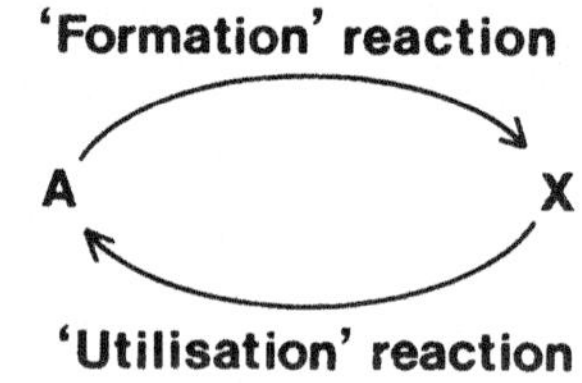

This system is analogous to the substrate cycles already discussed. Provided that the rates of both the formation and utilisation reactions were adequately regulated, it could result in very large yet controlled changes in repression concentration. A similar cyclic system has been described for the production of large changes in the concentration of adenosine, an important regulator of bloodflow in muscle and brain, and possibly also important as a modulator of neurotransmission in nervous tissue.[23,24] Large concentration changes are needed because it has to diffuse from one cell to another within a given organ in order to carry out its role as a local messenger or hormone.[23,24]

Ageing

While the process of ageing is not yet understood at molecular level, its effects can be seen in structural changes affecting some, possibly many, proteins[25] such as collagen and elastin. These structural changes may be caused by errors in the translation process, but it is also possible that they may arise during transcription and so become incorporated into the messenger-RNA. A central dogma of molecular biology lays down that genetic information is transferred unidirectionally:

DNA ——→ RNA ——→ protein

Consequently, any errors that arise in the synthesis of DNA or RNA will find their way into proteins, and this could result both in structural changes affecting cell constituents and in changes of enzyme activity. Such changes are likely to be detrimental to the wellbeing of the animal. So far, however, only one or two examples are known of changes in protein structure which can explain some of the very obvious macroscopic changes that characterise ageing (e.g. the changing protein structure of the lens which underlies deterioration in sight). There are sufficient grounds for speculation, however, and the following speculative hypothesis seeks to provide a molecular explanation for some of the characteristic macroscopic changes of ageing.

Failure of control systems during ageing. We have already seen that sensitivity in regulating the activity of enzymes that catalyse non-equilibrium reactions can only be improved by a limited number of mechanisms. Two of these could be described as dynamic, in that they depend upon the kinetics of an enzyme or enzymes, mainly or solely involved in regulation; they are the substrate cycle and the interconversion cycle. If the efficiency of these two separate cycles deteriorated with ageing, they would progressively fail to provide the high level of sensitivity required for normal metabolic control. This might come about in the following way.

The normal role of the substrate and interconversion cycles is to improve the sensitivity of the regulatory process, so that, when a regulator concentration alters, the change in enzyme activity will be sufficiently large to meet the demands of the new physiological situation. The regulator(s) could be operative within the cell (e.g. changed adenine nucleotide levels during exercise) or from outside (e.g. changed concentration of a hormone which mediates its effect through an intracellular secondary messenger). The high rate of the interconversion or substrate cycle will provide the necessary degree of amplification. However, if the maximum rates of these cycles are reduced during ageing, sensitivity to regulator changes could be very markedly reduced - with at least three consequences.

First, if the change in regulator concentration cannot produce a sufficient response from the metabolic system, then the physiological response will not be adequate. This can best be illustrated by an example: the energy for the contractile process in sprinting comes mainly from glycolysis, and the non-equilibrium enzymes in this process respond to changes in the concentration of certain regulators. If the sensitivity of the control mechanism is reduced, then the increase in the rate of glycolysis will not be sufficient to meet the energy demands of the contractile process. The rate of energy utilisation by the contractile process must then be curtailed, by the sprinter reducing speed or at least curbing acceleration. This is, of course, a well-known phenomenon of ageing.

Second, in an attempt to increase the rate of the metabolic process to meet physiological demand, the concentration of regulator may rise much higher than normal - to try and overcome the lack of sensitivity in the regulatory process. It is however possible that a very large increase in regulator concentration could be detrimental to the physiology of the particular tissue. We have already seen that large changes in metabolite concentration can disrupt the organised kinetic structure of a metabolic process; in addition, a large change in the concentration of a reactive intermediate could lead to the accumulation of side products which might be detrimental and even dangerous to the wellbeing of the cell. (For example, a large increase in the accumulation of intracellular glucose in a muscle - in an attempt to stimulate glycolysis and energy production - could lead to the accumulation of the less readily metabolised sugars, fructose and sorbitol via the polyol pathway. And there is evidence that the accumulation of fructose and sorbitol may be responsible for damage to nerves and possibly to the lens in diabetes mellitus).

Third, the substrate cycles discussed earlier as a mechanism for regulating the flux through metabolic pathways can be also involved in regulating the precise concentration of such things as intracellular ions (e.g. sodium and calcium ions). A reduction in the rate of such cycles could decrease the precision of regulation, to produce large fluctuations in the intracellular concentrations of such ions. This could cause detrimental changes in the rate of many important processes within the cell, such as might result in ionic and osmotic imbalance which could eventually lead to cell death.

The capacity of both interconversion and substrate cycles may be progressively reduced with age. In other words, the concentrations of the enzymes which determine the rate of operation of these cycles would be decreased during ageing. Alternatively, or perhaps in addition, it would be possible for the rate of such cycles to be reduced by impairment of the mechanism that responds to changes in regulation concentration. This could be as simple as a decrease in the affinity of an allosteric site on the enzyme that controls the rate of the cycle, or it could be as complex as impairment of the hormone receptor on the cell membrane. (Binding of hormone to receptor eventually brings about a change in the activity of the enzyme that controls the rate of the substrate or interconversion cycle). In either event the effect will be a reduction in the sensitivity of the regulatory system.

Since a large number of processes in all tissues of the body may be controlled by interconversion or substrate cycles, gradual impairment in the rate of such cycles with age could lead to a generalised decline in the responsiveness of tissues and of physiological processes within those tissues. This would produce a general deterioration in what might be termed the 'efficiency' of the many and varied physiological processes in the tissues and organs of the body.

We have discussed elsewhere[6] how a reduction in the rate of substrate cycles could, in particular, account for obesity; since this is common in middle and old age, it would be consistent with the hypothesis outlined above. Further, the syndrome of accidental hypothermia, which is very prevalent in debilitated elderly people in no more hostile an environment than their own home, could also be explained by inability to increase the rate of substrate cycles in response to hypothermia.[6] The energy normally expended in such cycles is released as heat, and this could well be one of the processes by which warm-blooded animals generate heat. A marked decrease in the capacity of such cycles, due to old age, would preclude adequate heat generation when they are stimulated.

DISCUSSION

The question of metabolic pathways an cycles that involve more than one tissue was taken up in discussion, with particular reference to the effect of introducing a new tissue like placenta. This might, for instance, affect the normal transfer of amino-acids between muscle and liver, and Hamish Munro enquired whether placental tissue diverts any of the alanine and glutamine released from muscle.

Certainly there are such effects, two of which were quoted by Maureen Young: a large amount of glutamine is transferred across the placental membrane, and glutamic acid is taken up by the placenta from the fetal circulation, for conversion into glutamine. More details of placental involvement in such processes are given in her own paper on techniques used in studying placental metabolism. Meanwhile, the next paper reviews the major metabolic processes that take place in the placenta and their relationships with both maternal and fetal metabolism.

A Personal note

Before giving her paper, Jean Ginsburg presented 'a brief vignette' about the symposium and its organiser. 'The story began 20 years ago when I went to Rome to learn some biochemistry and biochemical techniques from Professor Beaconsfield, who was then working with the Nobel laureate Daniel Bovet', she said. 'Twenty years is a long gestation, and the biologists here may feel that the fetus - the idea for this meeting - must have undergone facultative diapause a number of times in the process. That is in fact the case. Peter Beaconsfield tried more than once to interest obstetricians in the value of the placenta as a vehicle for various types of study and even wrote protocols for them, but they are faithful people who remained true to traditional views of the afterbirth. For them it remains something you incinerate or use to fertilise the roses. Yet thanks to Peter's tenacity and foresight, we are assembled here today. This symposium is his brainchild. He is a multifaceted individual whose intellectual curiosity has led him to have a finger in countless research pies since 1950. From tissue repair, tissue metabolism, and abnormal growth - all of which have engaged his attention over the years - it is only a step to feto-placental studies, and my own work here has been largely due to Peter's encouragement and participation. Those of you who know him will recognise his involvement in nearly all my publications. The paper I am presenting in a few minutes is his idea and construction, although I can take responsibility, and perhaps credit, for the tiresome chore of fishing out all the references - there are almost 200.

'The fact we are gathered here is proof that Peter's multidisciplinary concept, which he was one of the first to insist on, is now accepted as the route to progress in medical science. He is one of the few people who has always looked at research across the board, thinking horizontally to build up an overall picture, and only pausing for a vertical excursion into super-specialisation to solve particular problems.

'Ideas are the most precious things we have, and Peter has generated more - mostly for others to work on - than anybody else I know. Professor Pocchiari, who I am particularly glad to see sitting here, knows that what I am saying is correct. He was another member of that group generating ideas on biochemical processes in Rome 20 years ago - and he has never stopped either'.

CARBOHYDRATE, FAT AND PROTEIN METABOLISM IN THE PLACENTA: A CLINICIAN'S REVIEW

Peter Beaconsfield and Jean Ginsburg (Speaker)

'One man in his time plays many parts'

During its nine months of life, the placenta passes through the 'seven ages' of man, providing a multiple organ system which simultaneously serves fetal alimentary, pulmonary, renal,hepatic and endocrine functions at the various stages of development. The placenta is no passive filter. Yet the fact that it separates the maternal and fetal circulations anatomically, and that all exchange - gaseous, soluble or particulate, irrespective of the direction of transfer - takes place at this interface, long perpetuated the belief that the placenta functions simply as a filter barrier, albeit a specialised one. In recent years, however, this concept has been superseded by recognition that the placenta plays a selective and active role in transfer of substances essential for fetal development. The ability of the placenta to induce molecular modification of exogenous as well as endogenous material demonstrates its distinct metabolic identity, concerned with its own needs as well as those of the fetus.

Our clinical interest in the placenta is two-fold, as a regulator of the development and maintenance of the fetus and, second, to see what placental processes can teach us about corresponding physiopathological processes, from tissue rejection through cell replication to carcinoma. The placenta could serve as an excellent model system for such studies, but for the past ten years we have been unsuccessful in getting our obstetric colleagues to appreciate this fact and act on it.

The placenta takes nine months to develop, age, and be rejected, but who rejects who, and what controls the process? Since such biological processes are controlled by biochemical mechanisms, biochemistry offers one way of studying, understanding, and interfering with them. For full assessment of organ or gissue metabolism we need to know the metabolic pathways, the factors that control flux through then, the key intermediate metabolites and their turnover, and the ramic points which determine the direction of metabolic flow. This is the counsel of perfection. In reality the information available is seldom complete, and the precision attainable by the basic scientist is inevitably modified by the biological and ethical constraints imposed on the clinician. Equally a distinction must be made between the reasonable accuracy of controlled studies and the wide variations encountered in clinical practice.

These factors must be borne in mind when we consider the biochemical processes in the placenta, what influences them, and in what way this information could help explain - on one hand - the clinical problems of small-for-dates babies, toxaemia, and initiation of labour, and - on the other - the fundamental process of normal and abnormal cell replication, immunological response and rejection, and ageing. In the following outline, some points may appear to be oversimplified. This is deliberate; our aim is to review current knowledge, not present every detail. We may also seem guilty of biochemical blasphemy, but the blasphemy of yesterday has often become the gospel of tomorrow.

We are looking for parallels, for comparisons and for contrasts that may shed light on biochemical activity, immune responses, cell replication, and ageing in all body tissues. Rapid growth, energy consumption and various aspects of metabolism in the placenta have their counterparts in all replicating cells. This presupposes similar mechanisms of information transfer and feedback. But how is overall control exercised? Feedback mechanisms alone can be overwhelmed if confronted with too much information.

We know that metabolism is controlled by demand, by availability of substrate together with appropriate enzymes and co-factors which determine the activity of the pathways, and the turnover of intermediate metabolites. Rather than include all these factors, we want to look at the metabolic characteristics of the placenta, to note which are unique to it and which resemble processes in liver or other tissues. Both contribute to the placenta's potential as an experimental animal.

Placental transfer

The placenta behaves like a lipid membrane towards exogenous compounds such as environmental pollutants, drugs and other ingested chemicals. In the main, these cross in accordance with their concentration gradients, at rates related to their lipid solubility and degree of ionisation.[1] Other factors may also affect individual rates of transfer, the most important including relative protein binding, particular chemical groupings, and molecular modification by the placenta itself.[2,3]

By contrast, virtually all endogenous substances essential for fetal development (apart from the respiratory gases) cross the placenta against an electrochemical gradient. This is a process of considerable specificity. Gammaglobulin, for example, is transferred at a higher rate than albumin, despite its greater molecular size. Yet human chorionic somatotrophin (HCS) - which is of similar molecular weight and action, and produced by the trophoblast itself - is found only in minute quantities on the fetal side of the barrier.

Molecular transfer across the placenta is a more complex process than transfer across other cellular membranes, such as the blood / brain barrier. Transfer of proteins may involve passage through several placental cells with or without molecular modification in the process. The marked selectivity of placental transfer has important biological consequences. The immunoglobulins, as a group, cross faster than alpha- and betaglobulins, but there is further selectivity within the group, with discrimination against the IgM fractions.[4] The implications of this for maintenance of fetal immunological privilege are discussed in Section III.

In recognising and permitting protein entry into its cells, the placenta further differentiates between those proteins being transported through to the fetus and those which will undergo proteolysis in placental tissue. Whether some disturbances of pregnancy may be due to breakdown of these discriminatory mechanisms is open to discussion, as is the nature of the specific placental mechanisms which maintain immunological privilege for nine months, in contrast to graft rejection on one hand and with continued survival of carcinoma on the other.

The mechanisms responsible for placental transfer in general and the quantitative aspects of drug transfer in particular have been discussed in many reviews.[1-3,5] They will be considered here only in relation to placental metabolic processes. The selectivity of transfer and the active involvement of the placenta in the transfer of all compounds essential for fetal development is dependent on the energy produced by the placenta itself. How the placenta produces this energy by its own intrinsic metabolism and some of the factors which modify the pattern of placental metabolism is discussed below.

PLACENTAL CARBOHYDRATE METABOLISM

What drives the machinery?

Glucose is the pivotal point of intermediary metabolism. It is the main source of metabolic fuel and hence of energy; it provides the basis for reserve fuel stores, and by its catabolism yields a mosaic of intermediate metabolites - essential building blocks in the formation of structural and other cellular components. These three facets of intracellular glucose activity are also operative in the placenta, which has a very high basal metabolic rate. At least one-third of the oxygen and glucose provided by the maternal circulation for the conceptus is used to support the metabolism of the placenta itself[6,7] - the actual proportion depending on their relative size and respective metabolic activities of the fetus and placenta in different phases of gestation.

Monosaccharide transfer

The fetal liver supplies a small proportion of fetal glucose requirements, the major part coming from maternal glucose via the placenta, which it crosses in accordance with the concentration gradient. But the rate of glucose transfer is much greater than would be expected on physico-chemical grounds alone, indicating that its diffusion must be facilitated by special carrier systems. Several have been postulated for monosaccharide transfer[7,8,9,10,11] but little is known of their nature. They seem to be oxygen-dependent since maternal glucose levels, but not those of the fetus, increase if the mother becomes hypoxic.[12] The differential placental transfer of dextro-and laevo-isomers indicates stereochemical specificity of the carrier system: D-glucose and D-mannose are both transferred at a faster rate than L-glucose,[13] and fructose transfer is inhibited when glucose concentrations are increased.[14]

Although placental glucose transfer might be expected to vary at different stages of gestation in accordance with changes in placental and fetal growth, this aspect has not been studied in man. In the rat, the rate of tritium-labelled glucose transfer across the placenta has been shown to increase markedly towards the end of gestation[15] when there is a spurt in fetal growth.

Glucose uptake

Placental tissue has a high rate of glucose uptake, comparable with and even higher than that in the liver,[16,17] but the mechanisms regulating glucose uptake by the placenta and its subsequent metabolism through one or other of the alternative pathways of intermediary carbohydrate metabolism seem to differ in certain respects from those in the liver.[18] The early placenta has a high glucose uptake related to its rapid growth rate; at term, when placental growth has slowed, glucose uptake is less.[16,17]

Malignant tissues also have a high rate of glucose uptake[19,20,21] which is influenced in both placenta and tumors by the availability of oxygen.[16,17,20] Human placenta and carcinomata also both demonstrate the so-called Pasteur effect - increased glucose uptake in anoxic conditions[22] - but its mechanism and biological significance are not understood.[23]

Glucose phosphorylation

Glucose must be phosphorylated before it can take part in cellular metabolism. Glucose 6-phosphate is the ramic point whence a glucose molecule can be either degraded or converted into storage glycogen. In the liver there is a specific high-affinity hexokinase, glucokinase, which facilitates phosphorylation and probably acts as a controller in the minute-to-minute regulation of blood glucose.[21] In the placenta, however, only a non-specific hexokinase has been identified thus far.[25] Theoretically, this would imply rapid saturation of the mechanisms for placental glucose phosphorylation and hence reduced and regulated flux through one or other pathway of glucose metabolism. However, placental glucose utilisation is consistently high,[16,17,26] which seems to suggest that there may be an alternative mechanism for phosphorylation in the placenta. Is this an enzyme reaction as yet unidentified, or could it be an alternative pathway, as suggested by studies of intermediary metabolism in the liver?[27,28] The situation is similar in tumors where glucose uptake is also high[19,20,21] and the hexokinase has been shown in many instances to be a placental type iso-enzyme.[29] One of the distinctive features of the placenta is a high rate of lactate production[17,26] indicating a high rate of glycolytic flux, and this also occurs in tumors.

Pathways of glucose metabolism

The placenta has all the necessary enzymes and cofactors for operation of the two main pathways of glucose metabolism - the glycolytic Emden-Meyerhof pathway, associated with the Krebs'cycle, and the pentose phosphate pathway. Their continued operation provides energy as well as essential precursors for bio-synthesis of proteins, pyrimidines, and fats - among other compounds.

As in most adult tissues, the main route for glucose catabolism in the placenta is the glycolytic pathway.[18] Energy for multiple cellular purposes is generally provided by ATP resulting from stepwise degradation of glucose via the Emden-Meyerhof pathway and the Krebs' cycle, coupled with the mitochondrial cytochrome oxidative system.

The net gain of ATP as a result of substrate phosphorylation in the glycolytic pathway and through the mitochondrial oxidation of NADH is eight moles per mole of glucose;[30] completion of oxidation through the Krebs' cycle produces a further 30 moles of ATP, giving a total of 38 moles ATP from one mole of glucose in aerobic conditions.

The crucial factor for the cell's survival is availability of energy. Since ATP is the means whereby the cell gets its energy, an optimum supply must be maintained, and normally ATP formation is a fairly well controlled process. Glucose metabolism yields ATP, and this in turn is used in the synthesis of enzymes which catalyse ATP production - the process is autoregulatory and autocatalyic. Changes in the relative utilisation of the different pathways of glucose metabolism may alter this.

The precise quantative contributions of the alternative pathways of placental glucose breakdown depend on the stage of gestation. In the blastocyst, glucose breakdown is almost exclusively through the pentose pathway,[31] and only after implantation does the glycolytic route predominate.[32] Activity in the placental pentose pathway further declines in the course of pregnancy,[33] being estimated at some 10% of the total early in gestation and 5% at term,[18] with corresponding increases in the Emden-Meyerhof pathway. This shift in the relative utilisation of different metabolic pathways can be related to the relative rate of cell replication at different stages of gestation. Pentose shunt activity is elevated in all rapidly growing systems such as embryonic tissue, healing wounds, regenerating liver, neoplasia, and the early placenta.[33,34]

A parallel has been demonstrated between activity in the placental pentose phosphate pathway and rates of protein turnover and nucleic acid synthesis at different stages of gestation,[33] in keeping with the central role of the pentose shunt in providing D-ribose for nucleic acid synthesis. This is true of all cell replication, whether normal, such as regeneration, or abnormal as in cancer.

It has been suggested that a decrease in glucose metabolism by the pentose route results in decreased RNA formation and a general reduction in protein synthesis,[33] probably mainly as a result of reduced messenger-RNA synthesis. We know that slowing the pentose shunt slows down the rate of growth.

The perennial question then arises: why do some cells continue replicating and others not? Where is the breakdown or disturbance in relaying information in the metabolic process? We will return to this point later.

Lactate production

The placenta produces lactic acid, the end product of the Emden-Meyerhof pathway, in abundance throughout gestation, the rate being somewhat higher in the early placenta than at term.[17] The elevated rate of glycolysis may be linked with cell replication, and lactate production is also high in tumours where the rate of glycolysis correlates with the growth rate.[35] In this respect, the biochemical characteristics of the placenta parallel its initial invasive activity. Placental lactate production is increased in anoxic conditions, and under the influence of adrenaline.[17,36] Anoxia induces similar changes in tumour metabolism.

Why does the placenta produce so much lactate and what happens to it? The second question is the easier to answer. Being freely diffusible, lactate theoretically could cross the placenta in either direction but its passage seems to be selective towards the fetus. Lactic acid has been considered a metabolic 'cul de sac', but lactate from the placenta may be an important substrate for fetal metabolism, accounting for as much as 25% of fetal oxidative metabolism.[37] Excess lactate may also be oxidised by the placenta, presumably through the action of lactate dehydrogenase, and could then be used for amino-acid and thus protein synthesis.

As indicated above, operation of the glycolytic pathway as far as lactate results in less available useful energy than when glucose is oxidised through the Krebs' cycle. The parallels between tumours and placenta in respect of high lactate production may be related to their similar requirement of metabolites for tissue growth. Indeed the demand for products of the Krebs' cycle may be so great in both instances that full operation of the cycle to produce ATP is impeded. This interpretation is supported by Villee's finding that there is little net synthesis of ATP in placental mitochondria, although he gave different reasons for this.[38] Increased activity of the glycolytic pathway is required to make good the deficit, but since glycolysis up to pyruvate produces only a fraction of the amount of ATP obtained from completion of the Krebs' cycle, the rate of glycolysis, as judged by lactate formation, is markedly increased. So there could be a biological explanation of the somewhat bizarre biochemical pattern of both placenta and tumour tissue. We would be on much firmer ground in judging the true rate of metabolic activity had we been able to carry out turnover studies, instead of having to rely on measurement of changes in intermediate metabolites and other chemical compounds.

Glucose anabolism

1. Glycogen formation. It is 120 years since Claude Bernard first demonstrated glycogen in the rabbit placenta and suggested that this is the means whereby the placenta, 'un véritable organe hépatique', produced glucose for the fetus early in pregnancy pending functional maturity of the fetal liver. Placental glycogen levels are higher early in gestation than at term[16,17] in keeping with his concept.[39]

The attraction of the Claude Bernard hypothesis is that it provides a biological explanation, in terms of fetal requirements, of the observed biochemical changes in the placenta during gestation. However, this explanation ignores the fact that the placenta, and hence the fetus, has no problem in obtaining glucose at any stage of pregnancy so long as the mother is alive. There is no need to store glycogen in the placenta for this purpose since maternal glucose levels are maintained well above the concentration in the fetal circulation.

Placental glycogen is deposited in the walls and vicinity of the major fetal blood vessels, whereas glycogen concentration is low in the areas where nutritional transfer takes place.[40] Placental glycogen is therefore not sited where an emergency breakdown to glucose would be either advantageous or available to the fetus. The fetal liver is in fact much better equipped than the placenta to provide a fetal energy store, and it contains far more storage glycogen than the placenta.[40] In choriocarcinoma tissue there is also much more glycogen than in the placenta.[41] Decreased degradation of glycogen appearsto be responsible, rather than increased synthesis, since phosphorylase and glycogen synthetase activity are low. It is not to be expected that a rapidly growing tissue like cancer would also be a storage organ; it obtains its metabolic requisites from its host. Even in malignant hepatoma, glycogenic activity is decreased compared with normal liver.

What then is the function of placental glycogen and what are the factors determining its deposition? Although the site of deposition suggests involvement in placental vascular activity, the role of glycogen in such processes is not known. Glycogen may, under the influence of human chorionic gonadotrophin (HCG), provide the necessary energy and cofactors for aromatisation processes in placental steriod formation.[42,43] Glycogen degradation may also provide the energy necessary for continued amino-acid transfer to the fetus, even in anoxia.[44] Placental glycogen could therefore be considered as an energy source for placental metabolic activity and not as a provider of glucose for the fetus.

Glycogen synthetase activity in the placenta decreases towards term[45] and so does the placental glycogen concentration.[16,17] Activity of the phosphorylase which catalyses glycogen breakdown is greater at term than in the early placenta.[45] The inactive form phosphorylase <u>b</u> predominates at term and the active form <u>a</u> in early gestation. In the absence of turnover studies the significance of this is uncertain.

As might be expected, insulin increases placental glycogenesis,[46] apparently through an action on the enzyme regulating tissue glycogen synthesis, and glycogen levels increase further with increasing glucose concentration. Specific binding sites for insulin similar to those reported in other tissues are present in the human placenta[47,48,49] in greater quantity at term than early in gestation.[46] This may explain the greater effect of the hormone on placental glycogen synthesis at term,[46] which may be related in turn to an influence of insulin on tissue growth.

2. Glucose production by the placenta, whether resulting from gluconeogenesis or liberation of glucose from storage glycogen, is small by comparison with the amount of glucose received direct from maternal blood. The placenta can apparently produce glucose from pyruvate in the early weeks of gestation, but it is not thought to do so at term.[16,50]

The placental activity of enzymes associated with gluconeogenesis (such as phosphoenolpyruvate carboxylase and aspartate aminotransferase) does not fall in late pregnancy, but if anything increases, which suggests that glucose production de novo may be important even at term, but this has yet to be demonstrated. The absence of fructose 1-6 diphosphatase[25] in the placenta would, however, argue against gluconeogenesis being a major placental metabolic activity.

As regards glucose from glycogenolysis, adrenaline administration produces lactate in quantity from the placenta, rather than glucose. In this the placenta resembles skeletal muscle more than liver. Studying the effect of glucagon on the placenta should elucidate the mechanism of these differences. In the perfused placenta HCG has been shown to evoke the release of glucose into the perfusate.[42] This effect is reproduceable by dibutyryl cyclic-AMP and also by prostaglandins, but whether the glucose is derived directly and only from glycogen needs confirmation by radioactive studies.

What we really need to know is whether placental glucose, released by a glycogenolytic effect or produced by other means, is directly transferred to the fetus or used only by the placenta for its own anabolic activity, or if both, in what proportions.

3. Fructose formation in the placenta has been intensively studied ever since very high levels were found in the ungulate fetus (though not in that of man or rat). Placental transfer of fructose is much slower than that of glucose,[10,51] and the high levels in the sheep fetus result from placental production of this sugar.[51,53]

Since fetal fructose seems to be high in species where placental glycogen is low, and vice versa (as in man), it has been suggested that fructose may function as a reserve carbohydrate store for emergency use.[54]

It is not known why the human placenta produces fructose at all;[55] the only other human tissue which does so is the seminal vesicle. In the liver, dietary fructose has a greater capacity for triglyceride synthesis than glucose[56] but in the human placenta lipid synthesis from fructose is less than from glucose.

4. Lipid formation from glucose is thought to be responsible for only a small fraction of placental glucose utilisation and to contribute only a minor fraction of placental lipids. *In vitro* studies with the human placenta show that lipid synthesis from radioactively labelled glucose is less than that from palmitate.[58] Similarly, in rhesus monkeys, although labelled glucose was incorporated into placental (and also into fetal) lipids, palmitate is by far the more important precursor.[59] Although placental glucose utilisation is higher in early gestation than at term, monkey placentae at these stages show no difference in the proportion of glucose converted into lipid.[58,59] In fetal tissues however the relative distribution of glucose and palmitate between lipid synthesis and catabolism does change with age,[59] and presumably in relation to growth and differentiation.

CYCLIC-AMP and -GMP

Recognition that the nucleotides, cyclic adenosine monophosphate (cyclic-AMP) and cyclic guanosine monophosphate (cyclic-GMP), have specific intracellular roles has stimulated investigation of their involvement in cellular activity. Cyclic-AMP acts as a second messenger or intracellular effector of a variety of hormonal and metabolic events[60,61,62] while cyclic-GMP may promote opposing intracellular events, particularly in relation to cellular proliferation.[63,64]

An adenyl cyclase system responsive to catecholamines[64,65,66,67,68] and to HCG with simultaneous induction of placental glycogenolysis[42,69] is present in the human placenta. These effects can be reproduced by a cyclic-AMP analogue,[70] by certain prostaglandins,[43,69,71] and also by luteinising hormone (LH).[69]

A cyclic-AMP mediated role for HCG in placental steroid formation has been proposed, glycogenolysis being the first step, with production of glucose and also of NADPH.[42] By virtue of an action on placental glycogen levels and glucose production, HCG could influence placental metabolic energy. There seems to be a reciprocal relationship between HCG and cyclic-AMP in the placenta. At the same time as HCG activity is mediated by cyclic-AMP, placental HCG secretion is itself stimulated by dibutyryl cyclic-AMP[70,72,73] so that hormone action would, by increasing cyclic-AMP levels, create the conditons required for its own continued production. Could a similar mechanism operate with other placental hormones or with HCG production in tumours? Now that we can specifically measure HCG and other hormones in micro-concentrations, we could investigate the existence of similar reciprocal self-perpetuating mechanisms for proteins concerned in cell replication.

Placental cyclic-AMP levels and activity and their relation to placental and fetal development have not been investigated. Impairment of amino-acid transfer across the placenta in cases of 'small for dates' babies correlates with a lowered level of cyclic-AMP in the placenta - which suggests a causal relationship.[74]

Cyclic-GMP has been studied in tissues as disparate as psoriatic skin[75] and silkworm pupae,[76] but incredibly not even the level of nucleotide has been accorded the same attention in the human placenta.

PLACENTAL LIPID METABOLISM

Lipids are the major structural components of cell membrane, their characteristics modulating hormone and enzyme action, antigen-antibody reaction, and drug effects. The role of placental lipid metabolism in determining membrane characteristics is therefore relevant to cell replication and to immunological responses - which may be further affected by the changed pattern of blood lipids during gestation. Lipid solubility of drugs is the most important single factor governing their transplacental transfer, and the placental microsomal electron transfer system which metabolises drugs also participates in specific hydroxylation steps in steroid biosyntheses.

Lipids are also the body's major energy store. In the average man 100 000 kilocalories are provided by lipid from adipose tissue, but only 600 kilocalories from glycogen.[77] The total amount of lipid in the placenta is small by comparison with other tissues,[78,79] so it has been assumed to play a minor role in energy production. Studies of both placental lipid turnover and maternal fatty acid supply are necessary to clarify this assumption. Despite the importance of lipids in cell function, their metabolism is still the Cinderella of placental investigation, the only aspect extensively studied to date being their relationship to steriod hormone production.

The concentration of nearly all lipid fractions rises in maternal blood during pregnancy[80] with the exception of the phospholipid lysolecithin which falls.[81] The levels of most lipid fractions are higher in maternal than in fetal plasma, but there are marked differences in their relative concentration in placental tissue, maternal blood, and cord blood. Free fatty acid, free cholesterol, phospholipid, lecithin, lysolecithin, and sphingomyelin levels are much higher in placental tissue at term than in maternal plasma, but placental cholesterol ester and triglyceride levels are lower.[80] Linoleic acid concentration is relatively high, and arachidonic acid concentration low, in maternal blood, but the position is reversed in fetal blood.[80] These differences in relative concentration cannot be explained in terms of differences in phospholipid levels between blood and 'solid' tissue. The pattern suggests rather that the placenta plays an active role in fat transfer, synthesis, and catabolism.

The larger fat molecules such as lipoproteins and phospholipids apparently do not cross the placenta intact. Lipolysis is thought to occur in the placenta, with constituent fatty acids and other components being transferred to the fetal blood-stream while the larger fat molecules are resynthesised in fetal tissues.[82,83,84] The presence of the lipoprotein lipase which hydrolyses maternal serum triglyceride in the placenta[85] supports this view, as does the fact that there is no very low density lipoprotein (VLDL) in cord blood.[80]

Fatty acid transfer and metabolism

The ability of the placenta to transport fatty acids varies in different animal species. It is poor in rats[86] and sheep,[87] and appreciable in guinea pigs[88-9] rabbits,[90] and primates.[91-93] In contrast to fetal glucose and amino-acids, which are mainly supplied directly from maternal blood, only limited amounts of free fatty acids are thought to cross the placenta. Theoretically fetal fatty acids could be derived from two sources: from maternal plasma, in the form of free fatty acids or from placental breakdown of triglycerides and phospholipids,or from direct placental fatty acid synthesis.

In the human placenta, lipid transfer is usually in accordance with the concentration gradient, but perfusion of the human full term placenta after delivery has shown palmitate transfer against the concentration gradient.[92] In the same model the rate of placental fatty acid transfer increases with protein binding and with shortening of the carbon chain.[93] Transport of fatty acids in the reverse direction, i.e. from fetus to mother has also been demonstrated, both in laboratory animals[88-90] and in man.[92]

The selective nature of placental fatty acid transfer is indicated by the differential transfer rates for different fatty acids. Raising maternal free fatty acid levels by the administration of adrenaline does not produce a general rise in cord blood fatty acids.[94] Interpretation of this last study is complicated by the hormonal and metabolic response to the simultaneous rise in glucose and fatty acid levels induced by adrenaline. Linoleic acid transfer increases as pregnancy advances,[91] but since placental transfer of other acids has not been studied at different stages of gestation, we do not know if accelerated transfer occurs with other fatty acids at term. In rabbits, maternal fasting before delivery results in the young having larger fat stores with increased levels of triglyceride and free fatty acids and an increased metabolic response to cold thereafter.[95,96] In starvation, maternal lipid is presumed to be mobilised and transfer accelerated in utero. The implications of these results for human pregnancy are obvious; but many other changes induced by starvation might also affect maternal and placental metabolism.

Triglycerides from maternal plasma appear to be the major source of fatty acids for the fetus,[75] fatty acid synthesis being a minor metabolic process in the placenta in keeping with its low levels of acetyl coA carboxylase activity.[98] The placental contribution has been calculated to be about 2% of the total fatty acid requirements in fetal rats.[98] There are no comparable human data. A scheme has been proposed for fatty acid synthesis in the human placenta[99] but catabolism of fatty acid by the placenta has been little studied. However, palmitate is known to be oxidised by the human placenta linearly with time[100] and we may assume that other fatty acids are metabolised similarly.

Placental triglyceride and phospholipid metabolism

Placental triglycerides are apparently derived by esterification of fatty acids supplied either from the maternal circulation,[59,101,102] or produced as the result of de novo placental synthesis.[103] In the placenta, as in other tissues, triglyceride synthesis depends on continued provision of glycerophosphate, which in turn depends on the availability of ATP and hence on glycolysis. Thus, in vitro studies of the human placenta show triglyceride synthesis to be unaffected in the absence of exogenous glucose, and to fall slightly when tissue anoxia is induced by cyanide; there is also a marked fall in fatty acid incorporation after inhibition of glycolysis.[104] The presence of the lipoprotein lipase,[85] and the absence of VLDL in cord blood,[80] as mentioned earlier, indicates that triglycerides are not transferred as such to the fetus but that maternal triglycerides are degraded in situ. The precise fate of the residual components is not known. Despite the rapidity with which the placenta synthesises triglycerides, their overall concentration in it remains low, indicating that placental glyceride turnover must be high. Why is this so?

The concentration of phospholipids in the placenta is relatively high, representing about 75% of total placental lipids. This seems more likely to be the result of direct placental synthesis than uptake from maternal blood, since the fatty acid composition of placental phospholipids differs from those in maternal blood. At term the human placenta is able to perform all the necessary reactions for phosphoglyceride synthesis,[105] and comparable studies are needed on the early placenta. The available evidence suggests that placental phospholipid synthesis is higher in the later stages of gestation in human[106] and rat[107] placentae. This appears to parallel changes in arteriolar senescence.

It is difficult, however, to reconcile the higher overall rate of placental fat synthesis at term[106,107] with the finding of lowered placental pentose shunt activity[33] and NADPH levels[108] at this stage. This highlights our ignorance of the function of phospholipids in placental cellular economy. It has been suggested that they may be involved in transport of amino-acids across the placenta[109] and in the intravascular coagulation associated with toxaemia of pregnancy.[110] Further speculation is unwarranted until we know why their placental concentration is nearly three times that of maternal blood. Are phospholipids concerned with modulation of hormone action at the placental barrier? Do they provide a 'reserve' store for fetal requirements or for steroid biosynthesis? Are they involved in the regulation of RNA synthesis? Answers to some of these questions might also shed light on the genesis of atherosclerosis and on ageing of the immune system.

Placental cholesterol and cholesterol ester metabolism

Cholesterol is both transported across the placenta[111,112,113] and synthesised by placental tissue,[114,115,116] the latter being of particular importance in the production of steroid hormones. The fatty acid pattern of fetal cholesterol esters differs from that in maternal blood which suggests they are not transferred direct.[80] Placental tissue can synthesise cholesterol esters from fatty acids and cholesterol,[117] but the extent of this reaction and the subsequent fate of the cholesterol ester is not known. Neither is it known whether cholesterol esters can be catabolised by the human placenta; in other tissues, the enzyme responsible is a cyclic-AMP-dependent protein kinase, activated by a phosphorylase system.

Influence of lipids on placental function

The recognition that the placenta can synthesise triglycerides and phospholipids is generally discussed in relation to fetal requirements of these compounds. The importance of placental lipid metabolism for placental function itself is rarely discussed. Equally, we should consider the possible role of the placenta in determining maternal hyperlipidaemia and, vice versa, its possible influence on placental function. There is little evidence whether placental synthesis contributes to maternal hyperlipidaemia, though the fact that overall lipid synthesis in the placenta is relatively low might argue against this. The possibility that maternal hyperlipidaemia might influence placental function has not yet been studied.

Phylogenetically, as organisms become biochemically more sophisticated, peripheral tissues such as skeletal muscle increasingly burn fats, sparing glucose for tissues such as the brain, for which it is essential. The rise in maternal blood lipids has therefore been assumed to be a protective mechanism for the mother, whereby increased fat metabolism in peripheral maternal tissues would ensure that, despite division of glucose and gluconeogenic precursors by the placenta to the fetus, sufficient is available for essential needs such as the maternal brain. The fact that pregnant women are frequently ketonaemic would support this view. The increasing levels of HCS during pregnancy which stimulate lipolysis would provide an additional means of 'sparing' maternal glucose. In the light of the biochemical resemblances between the placenta and skeletal muscle referred to earlier, the placenta might similarly utilise fatty acids in preference to glucose. The relative utilisation of these two substrates by the placenta in different circumstances requires detailed investigation.

Lipids and immune responses

There is evidence from animal studies that lipids may influence immune responses to antigens and also immune defences against experimental neoplasia and transplantation,[118-120] and decreased immune responsiveness to antigens has been postulated in hyperlipidaemic states.[121] These findings obviously have important implications, yet the fact that no comparable studies have been performed with the human placenta shows how little importance has been given to the placenta except in its role of sustaining the fetus. Placental lipid metabolism may play a crucial part in the mechanisms conferring immune status on the conceptus.

PLACENTAL PROTEIN METABOLISM

Placental growth is dependent on protein metabolism. Proteins are responsible not only for the characteristic structure of the organ but for the enzymes which control both the growth process itself and the metabolic activity that provides the necessary energy. Protection of the fetus also depends on proteins - on those of the endoplasmic reticulum, on enzymes which modify foreign chemicals and environmental pollutants, and on the various placental proteins which may confer immunological privilege on the conceptus. In addition, the placenta synthesises a considerable quantity of proteins for 'export' - peptide hormones, certain globulins and enzymes - as well as for home consumption in its own structure and functions.

Protein synthesis is dependent on and controlled by nucleic acids. The process is similar in all forms of life - animals, plants and micro-organisms. In brief, the sequence of nucleotide bases in DNA determines the amino-acid sequence and hence the structure of individual proteins. Information from DNA is transferred to RNA which is then conveyed to the cytoplasm where the particular amino-acids are selected and directed to the ribosomes, the site of protein synthesis. The process is energy-dependent, and requires specific enzymes (which are themselves proteins) for the synthesis of individual proteins. Total protein production by the placenta has been calculated as 1.5 g per day at ten weeks, when the organ weighs only 50 g, and 7.5 g per day at term when it weighs 450 g.[122]

Protein synthesis can be studied by incubation of tissue slices and measurement of protein levels in tissue and medium, determination of labelled amino-acid incorporation into placental proteins after incubation, and protein production in cultures of specific cell lines from trophoblast tumours. Cell-free placental protein synthesis has also been studied, using free and membrane-bound polyribosomes obtained from human placentae.[123-4] and messenger-RNA extracted from placental polyribosomes.[124] The energy requirements for protein synthesis are considerable - four to five molecules of ATP for each peptide bond alone.[125] No wonder pregnant women get tired.

Changes in protein metabolism during pregnancy

Protein metabolism increases overall during pregnancy, not only in the areas where new tissue is being formed, and plasma protein turnover in particular is markedly increased.[126] The rate of protein metabolism is higher in the placenta than in any other tissue, including the liver.[126] In the first half of pregnancy the placenta grows faster than the fetus; in the second half the situation is reversed. Protein synthesis from both carbohydrate and amino-acid precursors is more than twice as high in human placentae before 16 weeks as it is at term.[33,127] The rate of placental protein synthesis at different stages parallels the rates of glucose metabolism via the pentose pathway and of RNA and DNA turnover, which are all significantly higher in the early rapidly proliferating placenta than at term. Pharmacologically induced changes in pentose shunt activity also induce corresponding changes in nucleic acid and protein synthesis in the placenta and other rapidly proliferating tissues.[33] These findings suggest that the availability of pentose sugars is a key rate-limiting factor in nucleic acid production, and hence in protein synthesis, and also support the view that protein synthesis in the early placenta is directed primarily towards fulfilling growth requirements while in later weeks it is directed mainly towards function. This makes the placenta a very suitable model for studying nucleic acid formation and protein synthesis in both replicating and differentiating cells.

Synthesis, uptake, transfer, and metabolism of amino-acids by the placenta

Amino-acids are the final precursors of proteins, the biological activity of a protein depending on the sequence of the amino-acids making its polypeptide chains. The amino-acids required for protein synthesis by both placenta and fetus are mainly derived from the mother. The placenta can synthesise some of them itself,[128] and can also presumably utilise amino-acids derived from degradation of plasma proteins. The relative contribution of these sources to placental protein synthesis has not been quantified, nor is it known how much, if any, of the placental amino-acid production passes to the fetus. The great increase in maternal plasma protein turnover in pregnancy suggests that placental degradation of plasma albumin could be responsible for a considerable proportion of the placenta's amino-acids. It is of interest that tumour tissue incorporates amino-acids derived from plasma proteins at a more rapid rate than normal tissue.[129]

The amino-acid concentration is consistently higher in the fetal than in the maternal blood, transfer to the fetus being against a concentration gradient.[130-1] This transfer is a complex process entailing three separate stages:

1. Transport from maternal blood into the placenta - necessarily a selective energy-dependent process

2. Amino-acid accumulation in the placenta and utilisation for protein synthesis or other biosynthetic purposes, and

3. Release of amino-acids into fetal blood.

The concentration gradient for this last process favours simple diffusion. Measureing the relative concentration of different amino-acids in umbilical and antecubital vein blood, which is frequently considered to indicate the extent of amino-acid transfer from maternal to fetal blood, cannot give an accurate picture of this process.

Much more is known about uptake of amino-acids than about their metabolism by the placenta. While it is important to understand the uptake mechanism, the value of such information is to know what the tissue does with the amino-acids thereafter - yet study of this has been comparatively neglected. How much amino-acid is transferred to the fetus? How much is used in the synthesis of enzymes and other proteins determining placental growth and function? How much is metabolised to form different amino-acids or other nitrogenous compounds, and what determines the relative proportions? What are the particular requirements at different stages of gestation, bearing in mind that the fate of different precursors entering a cell could provide an indicator of its subsequent function and rate of replication?

The characteristics of the transfer system and energy requirements for the process of uptake and transfer have been studied both by <u>in vitro</u> methods - such as incubation of tissue slices,[131,132,133] and perfusion of the isolated placenta[134] - and by <u>in vivo</u> perfusion of the placenta <u>in situ</u>.[134,135] Many of these studies have entailed the use of alpha-amino-isobutyric acid (AIB), an inert non-metabolisable amino-acid which, in other tissues, has been shown to have transfer mechanism characteristics in common with the essential amino-acids. The amino-acid transport mechanisms of the placenta are qualitatively similar to those in the kidney and other epithelial tissues in that they are energy-dependent, saturable, temperature sensitive, and stereochemically specific - i.e. individual amino-acids are transferred at different rates depending on their chemical characteristics.[132,137-141] Fetal protein synthesis is much higher in the later stages of gestation, when fetal growth is maximal.[142,143] Amino-acid transfer increases at this stage,[15] which could also be related to increased placental proteolysis of serum proteins.

The energy for amino-acid uptake and transfer is generally provided by aerobic mechanisms. Uptake and transfer continue in anoxia[144] but at a diminished rate. The energy for continued placental amino-acid transfer in these circumstances is thought to be provided by placental glycolysis with consequent increase in lactate formation.[44] Could this be part of the picture in 'snall-for-dates' babies?

Placental protein transfer

The placenta transfers certain maternal proteins directly to the fetus. The most important of these are the immunoglobulins, as apparently neither fetus nor placenta synthesise gammaglobulin[145] and antibody protection of the human fetus and newborn depends on maternal antibodies transferred across the placenta.[146] Placental transfer of the immunoglobulins is selective, with preferential transfer of I_gG compared with I_gM.[4] The mechanisms involved are discussed in Section III. But how does the placental cell differentiate between globulins for fetal protection, which must pass intact, and proteins which are to undergo proteolysis to supply amino-acids for placental and fetal growth? There are more questions than answers here, but raising them is a major purpose of this symposium.

Effects of hormones on placental protein synthesis

Protein synthesis in the placenta, as in other tissues, is influenced by hormones, but there has been no systematic study of their effects or of their primary sites of action in the placenta. Certain types of hormonal influence on the placenta have been identified, however. One example is oestradiol, which stimulates placental protein synthesis. It does so by increasing energy production as the result of a transhydrogenation reaction,[147] not through an influence on amino-acid incorporation. It is interesting that oestrone and oestradiol affect the stability of placental DNA,[148] but how this influences protein synthesis is not known. Large doses of oestradiol, and also of progesterone and testosterone, inhibit placental glycine incorporation and protein synthesis;[127,144] but these are probably pharmacological effects of unphysiologically high dosage.

The influence of insulin on placental AIB uptake is disputed,[132] but protein synthesis in the placenta is stimulated by insulin, irrespective of whether amino-acid uptake increases ot not. In addition to stimulating placental glycogenolysis,[42]

HCG also stimulates protein synthesis from both carbohydrate and amino-acid precursors.[149]

Protein degradation

The stages of protein degradation in the human placenta have not been studied in detail. Presumably, as in other tissues, peptide linkages are broken, with liberation of constituent amino-acids. The placenta possesses the transaminases, deaminases and other enzymes necessary for the further metabolism of amino-acids, but the relative proportions of amino-acid reutilisation by the placenta and diversion to glucose formation or other metabolic sequences are not known.

Does the placenta use maternal proteins for its own function? Certainly placental proteolysis of maternal proteins may provide amino-acids, but the amount involved is not known. Most of the so-called 'pregnancy-specific proteins' found in the placenta are produced there, while some originate in maternal liver.[150-152] Their placental deposition may relate to immunosuppressant and other actions concerned in maintaining immunological privilege for the fetus.

Placental growth and protein synthesis

In normal pregnancy the human placenta increases in size progressively until term. What determines the final placental size and its growth rate? How is the rate of cell replication in the tissue controlled? If we knew that we could answer a major question of developmental biology - what determines the final size of any organ or tissue and how is this regulated? Presumably by feedback phenomena - but then we have to ask what controls them. Placental growth seems to be regulated and predetermined, as with any other organ. The fetus, whether by virtue of size or number, does not apparently determine placental growth, which continues even after fetectomy.[153] The placenta therefore provides a very convenient medium for investigating the mechanisms responsible for normal tissue growth and the factors which determine and limit growth in an organ.

In vivo, the lifespan of the trophoblast is limited by the length of gestation in the particular species, but the factors which control the duration of gestation in different species, and hence the normal rate of placental growth, are not known. The inherent lifespan of placental cells in tissue culture is technically difficult to investigate; the available data suggest that the duration of placental growth is genetically determined and that intrinsic cellular processes, rather than the influence of extrinsic factors, are responsible for placental 'degeneration' *in vivo*. Fibroblast-like cells from early human placentae have a shorter lifespan and a decreased rate of incorporation of tritiated thymidine for DNA synthesis in tissue culture than cells from maternal skin or decidua.[154]

The relative contributions of cell replication and increased size of existing cells to placental growth has been assessed indirectly, as in other tissues, by determination of the total protein, RNA, and DNA content of the placenta. DNA levels are held to reflect cell number (and hence the rate of cell replication) and RNA cell size. Placental weight, total protein and total RNA content increase linearly until term.[155] The pattern of placental DNA changes during gestation is disputed. A progressive increase in placental DNA has been reported until 34-36 weeks in human pregnancy and up to day 17 in the rat, with constant levels thereafter,[155] and this has been held to indicate cessation of cell division before term. Placental growth in the later stages of gestation has therefore been presumed to result from enlargement of existing cells, and cell division has not been considered necessary for the placental maturation changes observed towards term. Accordingly, growth in the early placenta is considered mainly proliferative and that in the later stages mainly hypertrophic. Supporting evidence includes the apparent absence of mitoses in human placentae after 36 weeks[156] and autoradiographic studies in rats and man reporting reduced DNA synthesis towards the end of gestation.[157,158] By contrast, a more recent study[159] reports a linear increase in human placental DNA from 25 weeks onwards with no levelling off near term, with a similar trend in rats, unless litter size is exceptionally large - which indicates continuing placental cell replication until the end of gestation.

Hormone influences of placental growth

Placental growth, like that of some human tumours, is influenced by the ovary. The placenta hypertrophies after ovariectomy in rodents when physiological doses of progesterone and oestradiol are given by way of replacement therapy,[160] the increase in placental size being attributed to hyperplasia rather than enlargement of existing cells. The placenta also hypertrophies after ovariectomy in rabbits.[161] Placental growth in these animals appears to be restricted normally by an ovarian factor that is neigher oestradiol nor progesterone. In rats, surgical reduction of litter size in the first half of pregnancy results in enhanced growth of the surviving placentae and fetuses, but if litter number is reduced later in pregnancy there is no growth enhancement in either. The placentae left behind after fetectomy apparently continue to grow but the remaining placentae and fetuses exhibit no growth enhancement.[162] Neither the mechanism of this nor its relationship to the ovarian factor that normally influences placental growth in animals are known.

Do the ovaries modify placental growth in man? There is no direct evidence, but cultures of full-term human placenta implanted subcutaneously into rats proliferate and produce HCG.[163] The growth pattern and cellular morphology of these cultures depend on the maturity of the rat and on whether the ovaries are present. In the normal adult females, the placental implant becomes multi-layered and shows epithelial cell development. In ovariectomised adult rats, only monolayers develop in the implant, whilst in the immature female placental proliferation is decreased compared with the other two groups.[163] When similar studies are performed with choriocarcinoma, the growth rate of the implanted tissue is independent both of the rat's maturity and of the presence or absence of the gonads.[164] In this respect human placental growth differs from that of neoplastic tissue.

Protein deprivation

The finding of a positive nitrogen balance in pregnancy led originally to the belief that it is associated with protein storage - in the placenta for emergency use by the fetus and in the tissues for lactation. But recent studies[165] have shown no evidence of protein storage in the placenta such as might be available to the fetus in time of need. In fact when maternal protein is limited, there is a fall in placental amino-acid transfer to the fetus, as indicated by AIB levels,[166,167] and the release of amino-acids from the placenta is reduced. The fetus does not apparently take precedence over the placenta, which regulates transfer in accordance with its own requirements rather than with those of the fetus.

Animals on a protein-free diet supplemented by the essential amino-acids show no significant reduction in the weight of their placentae,[168] but the fetuses are smaller with a disproportionate reduction in brain size.[169] Whether these findings reflect a biochemical abnormality in the placenta or in the fetus is not known. It would be interesting to find out if placental protein and water content remain constant in these circumstances. That the placenta gives priority to its own needs - not those of the fetus - when protein is limited parallels the behaviour of tumours, which continue to grow and synthesise new proteins, irrespective of the nutritional state of the host.

In the total absence of dietary protein, rats resorb their litters[170] unless oestrogen and progesterone are given from days five to nine,[171] at which stage the placenta is presumably producing enough steroids itself. The pregnancy-maintaining effect of oestrogen and progesterone appears to be due to mobilisation of protein from maternal skeletal muscle,[172] and consequent provision of amino-acids for placental biosynthetic activity. This supports the view that de novo placental amino-acid production is limited. Pregnancy can also be maintained in a high proportion of rats on a protein-free diet by the administration of reserpine,[173] an effect attributed to the drug promoting prolactin release from the pituitary with a consequent increase in ovarian hormone production. These animal studies illustrate the importance of continued provision of protein precursors for placental and fetal growth; even small supplements may help redress the balance and minimise the effects of malnutrition. The addition of a protein supplement in early pregnancy to rats subsequently deprived of protein throughout the rest of pregnancy results in a substantial increase in the weight and cellularity of both placentae and fetuses at term compared with those not given such supplements.[174] The obvious implication of this animal work is that protein deficiency in human pregnancy should be taken seriously, pending more specific evidence of its effects in man.

In animals, protein-calorie deficiency is associated with a reduction in cellular RNA in organs with a high protein turnover and stable cell population, and with a reduction in DNA synthesis in tissue with a high cell turnover.[175] In human malnutrition, paradoxical changes in placental protein and nucleic acid content have been reported, however. While placental weight, total protein and DNA are decreased compared with normal, RNA is reported to be increased.[176] This has been attributed to a decline in cell numbers,[176] but since the turnover of RNA in these circumstances has not been studied, other interpretations are possible. Placental RNase activity is increased in malnourished women,[177] but the significance of this finding remains obscure.

Who is in the driving seat - placenta or fetus?

Because placental size generally correlates with fetal size and number, the requirements of the fetus have usually been considered the dominant driving force for placental growth. However , the studies discussed above suggest that placental growth is not directed by the fetus. In particular, the placenta continues to grow after fetectomy[153] and will continue to produce specific hormones even in the absence of a fetus.[153] The placenta seems to dominate the fetus, determining its growth and intrauterine lifespan and control lies more with it than the fetus.

METABOLISM DURING PLACENTAL AGEING AND IN ABNORMAL PREGNANCY

Ageing

The evidence for placental ageing towards term is chiefly morphological, but the observed structural changes are difficult to relate to altered placental function towards the end of pregnancy. Ageing is generally assumed to be responsible for the decreased ability to adapt to a changing environment, as demonstrated, for example, in the impaired response to anoxia. The reduced efficiency of oxidative phosphorylation in full-term placentae[38] might contribute to the problems of the postmature fetus or small-for-dates baby. Similarly, an age-related breakdown of the placental immunological mechanisms which have prevented rejection of the placental graft thus far might be an important factor in the onset of labour.

There is some evidence of a metabolic decline with advancing pregnancy in the falling rate of certain processes and the lower activity of some key regulatory enzymes in the placenta towards term. Oxygen consumption,[178] glucose uptake, lactate and pyruvate production[16,17,36] and pentose shunt activity[33] are all higher in earlier placentae than at term. Glycogen concentration, glucose-6-phosphatase activity, and the specific activity of the key enzymes regulating glycolysis, gluconeogenesis, glycogenesis, NADPH generation, and fatty acid synthesis are also less at term.[51] As noted earlier, RNA turnover from glucose and protein synthesis from glycine are both reduced to less than half at term, compared with tissue examined before 16 weeks of gestation.[33] In fibroblasts, ageing is associated with qualitative changes in the activity of the first two enzymes in the pentose pathway.[179] Does this also occur in the placenta when the pentose pathway activity falls at term, and could it be related to any of the structural changes? These are questions which need investigation.

In contrast to the metabolic processes that decline, production of placental steroid and of HCS and certain enzymes increases progressively during gestation, and transport of water and ions such as sodium and iron reaches a peak near term. Moreover, there is little if any evidence that transfer of amino-acids or of other compounds essential for fetal growth is less efficient at term.

Abnormal pregnancy

There are only fragmentary studies of placental metabolism in abnormal pregnancy - notably in toxaemia, diabetes, and intra-uterine growth retardation (IUGR).

Pre-eclamptic toxaemia is associated with increased rates of placental lactate production and glucose uptake, both being higher than in normal pregnancies or in patients with essential hypertension.[180] This suggests that placental glycolysis must be increased in toxaemia. Maternal lipaemia[78,181] and total placental lipids are also increased[80,182] - the latter apparently being due to a rise in triglycerides,[80] since placental phospholipid synthesis is depressed in severe toxaemia.[106] This contrasts with normal placenta where phospholipid synthesis is increased at term.[80] Placental prostaglandin E content is reduced in toxaemia[183,184] and its metabolism impaired, with transformation into prostaglandin A decreased - apparently in direct proportion to the severity of the disease.[185] Placental amino-acid transfer is also impaired,[186] and amino-acid incorporation into protein and RNA in subcellular fractions of toxaemic placentae reduced compared with normal.[187] While impaired fetal growth and morbidity in toxaemia are logically related to a reduction in placental protein, it is not known how the various changes in placental metabolism are triggered, nor how they are related to the altered vascular responses and arteriosclerotic lesions of toxaemia.

Diabetes is accompanied by higher placental glycogen levels than are normal for the stage of gestation,[188] and placental lactate production is increased.[189] Surprisingly, glycogen synthetase activity is lower than normal and phosphorylase activity higher in placentae from diabetic patients[190] - which suggests that placental glycogenesis may in fact be limited and glycogen breakdown increased in these circumstances. In explanation of these paradoxical findings it has been suggested that initially, maternal hyperglycaemia induces a rise in placental glycogen by increasing synthetase activity and lowering that of phosphorylase.[190] Then, as placental glycogen concentrations rise, synthetase activity is inhibited and phosphorylase activity increased by a feedback mechanism.[190]

The disturbance of carbohydrate metabolism observed in the diabetic placenta - which may reflect metabolic feed-back similar to that demonstrated in cardiac muscle in diabetes[191] - could result from the difficulty of maintaining round-the-clock glucose control in pregnancy. Alternatively, these findings might be due to a generalised metabolic disturbance in diabetic subjects, analogous to retinopathy and peripheral vascular disease, and not necessarily prevented by administration of exogenous insulin. If we knew what the basis of the placental biochemical disturbance was we might have a better understanding of the cellular disturbance produced by diabetes itself. However, these changes in placental metabolism do not explain fetal morbidity and mortality in diabetes. The fetal adiposity is now attributed to the increased level of maternal fatty acids and their subsequent transfer, esterification and incorporation into the fetal triglyceride pool[192] and not, as formerly, to increased fetal fat in consequence of raised glucose levels.

Intra-uterine Growth Retardation (IUGR) results in a fetus with little subcutaneous fat and decreased hepatic glycogen. The placental glycogen concentration is similar to that in normal pregnancy,[193] but the total placental glycogen content is significantly reduced,[193] these placentae being smaller than normal. Placental glycogen utilisation is increased in IUGR,[193] as are the specific activities of enzymes critical for the regulation of glycolysis, glyconeogenesis, NADPH generation and fatty acid synthesis. This last finding has been attributed to an arrest of placental ageing, since activity of these enzymes normally decreases during gestation.[51] The altered enzyme activity may also result from a primary disturbance of placental biochemical homoeostasis in IUGR with consequent imbalance of energy relationships for the placenta and hence for placental and fetal growth.

Altered placental protein metabolism would be expected in IUGR but this has not been studied. Impaired amino-acid uptake has been reported in placentae from 'small-for-dates' babies not associated with maternal disease such as toxaemia or hypertension, as have lower levels of placental cyclic-AMP.[74] Attempts to reproduce IUGR in animals through ligation of the uterine arteries supplying one uterine horn or by injection of HCG to prolong gestation have resulted in smaller fetuses and placentae for the stage of gestation, with lower concentrations of hepatic glycogen and circulating glucose in the growth-retarded fetus.[194] No parallel studies of biochemical changes in the placenta were carried out, demonstrating once again the extraordinary intellectual dichotomy of workers in this field. Their interest in the fetus contrasts with their lack of interest in the placenta - be it for the sake of the fetus or for its own sake.

Placental metabolism in abnormal pregnancy differs from normal in respect of every measurement made to date. However, the haphazard manner in which these processes have been studied does not yet enable us to say what the biochemical lesion is in particular conditions, or to explain clinical pathology in terms of disturbed placental metabolism.

Malignant trophoblast

While hormone production from the malignant trophoblast has been studied extensively, there have been only a few metabolic studies in choriocarcinoma. It is however known that tissue glycogen decreases in both the normal placenta[17,26] and in choriocarcinoma [195] when extracellular glucose levels are lowered, and also in anoxia. If glycogen-depleted choriocarcinoma cultures are refed with glucose, consumption increases and cellular glycogen accumulates again, but the rate of glycogen synthesis appears to be independent of the extracellular glucose concentration.[195] In the normal placenta[16] and in the liver[196,197] glycogen synthesis is glucose-dependent, and rises with increasing glucose concentration. Since the maximum glycogen storage rate in the malignant placenta seems to be regulated internally, its mechanism for controlling glycogen deposition may be unique - contrasting with the behaviour of other neoplasms[198] and with normal placenta.

Prostaglandin synthesis from arachidonic acid can be demonstrated in choriocarcinoma cultures (by means of isotope studies) only if serum has been added to the cell culture at least 24 hours previously.[199] It has therefore been suggested that trophoblast cells in long-continued cultures lose their ability to synthesise prostaglandins and have to 'learn afresh'. Experimental conditions may also explain the apparent absence of prostaglandin synthesis in the malignant trophoblast: in investigations of prostaglandin synthesis adrenaline was added to the medium for studying normal placentae[200] but not for similar studies of choriocarcinoma. Prostaglandins have been shown to stimulate adenyl cyclase activity and HCG secretion in normal placentae[42] but not in malignant trophoblast cultures.[201] While this may be due to continuous culture, a basic difference between normal and malignant placenta could be at least partly responsible.

All this evidence suggests fundamental differences in metabolic behaviour between choriocarcinoma and normal placenta - limiting their biochemical comparability. Choriocarcinomata also differ from other neoplasms in their responses, and this must cast doubt on the validity of using choriocarcinoma cell cultures as 'a model for cancer research'.[202] Similarly, the malignant trophoblast is a questionable model for explaining normal trophoblast behaviour.

DISCUSSION

Since rapidly proliferating tissues like the placenta are critically dependent on sufficient fuel supply to maintain their normal growth rate, accurate methods of measuring fuel utilisation are needed in the study of tissue growth. The activity of enzymes concerned in glycolysis can provide this information, but those studied are usually chosen because they are the simplest to measure: lactic dehydrogenase, glyceraldehyde-3-phosphate dehydrogenase, or even pyruvate kinase. Although these give some evidence of glycolytic capacity, they do not provide any quantitative information. Their maximum activities, as measured in vitro, bear no relationship to flux through the glycolytic pathway in vivo. Drawing attention to this, Eric Newsholme reported development of specific enzyme markers for use in vitro as quantitative indices of fuel utilisation. This means, for example, that maximum glycolytic capacity - from glycogen to lactate - can be studied using phosphofructokinase as indicator. For measuring entry to the citric acid cycle, which is really the oxidative capacity, pyruvate dehydrogenase provides a good index, particularly if the inactive b-form is converted into the a-form. Oxoglutarate dehydrogenase is a very good quantitative index of the citric acid cycle. And the level of fatty acid oxidation can be measured by means of choline acyltransferase, the enzyme responsible for transport of fatty acids across the mitochondrial membrane. However, nobody appears to have studied the maximum activities, under optimal in vitro conditions, of phosphofructokinase, pyruvate dehydrogenase, oxoglutarate dehydrogenase, or choline acyltransferase, with particular reference to the placenta.

Why does placental metabolism produce so much lactate? In response to this question, Claude Villee suggested that the placenta exports lactate to the fetus, which uses it as an energy source. This appears to be an alternative way of getting carbohydrate substrate to the fetus to supplement the glucose pathway. Measurements in the sheep have shown that lactate accounts for something like 25-30% of the energy used by the fetus. The tissues utilise it directly, and Jean Ginsburg reported that about 50% of fetal energy comes from glucose, while amino-acids provide the remaining 25% or so.

Do measurements of enzyme activity give any idea of substrate turnover? Raising this general question, Francesco Pocchiari expressed the view that measurements of substrate turnover provide a more accurate guide than enzyme determinations of pathway activity. In measuring phosphofructokinase, he asked has anyone also measured the turnover of fructose-1-6-diphosphate, to see if it increases or subsides. Such problems open up the whole question of cell compartments in which particular reactions and/or substances may be relatively isolated. So what can in vitro measurements of enzyme activity tell us about processes actually taking place in cells?

This is what Claude Villee described as a'second order' question - concerned not only with enzyme activity but also with what controls it and how cells communicate with one another. Is the mechanism hormonal, or are the substrates themselves able to evoke changes? Such uncertainties make it all the more important to check the relevance of data on enzyme activity by other methods, and Eric Newsholme agreed with Professor Pocchiari that the activity of an enzyme did not necessarily reflect the flux through a particular pathway. Nevertheless, work in his department, particularly on comparative studies, has demonstrated quantitative correlations between measurements of enzyme activity and the maximum capacity of the system in the living cell. Studies of muscle, for example, to determine the maximum rate of fuel utilisation in the living animal when it is running at full speed correlate well with measurement of glycolytic activity. As a result, it is now possible to measure glycolytic activity in a biopsy sample of muscle, and to forecast its glycolytic capacity when sprinting. There is no need to measure lactate production; it can be accurately predicted by determination of enzyme activity - but Dr. Newsholme stressed that such correlations need to be checked, not taken for granted.

In the placenta, as Claude Villee pointed out, many systems are not operating at capacity, their actual rates not necessarily correlating with measurements of enzyme activity yet plainly under effective feedback control. This is of course true of most metabolic systems, in the placenta and elsewhere, most of the time; there has to be a reserve. The placenta normally operates at levels which may be optimal, but are certainly not maximal. That changes in the activity levels of certain enzymes take place during the development of the placenta was indicated by Marcellino Dianzani. The fact that growth arrest coincides with increased activity of lysosomal enzymes in various tissues is just one example that might well be relevant to the placenta, in which lysosomal enzymes are known to be present. Does their activity increase when placental growth ceases? Nobody seems to know. Such questions have not been adequately studied; much of the literature is piecemeal, and there has been no comprehensive study of the different enzyme activities during the stages of development. The most comprehensive studies, quoted by Jean Ginsburg, have been devoted to alkaline phosphatase isoenzymes in placental tumours. More work is needed, especially on the activity of regulatory enzymes and their changes during development.

Discussion then turned to proteolysis in the placenta as a source of amino-acids both for its own development and for the fetus. While there is good evidence of such proteolysis in yolk-sac placentae, it is uncertain whether this really takes place in the human chorioallantoic placenta or,particularly, in the syncytiotrophoblast. No studies have been done by modern techniques. Nevertheless, it is reasonable to infer that proteolysis does take place, from what is already known of high maternal turnover of plasma proteins, coupled with the high amino-acid requirements of the placenta - bearing in mind that it has to supply the fetus as well. The aim of research should be to construct a metabolic balance sheet for amino-acids and proteins showing how much goes to the fetus, and how much the placenta uses itself and in what way.

The need for more information on placental protein metabolism was also stressed by Arthur Wild, who wanted to know if the syncytiotrophoblast could take up, non-selectively, a wide range of proteins other than immunoglobulin. We may be in danger, as he went on to point out, of overgeneralising about the placenta, when we should distinguish between syncytiotrophoblast, fetal endothelium and mesenchymal cells, for example, and always specify the particular tissue studied. The timing of studies must also be taken into account in the placenta, where the kinds of cells present change between early and late gestation. Working with an organ in such a state of flux is a great challenge, but Claude Villee stressed that its value as an experimental model is all the greater on that account. The need to distinguish between the cell and tissue types in an organ is not, as he also emphasised, confined to the placenta. Earlier speakers had referred to 'the' muscle - which contains several different kinds of cells; similarly we all talk glibly about another complex organ as 'the' liver. Yet at the opposite extreme, we should ask ourselves if studies of single cells, perhaps even cloned cells, from a tissue give results which really represent what happens in the intact organ. It is vital, in Claude Villee's view, to put the pieces together, so that cell and organ studies can complement each other to make overall sense. The need is clear, yet the long-established dichotomy persists - not only between cell and organ studies but also in the way they are regarded. All great medical advances, said Peter Beaconsfield, have come from study of organs, but all Nobel Prizes in medicine are won for study of cells.

Finally, discussion turned to two examples of biochemical changes peculiar to the placenta and/or particular phases of gestation. As regards catabolism of maternal immunoglobulins, Arthur Wild reported that something like 90% of I_gG experimentally injected into the uterine lumen is broken down to amino-acids during transport in the case of yolk-sac placentae. Only about 10% actually reaches the fetus. Although no comparable data are available for the human chorioallantoic placenta, it seems that - as with neonatal intestine - special vesicular uptake and transport mechanisms enable immunoglobulins to be identified and actively transfered. But which cells are involved, at what stage of gestation, with handling of which immunoglobulins? It is necessary to consider all these variables, as Willi Hijmans pointed out, not simply talking about antibodies in general but, for example studying which subclasses of I_gG are catabolised more than others, at what stage and by what tissues - a subject covered more fully in Section III. Similar considerations apply to carbohydrate metabolism, where the placental glycogen concentration is quite high early in human pregnancy but then decreases until after about 15 weeks there is little present. Again, as Claude Villee concluded, it is necessary to specify early, middle or late placenta - and which cells are concerned. All such changes are of course under genetic control, the subject of the following paper.

NUCLEIC ACIDS AND PLACENTAL DEVELOPMENT

Hamish N. Munro

The human placenta is a genetically programmed organ, mainly of fetal origin, with a predestined life-cycle of nine months. Its programming is expressed in its capacity for growth, in the changing proportions of its various constituent cells during development, and in the secretion of hormonal and non-hormonal peptides into the maternal blood in a defined sequence. Such processes are controlled by DNA, RNA and the whole series of mechanisms regulating protein synthesis, but study of their role in placental development and function is made difficult by the complexity of the placenta itself. The trophoblast, for example which is responsible for secretion of proteins and peptide hormones, represents only 13% of the placental mass at term.[1] Nearly all biochemical preparations made from whole placenta include the components of several tissues. However, this is probably not as great an impediment as may at first appear, because the trophoblast is the tissue most actively involved in protein synthesis; two-thirds of the remaining placental mass consists of connective tissue, fibrous septa, and blood present in the intervillous spaces.

Assessment of placental growth

Growth in most tissues follows the sequence of initial hyperplasia (cell division), then hyperplasia with some hypertrophy, (cell enlargement), and finally hypertrophy alone. These phases can be studied by the pattern of accretion of DNA, RNA and protein. In hyperplasia, the increasing DNA content of a tissue keeps pace with the increase in total protein. In hypertrophy, since no new DNA-containing cell nuclei are being formed, the total protein continues to rise, outstripping the DNA content. Figure 1 shows the rapid increase in weight (corresponding to total protein) of rat placenta from days 14 to 20 of the 21-day pregnancy, related to

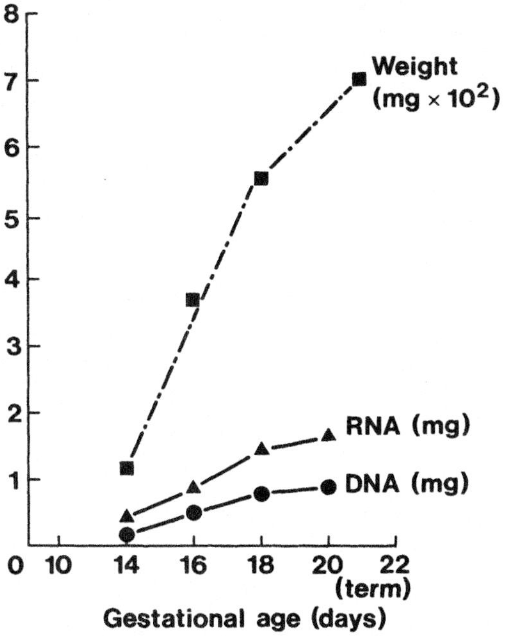

Fig. 1. Total weight, and RNA and DNA content of rat placenta from 14 to 20 days of pregnancy.[2]

nucleic acid levels.[2] Accumulation of DNA is equally rapid at first, indicating hyperplasia, but falls off towards the end of this period. This was originally shown by Winick and Noble[3] to be due to cessation of DNA synthesis, when they found that uptake of ^{14}C-thymidine ceases after day 16, and subsequently confirmed by the finding that placental DNA-polymerase activity falls from day 13 to day 19 of rat pregnancy.[4] In human placenta DNA synthesis ceases around 36 weeks.[5,6]

The question of hyperplasia versus hypertrophy can be studied in detail by computing the relative weights of placental tissue and DNA. This has been done for both rat and human placenta, as shown in Table I. In addition to hyperplasia, rat placenta appears to undergo some hypertrophy (presumably after DNA synthesis has ceased) in the course of its rapid development between days 14 and 20, since the total weight of tissue rises faster than its DNA content - as shown in two of the three studies quoted.[2,3,7] By contrast, the mean cell weight of the human placenta

TABLE I

RNA and DNA content of human and rat placentas at different stages of development

Sources	RNA (mg/g)		DNA (mg/g)		Placental Weight/DNA (mg/mg)		RNA/DNA (mg/mg)	
Rat Placenta (days)	14	20/21	14	20/21	14	20/21	14	20/21
Winick and Noble[3] (1966)	5.5	3.5	2.3	1.3	430	770	2.4	2.7
Butterstein and Leathem[7] (1974)	6.5	4.9	2.9	1.9	350	520	2.2	2.6
Mozayani et al[2] (1978b)	2.9	2.3	1.1	1.1	910	910	2.5	2.1
Means	5.0	3.6	2.1	1.4	560	730	2.4	2.5
Human placenta (trimesters)	I	III	I	III	I	III	I	III
Brody[19,20] (1952,53)	1.7	1.5	1.2	1.7	830	580	1.4	0.8
Stark and Klinkherst[23] (1956)	2.0	2.3	1.9	3.1	520	320	1.1	0.7
Mori[22] (1965)	2.3	1.9	1.3	2.5	770	400	1.7	0.8
Winick et al[6] (1967)	1.0	1.4	2.0	2.6	500	380	0.5	0.5
Laga et al[21] (1973)	3.9	3.5	2.5	2.9	400	340	1.6	1.2
Kusamran et al[17] (1978)	2.4	1.4	3.1	3.2	320	310	0.7	0.4
Means	2.7	2.0	2.0	2.8	560	390	1.2	0.7

actually falls in relation to its DNA content by the end of the third trimester (Table I). The different course of placental development in rat and man may be related to their differing maturity at birth; the rat is known to be less mature in brain development[8] and in antibody transfer[9] and may therefore have a less mature placenta.

The amount of RNA in the average cell (expressed as RNA/DNA ratio) changes between early and late pregnancy, and also differs between man and the rat (Table I). Almost all observers find that the RNA/DNA ratio is less in the mature than in the early human placenta, whereas the rat does not show a reduction in the ratio at the end of pregnancy. This difference is consistent with continuing hypertrophy in rat placenta but not in human placenta, after cessation of DNA synthesis. It is also to be noted in Table I that the RNA/DNA ratio is always higher in rat than in human placenta. In general, the RNA content of a tissue reflects the intensity of protein synthesis, the smaller species of mammal having a higher RNA content because their synthesis of proteins is generally more rapid.[10] The higher RNA/DNA ratio of rat placenta is therefore consistent with fetal protein synthesis generally being more intense in rats than in man. Human placenta contains more fibrous tissue, and fibroblasts contain relatively little RNA.[3]

Although the rat placenta is still undergoing some hypertrophy at the end of pregnancy, its rate is low. When rat gestation is artificially prolonged from the customary 21 days to 23 days by administration of progesterone (Fig. 2), the protein and DNA content remain unchanged, indicating that the cell mass is now constant, whereas the amount of RNA per unit of DNA declines with each day past 21 and the ribonuclease level rises.[11] In addition, the polyamine concentration falls,

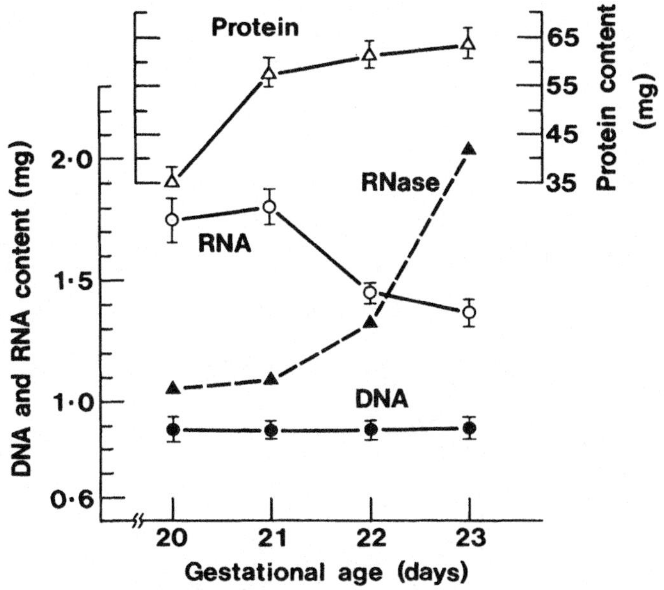

Fig. 2. Protein, DNA, RNA and RNase content of rat placenta near term and during progesterone-induced prolonged pregnancy.[11]

indicating reduced synthesis of RNA.[11] Thus the end of pregnancy in the rat coincides with a period of reduced RNA synthesis, and presumably of protein synthesis, heralding the end of the hypertrophic phase of placental growth.

Protein synthesis by the placenta

Proteins are synthesised on polyribosomes either free in the cell sap (for proteins retained in the cell) or attached to the membranes of the endoplasmic reticulum (for secreted proteins). The placenta makes both classes of proteins, and the cytotrophoblast contains both types of polyribosomes in abundance. In the case of the rat, we have quantitated these populations of ribosomes and shown that 60-70% of them are membrane-bound, at both 14 days and 20 days of gestation.[12] Most protein synthesis in the placenta thus appears to be associated with secretion of proteins.

In man, we have estimated the proportions of secreted hormones and of total synthesis by early and by full-term placentas.[13] The polyribosomes were separated from these placentas and the messenger-RNA (m-RNA) extracted. By incubation in suitable systems, the amounts of human chorionic gonadotropin (HCG) or human placental lactogen (HPL) made at different stages of gestation could be measured as a percentage of total protein synthetic capacity. Table II shows that the early placenta makes mainly HCG, whereas the late placenta manufactures more HPL and less HCG. Furthermore, the proportions of alpha and beta chains of HCG made by the polyribosomes change as the placenta matures.[14] From these data, we can conclude that

TABLE II

Synthesis of placental peptide hormones compared with plasma levels in early and late pregnancy

Hormone	Site	Early pregnancy	Late pregnancy
HCG	Placental synthesis[13] (% total synthesis)	10.6%	2.6%
	Plasma level (μg/ml)[14]	2.5	0.5
HPL	Placental synthesis[13] (% total synthesis)	0%	7.7%
	Plasma level (μg/ml)[14]	trace	6

the m-RNA changes in type during the course of placental development, and that the abundance of each m-RNA type determines how much of each peptide hormone will be secreted, since the plasma level of HCG is maximal at 10 weeks of gestation, whereas HPL output increases progessively until near the end of pregnancy.

Recently we have examined[2] the effects of protein deficiency and of ethyl alcohol administration during pregnancy on the output of rat chorionic mammotropin (RCM), the hormone secreted by the rat placenta during the latter half of pregnancy and corresponding to HPL in the human. Table III shows that feeding 5% protein in the diet of the rat from day ten to day 20 of pregnancy significantly reduces birth weight compared with mothers fed an 18% protein diet. Consumption of one-third of

TABLE III

Effect of protein deficiency or alcohol consumption on maternal food intake of rats, on fetal weight, on total placental content of protein, RNA and chorionic mammotropin (RCM), and on plasma concentration of RCM[12] (percentages of 18% protein group in parentheses).

Measurement	18% protein group	5% protein group	18% protein + alcohol group
Food Intake			
Energy (Kcal/day)	61	49	62
Protein (g/day)	2.8	0.6	1.8
Fetuses			
Weight (g/fetus)	3.31 (100)	2.62 (79)*	2.96 (89)
Placenta			
Weight (mg)	590 (100)	470 (79)*	560 (95)
Protein (mg)	46 (100)	18 (33)*	37 (80)*
RNA (mg)	1.52 (100)	0.93 (61)*	0.96 (63)*
RCM (μg)	14.5 (100)	7.6 (53)*	7.5 (52)*
Serum			
RCM (μg/ml)	4.5 (100)	1.5 (33)	2.7 (60)

* Mozayani et al.[12]

the calories as alcohol along with the 18% protein diet also reduced birthweight, to just above the level of significance. Placental weight was reduced only in the low-protein group, but the total protein content of the placenta was less in both the low-protein and the alcohol groups, and the placental RNA content in both restricted groups was only 60% of that in the group receiving 18% protein. Similarly, the amount of RCM in the placentas of the two malnourished groups was only half that of the controls, and the concentration of RCM in the serum was also much lower in these two groups. Comparison of the reduction in placental RCM content and in RNA content for the three dietary groups shows close parallels, suggesting that capacity to form and release this peptide hormone is determined by the amount of placental RNA, most of which is in the form of ribosomes. Elsewhere,[15] we have used the ribosome content of the human full-term placenta to compute total capacity for protein synthesis and peptide hormone secretion, and this gave data in good agreement with the known daily output of HPL. Thus the primary lesion in malnutrition may well reside in placental RNA formation.

Control of placental protein synthesis

The control of messenger RNA availability at different phases of placental growth is likely to be due to changes in chromatin for transcription. We have examined the capacity of chromatin from rat placentas and human placentas at different phases of their growth to act as templates for RNA polymerase.[16] Figure 3 shows that transcription of rat placental chromatin by a constant amount of rat liver RNA polymerase II yields progressively less new m-RNA as the placenta ages from 14 to 20 days. However, total RNA polymerase activity increases during this period while ribonuclease activity remains low throughout (results not shown). We may conclude that template availability probably becomes rate-limiting for RNA synthesis as the placenta ages. We have made similar observations of decreased template availability, slightly increased RNA polymerase activity and little RNase content for human placentas as they grow from 3 months to full term.[17]

In order to examine the consequences of these changes for control of placental proteins, we have begun to isolate messenger-RNA particles released by nuclei incubated in vivo. Nuclei isolated from human placenta have been incubated with (^{3}H)-UTP, and the labelled RNA released from the nuclei passed through an oligo-dT affinity chromatography column (Fig. 4). Ribosomal and other RNA without stretches of polyadenylic acid is eluted first, followed at 2°C in low salt concentration by m-RNA containing polyadenylic acid, then at 45° C by m-RNA combined with protein (m-RNP), part of which also eluted with formamide. We have verified by various techniques that the product released by these last two conditions of elution has the characteristic of m-RNP.

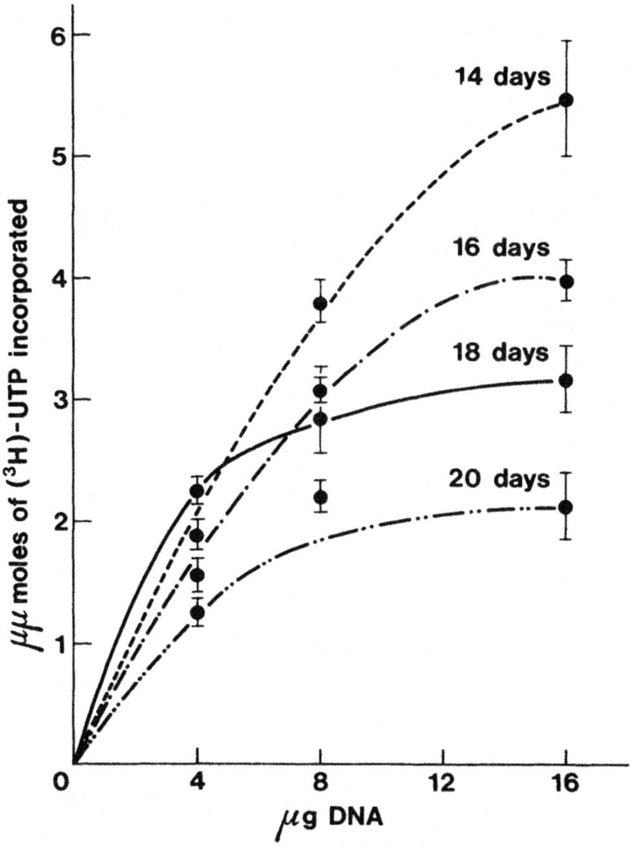

Fig. 3. Template capacity of rat placental chromatin at different days of pregnancy. Various quantities of the isolated chromatin were incubated with rat liver RNA polymerase II. The figure records the amount of (^{3}H)-UTP incorporated into RNA.[16]

This procedure enables m-RNP to be obtained from placental nuclei at various phases of growth. The messages carried by these m-RNP particles can then be translated in a cell-free system and the products identified as indicated above (Table II), and described in more detail elsewhere.[13,15] In this way it may be possible to determine whether m-RNA formation by the nuclei of the syncytiotrophoblast is controlled by factors similar to the hypothalamic releasing factors regulating anterior hypophyseal hormone secretion. There is some evidence that thyrotropin releasing factor and luteotropin releasing factor[18] or their anologues are present in the placenta, probably in the cytotrophoblast cells. A schematic representation of such a control mechanism is proposed in Figure 5. If this mechanism is correct, then programming of the placenta may reside primarily in changes in the cytotrophoblast cells.

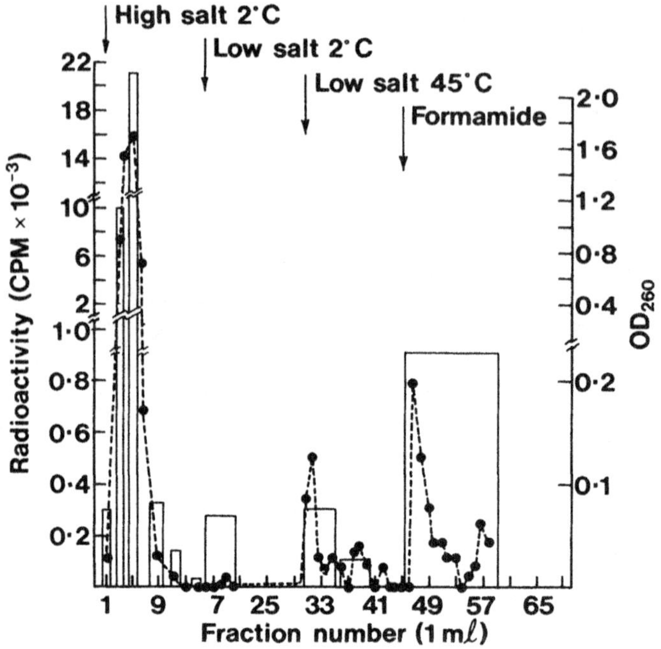

Fig. 4. Release of messenger ribonucleoprotein (m-RNP) particles by human placental nuclei incubated in vitro. Following incubation of isolated nuclei with (^{3}H)=UTP for 3 hours at 29°C, the RNA released by the nuclei was passed through an oligo-dT column to yield ribosomal RNA (high salt fraction), free messenger-RNA (low salt at 2°C, none obtained), messenger-RNP (low salt at 45°C) and further messenger-RNP (formamide).[18]

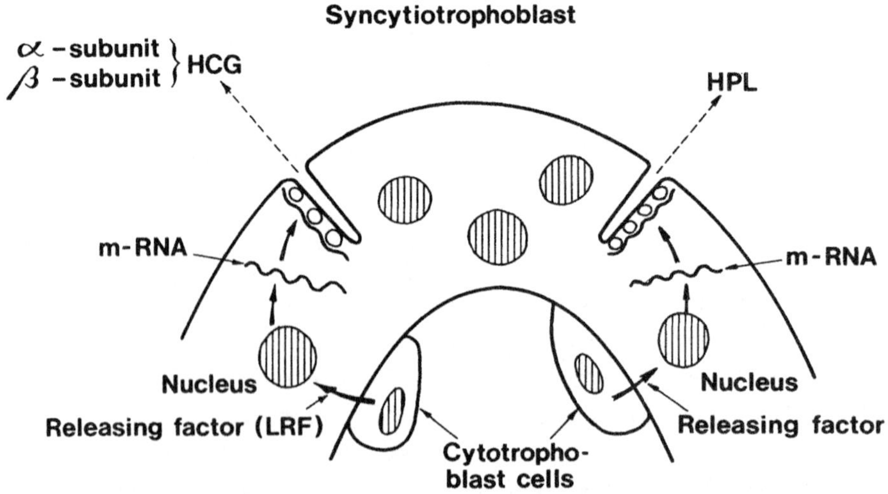

Fig. 5. Hypothetical scheme for control of synthesis of placental peptide hormones in the syncytiotrophoblast through changes in releasing factors from cytotrophoblast cells.

DISCUSSION

The comprehensive range of processes referred to in this paper led Claude Villee to comment that the placenta combines many of the characteristic functions of other tissues - from liver and skeletal muscle to the hypothalamus and pituitary. Agreeing that this is indeed the case, Hamish Munro mentioned the isolation of a corticotrophin, a vasoactive peptide, and several other hormones from placenta. In his view, the capacity of the syncytiotrophoblast to synthesise peptide hormones might well considerably exceed those of primary organs like the pituitary which had previously been regarded as the most prolific source of biochemical precursors.

Discussion then turned to the releasing role of the cytotrophoblast, and E. C. Amoroso pointed to the need to reconcile this phenomenon, as evidenced in the human placenta, with the conditions in other placentae with the same capacity for secreting chorionic gonadotrophin, in which there is no syncytiotrophoblast but only cytotrophoblast. In the evolutionary history of the trophoblast from the chorion, the first attribute of the cytotrophoblast might not have been to produce releasing factors but to synthesise chorionic gonadotrophins itself. These protein hormones may, in Prof. Amoroso's view eventually prove to be a universal characteristic of the trophoblast in all mammalian placentae and in some marsupials. Most of the latter have yolk-sac placentae, only one or two marsupial species having learnt the trick of providing a chorioallantois . There is now evidence that those marsupial placentae, in which the allantoic mesenchyme plays an important part in vascularising the chorion, secrete a chorionic gonadotrophin. There is also evidence, reported by Gerald Easty on the basis of a limited in vitro study, that human cytotrophoblast cells (virtually uncontaminated, with less than 0.01% syncytiotrophoblast cells) have the ability both to synthesise and to secrete HCG. This is a matter of controversy, however.

On one hand, if human placental tissue survives in culture, it will always be the cytotrophoblast - not the syncytiotrophoblast, which is not self-perpetuating. It has lost the ability to undergo mitotic division, except perhaps on very rare occasions; maybe one mitotic spindle observed in several hundred placentae, according to E. C. Amoroso. Hormone production from placental tissue culture is therefore virtually certain to come from proliferating cytotrophoblast cells. On the other hand, as Harold Fox put it, while there is no doubt that the cytotrophoblast can synthesise HCG in vitro, it does not do so in vivo - where the syncytiotrophoblast is responsible. He also queried the suggestion that LH and releasing hormone may be produced by the cytotrophoblast. If that were so, conditions such as pre-eclampsia, where there is a considerable increase in the cytotrophoblastic cell content and activity of human placenta, might be expected to show increased levels of maternal HCS. In fact. they are decreased. But Hamish Munro thought this could be due to the syncytiotrophoblast, which is responsible for producing the hormone, not operating under optimal conditions. Releasing factors might then knock at the door, as it were, but not get an answer.

As regards the controversy about secretion of HCG by the cytotrophoblast, he postulated that cell division and hormone secretion might be incompatible - except in malignant tissue where they sometimes coexist (though not necessarily in the same cell simultaneously). It is generally agreed that the syncytiotrophoblast comes from cytotrophoblast cells, but what makes the syncytiotrophoblast an active producer, while the cytotrophoblast in vivo appears not to be? Perhaps the capacity for secretion develops with cessation of cell division, as a result of nuclear programming. In choriocarcinoma, that programming has gone awry to create the hormone producer par excellence, which is also replicating - though not as fast as the placenta, the growth rate of all tumours being slower. A possible explanation was put forward by E. C. Amoroso. In choriocarcinoma with widespread metastases in the lungs, removal of the primary growth is sometimes followed by spontaneous regression of the metastases. In those cases that spontaneously regress in this way, the metastases may have consisted mainly or wholly of syncytiotrophoblast cells, capable of secreting for a while before reaching the end of their limited lifespan. They can then no longer produce the chorionic gonadotrophin and other hormones which may have been acting as immunosuppressants and lymphocytes can attack the metastases. Where there is no such regression, the metastases might be composed not only of syncytiotrophoblast but also of laggard remnants of cytotrophoblast. There is no way in which their mitotic activity can be inhibited, so they continue to produce syncytiotrophoblast, which secretes HCG and other hormones that - among other things - might act immunosuppressively.

Hormone production by the syncytiotrophoblast might also explain the failure of the maternal organism to recognise her baby as non-self. This is not due to the abrogation of any maternal competence or immune mechanisms, or to fetal immaturity; nor is the uterus a privileged site. In Prof. Amoroso's view, the syncytiotrophoblast may be responsible. By producing not only chorionic gonadotrophin and HPL but also ACTH, TSH, growth hormone, mammotropin, corticosteroids, oestrogens and progesterone, it may ensure the maintenance of pregnancy and the integrity of the fetus. If the source of progesterone is removed in any mammalian female, she will abort or reject her fetus. There is no reason to exclude the possibility that hormones from the syncytiotrophoblast interfere, in some as yet unknown way, with the immunological mechanisms of rejection.

Moreover, as Prof. Amoroso went on to point out, there is an anatomical interesting situation in the human placenta, which has surface cells on the chorionic villi exposed to circulating maternal blood, and a basal plate attached directly to the decidua. Its blood supply comes from the latter via spiral arteries, producing turbulence in the maternal blood space. Any hormones produced on the surface of the chorionic villi will therefore tend to be leached into the maternal circulation and cannot be recycled back onto the villi, so they are excreted in quantity - which probably explains the large quantities of chorionic gonadotrophin constantly formed in human pregnancy and excreted in the urine. This does not happen to the same degree in the guinea pig, where the placental relationship is similar, with the chorionic surface bathed by circulating maternal blood. But there is one important difference. In the guinea pig placentae - and the same applies to the rabbit and rat - blood circulates smoothly through a labyrinth of canals without turbulence; the flow is laminar. There is therefore less surface leaching of hormones secreted by the chorionic spithelium and no need for constant production at such high levels as in man. Assuming that these hormones, principally progesterone and the protein hormones possess immunosuppressive properties, then a coating of them could prevent circulating maternal lymphocytes from making contact with the antigenic surface and thus avert any immune rejection. However, Guy Voisin took a rather different view, further elaborated in Section III. The mother, he said, is known to react immunologically against fetal or placental antigen, but the form that immunoreaction takes might be incapable of inducing rejection. The role of the placenta may well be to divert the immune reaction into other channels. Nevertheless, Hamish Munro expressed interest in the possible immunosuppressant role of syncytiotrophoblast hormones - which is supported by some, admittedly disputed, studies on lack of immunological attack.

The discussion concluded with three brief references to nuclear control in the placenta and the mechanisms by which it is exerted. On the role of releasing factors, Hamish Munro said that LH, RH and TRH had all been demonstrated by fluorescent antibody techniques and that other releasing factors might also be present in cytotrophoblast cells. The question of the regularity of HCG release from the placenta was then raised by Robert Aitken: is it secreted in tonic fashion or in pulses, or from the pituitary? This might have important consequences for the target organ, the corpus luteum. In the male rat, for example, the reason why LH is released from the pituitary in pulses, rather than tonically, is that if LH were present continuously, the gonadotrophin receptors on the surface of the testis cells would be destroyed. Similarly, high tonic levels of HCG, which are released in the first trimester of pregnancy, might be expected to induce luteolysis - which does ultimately happen - by destroying the receptors on the surface of the luteum cells. Finally, Richard Gardner suggested that a change might take place in the nuclear/cytoplasmic ratio when the cytotrophoblast is transformed to syncytiotrophoblast, but the only present evidence - from Gerald Easty's work - consists of observation that the nucleus shrinks at the stage of amitosis or fusion, when HCG first appears. The biosynthesis and functions of that and other placental hormones are outlined in the next paper.

ENDOCRINE FUNCTIONS OF THE PLACENTA

Dorothy B. Villee

Although the placenta was at one time thought to function almost exclusively in the transfer of nutrients and oxygen to the fetus we know now that it possesses many other functions as well. Among these is that of hormone production. From the earliest days of pregnancy trophoblastic cells are veritable factories turning out a variety of hormones. This endocrine function is particularly evident in the human placenta, which produces protein and steriod hormones in large amounts, there being tremendous species variation.[1] For example, virtually no progesterone is synthesised by the placenta in goats, where the corpus luteum provides this important hormone. In contrast, most progesterone in primates is produced by the placenta. Oestrogen is not formed in the placentas of rat, rabbit or guinea pig,[1] whereas most other species have placentas capable of forming oestrone, oestradiol, and in some instances, oestradiol-17 alpha or oestriol.

The pioneer work of Aschheim and Zondek[2] on human chorionic gonadotrophin (HCG) paved the way for the discovery of a succession of placental protein hormones, including the discovery of human placental lactogen (HPL) by Josimovich and MacLaren[3] in 1962 and more recently the description of thyrotropic[4] and corticotropic[5] placental hormones. The biosynthesis of these and other hormones by the placenta and regulation of the process concerned are reviewed below, with notes on some of the functions of placental hormones during pregnancy.

THE EARLY PLACENTA

Viviparity entails a parabiotic union between two different organisms of dissimilar genetic construction. In mammals, the trophoblastic cells of the fetus are in direct contact with, and actually bathed by, maternal blood, Thus the conceptus is a natural allograft, and yet rejection does not take place. When allogeneic blastocysts have been transferred under the kidney capsule of a previously immunised mouse host,[6] this preimmunisation does not interfere with trophoblastic proliferation, but embryonic tissue does not grow. Therefore trophoblastic cells appear to lack sensitivity to cell-mediated immune mechanisms. Amoroso et al[7] suggest that during gestation there is an immunological buffer zone at the interface between maternal and fetal tissues. Since trophoblastic cells have HLA-antigens it has been suggested that some form of immunologically inert material, closely associated with the maternal surface of the trophoblast, masks histocompatibility antigens.

In humans, HCG is localised on the cell membrane of the syncytiotrophoblast facing the maternal blood stream.[8] Wiley,[9] using antiserum to HCG and indirect immunofluorescence has detected a luteinizing hormone (LH) or HCG-like substance ('embryonic gonadotropin') on the cell surfaces of live mouse preimplantation embryos. Before the eight-cell stage little or no gonadotropin was detectable on cell surfaces, whereas in the morula stage these surfaces were strongly positive for gonadotropin and remained so through blastocoel formation.[9] Haour and Saxena[10] analysed the fluid from disrupted six-day rabbit blastocysts. They found HCG or LH-like material in concentrations of 87 $\pm$17 ng/ml. These values far exceeded those obtained for plasma from five to six day pregnant (6-8 ng/ml) or non-pregnant rabbits (<3 ng/ml). Thus gonadotropin is formed very early in differentiation of the trophoblast and by its presence on the surface of the implanting organism may act as an immunological barrier. It has been shown that HCG is capable of inhibiting immune response of the lymphocyte to phytohaemagglutinin (PHA).[11] More recently Finn et al[12] isolated a glycoprotein from placenta which depressed PHA-induced lymphocyte transformation. This protein was distinct from HCG and alpha-fetoprotein. It is of interest that lymphocytes obtained from the mother at the time of delivery are capable of increasing HCG production by trophoblastic cells of her offspring's placenta *in vitro*.[13] Maternal lymphocytes from unrelated donors had no effect.

The early embryo and/or trophoblast can synthesise steroid hormones as well as HCG. Pig blastocyst incubated with labelled dehydroepiandrosterone or androstenedione formed oestrone and oestradiol by days 14-16 of gestation;[14] on day ten there was no significant transformation of androgens into oestrogens. Conversion of labelled progesterone to oestrogen also took place after day 14-15. From these studies the authors conclude that blastocyst tissue has aromatase, 17-20 desmolase, and 3 beta-hydroxysteroid dehydrogenase-isomerase. They also suggest that the presence of unconjugated oestrogen and progesterone in blastocyst tissue results from synthesis _in situ_ and these hormones may play a role in implantaion. Definitive attachment by interlocking microvilli is not seen in the pig until about 18 days after copulation.

Histochemical studies of pre-implantation rat embryos also gave evidence of the presence of 3 beta-hydroxysteroid dehydrogenase early in development.[15] The enzyme was not present in the three-day embryos (2-5 cell stage) but was strongly positive in half the four-day embryos (4-8 cell stage) and in all the five day embryos (blastocysts). Implantation in the rat begins late in the afternoon of day five. The authors suggest that transformation of morula to blastocyst and subsequent implantation of the blastocyst may depend in part on local influences of steroid hormones produced by the early embryo.[15] Steroid synthesis has also been demonstrated in the rabbit preimplantation blastocyst.[16-18]

PROTEIN HORMONES OF THE PLACENTA

The first protein hormone of the placenta, HCG, was described over 50 years ago.[2] Since then new placental products have been discovered and characterised, and a picture has unfolded of protein hormones made in the placenta that are remarkably similar to their pituitary counterparts. It is these hormones that we shall discuss; it should however be remembered that the placenta makes many proteins,[19] some of which possess growth promoting activities.[20]

Human chorionic gonadotrophin

HCG is synthesised in the placenta from the earliest stages investigated. Labelled hormone has been isolated from placental cultures maintained in media containing labelled amino-acids and its biochemical characteristics been investigated.[21] Like other glycoprotein hormones (FSH, LH, TSH) HCG consists of alpha and beta subunits bound non-covalently to each other.[22] The primary structure of all alpha subunits of all human glycoprotein hormones are nearly identical, whereas the beta subunits are distinctive. The beta subunit of HCG, for example, has an additional 30 amino-acid residue at the carboxyl end which is not present in the beta subunits of the other glycoprotein hormones.[22] Using anti-beta-subunit antibody Naughton[23] was able to localise HCG as a continuous layer on the surface of syncytiotrophoblastic cells.

Heterogeneity of the HCG molecule has been described, some of it due to microheterogeneity in amino-acids at the amino terminal end and some to differences in carbohydrate content.[21] Removal of the sialic acid decreases the biological activity of HCG[24,25] and shortens the half-life of the hormone. Thus the sialic acid may protect HCG against metabolic degradation _in vivo_.

Immunochemical studies have shown that HCG is produced and secreted by the syncytiotrophoblast. Using peroxidase antibody to HCG several investigators have shown that it is located in the syncytiotrophoblast of both early and full-term placentas,[26,28] though this technique for localising placental hormones has been called into question recently.[29]

HCG is detectable in blood and urine as early as 9-12 days after fertilisation,[30] rising in concentration thereafter to reach a peak about seven to ten weeks after the last menstrual period. By mid-pregnancy HCG levels decline and remain at this lower level until term. Trophoblastic cells in embryos around the time of implantation appear to synthesise more HCG than do cells from older embryos.[31] Boroditsky et al[32] have shown a fetal sex difference in the levels of HCG during pregnancy. Women bearing female fetuses have higher serum concentrations of HCG in the last trimester than do women bearing male fetuses. It is possible that the lower level of HCG in the latter represents a response to an inhibitory influence of testosterone from the fetal testis. In twin pregnancies both HCG and HPL concentrations in serum are elevated.[33]

Free alpha and beta subunits of HCG have been identified in small amounts in the plasma of pregnant women.[34,35] Large quantities of free HCG alpha are present in normal placenta tissue obtained from all trimesters of pregnancy.[35] With progression of pregnancy there is a marked excess of HCG alpha relative to HCG beta, an increasing proportion of alpha subunits relative to beta subunits being synthesized on placental ribosomes during pregnancy.[36] The evidence suggests that the production of the two chains is not necessarily coordinated and that the amount of complete HCG secreted into the plasma may be limited by availability of the beta chain.

Regulation of the HCG biosynthesis is still under intense investigation. Several investigators have observed that cyclic-AMP is capable of stimulating the synthesis of HCG by trophoblastic cells in culture.[37-39] Cells grown from trophoblastic and non-trophoblastic tumours appear to differ in the regulation of HCG synthesis. For example, 5-bromo-2'deoxyuridine induced HCG alpha synthesis in non-trophoblastic tumour cells, but did not affect intact HCG synthesis in these cells.[40] In contrast, this compound inhibited the synthesis of both intact HCG and HCG alpha in trophoblastic cells.[40] Gibbons et al[41] have identified a LHRH-like product of the placenta. Such a hormone could bring about the formation of more cyclic-AMP, which could induce HCG synthesis. Thus the placenta might regulate its own synthesis of HCG via a placental releasing factor analogous to hypothalamic LHRH.

It is interesting that cyclic-AMP may not only induce HCG synthesis, but also may act as a second messenger in the action of gonadotropins on placental metabolism.[42] HCG as well as LH and prostaglandins induce a marked increase in the intracellular cyclic-AMP concentration in perfused human placenta.[43] HCG also stimulates placental oestrogen production.[42] There is a striking parallel between the amount of the cyclic-AMP accumulation in the tissue and the aromatisation process elicited by HCG.[43]

HCG has other actions as well. It helps maintain the corpus luteum of pregnancy, ensuring a continual production of progesterone. Indeed, granulosa cells are remarkably sensitive to HCG in regard to progesterone production.[44] Small amounts of HCG reach the fetus and may play a role in the early development of steroid synthesis in the fetal adrenal and testis.[45] As already noted, HCG also has a possible role in protecting the fetal allograft from rejection.

Human placental lactogen

The synthesis of HPL was first demonstrated in slices of first and third trimester placentas by Grumbach and Kaplan.[47] Friesen et al[48] concluded, from studies using slices of human placenta or the perfusion of monkey placentas with tritiated leucine, that HPL is the major protein synthesised by the primate placenta near term; it accounts for as much as 10% of the protein released from slices of human full-term placenta.

Polysomes and messenger-RNAs isolated from placental tissue and incubated in vitro have synthesised HPL.[49] In a cell-free system containing placental polysomes, a cell sap fraction from Krebs ascites tumour cells and S35-methionine, HPL was synthesised in vitro and identified by tryptic 'fingerprints'.[50] HPL is preferentially synthesised on membrane-bound polyribosomes and greater amounts of HPL are synthesised by 40-week than by 20-week placentas.[51,52] Heterogeneity of HPL has been demonstrated[53,54] which may reflect a precursor form.[55] Szczesna and Boime have shown that m-RNA from full-term placenta directs the synthesis of a protein that is larger (mol.wt. 25 000) than HPL (22 000).[56] Cleavage of this precursor molecule occurs on ribosome-bound nascent peptide chains.[56]

Structurally, HPL bears a marked resemblance to human growth hormone (HGH), about 80% of the amino-acid residues being identical in the two molecules.[57,58] Observation of internal sequence homologies among pituitary GH, prolactin, and HPL suggest that these polypeptide hormones may have evolved by genetic reduplication from a smaller ancestral peptide.[57,58]

Evidence suggests that the synthesis of several types of peptides in the placenta is regulated primarily by the availability of messenger-RNA. Both HCG and HPL are rapidly released from placental slices after synthesis - as judged by the kinetics of the appearance of peptides containing labelled amino-acids.[59,60] Evidence that there may be control mechanisms specific for the synthesis or release of HPL is provided by the observation that placental slices incubated in vitro rapidly lose their ability to synthesise HPL but retain their ability to synthesise HCG.[61]

The regulation of HPL synthesis, like that of HCG, remains an enigma. In general the amount of HPL formed is related to placental size, but other factors such as the ionic environment[62] may also contribute. It is of interest that rapid administration of intravenous glucose to pregnant women brings about a decrease in plasma HPL, whereas intravenous arginine raises plasma HPL levels.[63] The amounts used were comparable to those used in growth hormone challenge tests, and the results provide additional evidence of similarity between HPL and HGH. Oral glucose or continuous intravenous glucose failed to modify plasma HPL levels suggesting that only sudden changes in maternal plasma glucose can exert a regulatory effect on HPL secretion.[63] Other investigators have also noted a relationship between blood glucose concentration and HPL levels.[64–66] In addition to ionic and nutrient variables, HPL secretion may be regulated by some placental factor analogous to the hypothalamic factor controlling GH release by the pituitary gland. Other releasing factors have been described for the placenta,[41] making this type of regulation an attractive hypothesis.

HPL undoubtedly has a multitude of actions during pregnancy. Josimovich and Archer have summarised these recently.[67] HPL possesses lactogenic activity in rabbits and pigeons and luteotrophic action in the rat. It may also potentiate the ability of HGH to cause growth of the tibial epiphyses in hypophysectomised rats.[68] Chondrocytes isolated from human fetal cartilage showed no direct response to HPL in vitro though somatomedin brought about increased incorporation of thymidine into DNA in these cells.[69] Small amounts of HPL do appear to reach the fetus[70] though the role of this hormone in fetal development is unknown; its effects on maternal metabolism may be of greater significance. The lipolytic action of HPL is thought to be important in conserving carbohydrate during pregnancy. In the pregnant woman the basal and the HPL-stimulated rate of lipolysis in adipose tissue is higher than that in the non-pregnant woman.[72]

Though we have discussed only human placental lactogen it should be remembered that lactogenic placental hormones are found in other species as well. Rodents whose placentas form a lactogenic hormone include the rat, mouse, hamster, chinchilla and guinea pig.[72] Among the Artiodactyla, placental lactogens are found in goat, cow, sheep, fallow deer but not in pig. Immunologically and electrophoretically related molecules are formed in the monkey, cat, dog, pig, horse, sheep and rabbit. In general, the greatest lactogenic activity is found in the primates, with lesser amounts in the Rodentia and least in the Artiodactyla.[72]

Human chorionic thyrotropin (HCT)

A chorionic thyrotropin was isolated from human full-term placentas by Hennen[73] in 1965. Like pituitary TSH, HCT stimulates the secretion of thyroid hormone when injected into mice, but it is chemically and anti-genically distinct from TSH,[74] and has a much lower carbohydrate content (3.5%) than HCG. There is some dispute as to the existence of a separate chorionic thyrotropin because of the known thyropic activity which resides within the HCG molecule.[75] Nevertheless HCT preparations have been shown to stimulate cyclic-AMP formation in slices of guinea pig thyroid gland; purified HCG did not have this action.[21]

The role of HCT in pregnancy is unknown. The mother is not hyperthyroid, though the thyroid gland is enlarged in pregnancy secondary to increased clearance of iodine by the kidneys simulating an iodine-deficient state. HCT may reach the fetus in small amounts and play some role in the fetal thyroid which traps iodine and synthesises thyroid hormone prior to production of TSH by the fetal pituitary.[76]

Human chorionic follicle-stimulating hormone (HCFSH)

Tojo and his colleagues[77] have presented evidence of a separate HCFSH, present in maximum amounts in first trimester placentas. This hormone, like pituitary FSH, stimulates cell division in the ovary. In vitro studies with placental explants have shown synthesis of HCFSH.[78]

Human chorionic corticotropin (HCC)

Evidence for the synthesis of a chorionic adrenocorticotrophic hormone has been provided by Genazzani et al;[5] its content in placental extracts has been estimated to be about 7 μg per placenta, much less than the amounts of HCG and HPL that can be recovered from placentas.[79]

STEROID HORMONES OF THE PLACENTA

During pregnancy in humans there is a gradual increase in urinary excretion of progestins and oestrogens. This change in steroid metabolism with gestation is secondary to the biosynthesis of steroid hormones by the placenta and the fetus.[80] Diczfalusy coined the term 'fetoplacental unit' to signify the collaborative effort of two incomplete steroid synthesising tissues (placenta and fetus) in the biosynthesis of oestrogens.

Progesterone

The human placenta synthesises large amounts of progesterone, utilising maternal blood cholesterol as principal substrate,[81] while the fetus contributes very little to total progesterone production.[82] Near term the human placenta is producing about 250 mg progesterone daily of which 75 mg are delivered to the fetus.[83,84] Placentas from other species also form progesterone.[85–87]

A beta-hydroxysteroid dehydrogenase-isomerase system catalyzes the conversion of pregnenolone to progesterone. Small but detectable amounts of pregn-5-ene-3,20-dione have been isolated during this conversion, suggesting that the oxidation of the 3 beta-hydroxyl group of pregnenolone may occur first.[88] The 3 beta-hydroxysteroid dehydrogenase has been found in placental microsomes and mitochondria;[89] it is inhibited by the products of the enzyme system and by high concentrations of cyclic-AMP. Other strong inhibitors include oestradiol and androstenedione.[89] The conversion of dehydroepiandrosterone to androstenedione is not inhibited by progesterone or oestradiol but is inhibited by androstenedione. Two different 3 beta-hydroxysteroid dehydrogenases may therefore be present in the placenta,[89] one specific for 21-carbon substrates and another for 19-carbon substrates. Both NAD and NADP may serve as cofactors for the microsomal enzyme.[90]

There is relatively little metabolism of progesterone by the placenta. Quantitatively the most important product is 20 alpha-dihydroprogesterone. Because the human placenta lacks a 17 hydroxylase and a C17-20 desmolase neither androgens nor oestrogens are formed from progesterone.[45] It is therefore an incomplete steroid synthesising organ, producing large quantities of progesterone and oestrogens but lacking the capacity to convert progesterone into oestrogens; it can, however, supply progesterone to the fetal adrenal for the biosynthesis of steroid hormones.[45]

The mechanism regulating progesterone synthesis is unknown. A positive correlation has been noted between the concentration of prostaglandin dehydrogenase and that of progesterone in the 14-week human placenta.[91] It has also been suggested that the concentration of tricarboxylic acids within placental mitochondria may play an important role in progesterone formation.[92] The rate of conversion of progesterone to 20 alpha-dihydroprogesterone may help regulate the amount of progesterone secreted by the placenta. The activity of 20 alpha - hyroxysteroid dehydrogenase is increased fivefold in full-term placentas compared to those from the first half of pregnancy.[93] Fetal hormones may alter progesterone synthesis in the placenta. Hagemenas et al[94] have shown that placental slices from pregnancies of decapitated rhesus fetuses secreted significantly less progesterone in vitro than did comparable slices from intact pregnancies. They also found that placentas from female fetuses secreted more progesterone than those from males. HCG has been shown to increase progesterone production in rat placentas.[95]

Oestrogens

The other major steroid hormones produced by the human placenta are oestrogens: oestrone, oestradiol and oestriol. The placenta lacks 16 alpha-hydroxylase and can form oestriol only from 16 alpha-hydroxylated precursors. In general, sulphurylated dehydroepiandrosterone and its 16 alpha-hydroxylated product serve as precursors for the oestrogens.[45] The first step in placental biosynthesis of oestrogens is removal of the sulphate group from dehydroepiandrosterone sulphate. In contrast to the fetus, which possesses very active sulphokinase activity and little or no sulphatase, the human placenta can rapidly cleave the sulphate group releasing free dehydroepiandrosterone or 16alpha-hydroxydehydroepiandrosterone for conversion to oestrogens. Placental steroid sulphatase deficiency is an unusual cause of low oestrogen production in pregnancy.[96]

The further steps in oestrogen production have been studied using in vitro techniques. Extensive aromatisation of dehydroepiandrosterone, androstenedione and testosterone was documented in human placentas perfused in situ with tracer amounts of labelled steroids.[97] Varangot and colleagues[98] perfused placentas and found that the maximum yield of oestrogens was obtained with 19alpha-hydroxyandrostenedione as substrate. The placental oestradiol-17 beta dehydrogenase maintained an equilibrium ratio between oestrone and oestradiol of about three to one in these studies. HCG increased the yield of oestrogens from other substrates but not from 19 alpha-hydroxyandrostenedione.[98] More recent perfusion studies by Wolf et al[99] using dehydroepiandrosterone sulphate as the substrate showed, first, a rapid rise in concentration of androstenedione, followed by a slower increment in concentration of oestrone in the perfusate. Similarly the slower rise in oestradiol levels was preceded by a surge of testosterone. Thus the human placenta can convert delta5-3 beta hydroxy steroids to delta4-3 ketone steroids (3 beta-hydroxysteroid dehydrogenase-isomerase) rapidly followed by aromatisation of these androgens.

The aromatisation system of the human placenta, which is present very early in gestation,[100] has been studied extensively. This conversion of androgens to oestrogens occurs in the microsomes and involves two successive oxidations of C19, removal of C19 as formic acid, and loss of the 1 beta and 2 beta hydrogen atoms.[101] In the process of aromatisation of one mole of androstenedione, three moles of oxygen and three moles of NADPH are consumed with sequential formation of 19 alpha-hydroxyandrostenedione, 19-oxoandrostenedione and oestrone.[102,103] Both 19 alpha-hydroxyandrostenedione and 19-oxoandrostenedione are competitive inhibitors of aromatisation of androstenedione; both compete with and form common binding sites in placental microsomes.[104] Each of the oxidation steps is catalysed by a microsomal cytochrome P-450.[105]

Oestrogen synthesis in the human placenta is known to be stimulated by HCG[98] LH,[106] and HPL.[107] This effect is probably mediated by cyclic-AMP. LH, HCG and prostaglandins E_1 and F_{2alpha} induce marked increases in the intracellular cyclic-AMP concentration of perfused placenta.[43] The placenta may therefore regulate its oestrogen synthesis via its own protein hormones. This, coupled with the releasing factors of the placenta,[41] suggests that it may maintain its own regulation of hormone synthesis with relatively little control from extraplacental influences.

Oestrogen have widespread effects upon various organs and tissues.[108] These include specific effects on target organs (growth of uterus and breasts), inhibition of the synthesis of FSH by the pituitary, and metabolic effects (decreased capillary wall strength, increased synthesis of liver proteins, decreased plasma cholesterol). All of these actions occur during pregnancy and, since oestrogens cross the placenta and reach the fetus, the latter is also subjected to oestrogenic effects. The fetal liver has many hydroxylases, especially 16 alpha-hydroxylase, which modify oestradiol (the biologically active oestrogen) to render it biologically inactive. Oestriol, which is formed in large amounts during pregnancy, is a 16 alpha-hydroxylated oestrogen of low biological activity. It is uncertain what if any role this steriod may have in pregnancy other than serving as an idicator of fetal wellbeing.

Liggins[109] has shown that in sheep relatively high concentrations of cortisol act on the placenta to reduce the secretion of progesterone and to increase the secretion of oestrogen. These steroid changes may be secondary to the induction by cortisol of 17-hydroxylase and desmolase in the placenta. Oestrogen causes prostaglandin release from the placenta, whereas progesterone inhibits it. Thus the decrease in progesterone and the increase in oestrogen produced by cortisol enhances prostaglandin release, and this in turn promotes uterine contractility. Liggins believes that glucocorticoids from the fetus initiate this process in sheep, thereby regulating the onset of labour. It is unknown whether or not a comparable mechanism may be involved in the onset of human parturition.

Conclusion

The human placenta forms many hormones mimicking in many ways the functions of the pituitary, hypothalamus and gonads. By these diverse functions it becomes more or less self-regulatory. It is, however, dependent upon the fetus for substrates for oestrogen synthesis, and it may well be the fetus who calls the tune to end the pregnancy and thus destroy the placenta.

DISCUSSION

Following her formal presentation, Dorothy Villee opened the discussion with a general review of the findings reported, as seen from an endocrinologist's standpoint. In the adult organism, she said, we are accustomed to separate endocrine glands each producing their own specific hormones - tissues of mesothelial origin adrenals and gonads making the steroid hormones, and those of ectodermal origin making for the most part, the protein hormones. But in the placenta there is a prolific mix of very active steroid synthesis with production of many protein hormones going on simultaneously in a single complex organ. Not surprisingly, there are other differences too. The similarities between placental and some pituitary and hypothalamic functions should not be allowed to obscure the fact that for instance, the beta subunit of HCG differs from the beta subunit of LH, producing a distinctive polypeptide chain. Although HPL is structurally very similar to growth hormone and prolactin from the pituitary, there are nevertheless definite differences. Just because the placenta can make protein hormones that are biologically very similar to their endocrine counterparts, and have many homologous areas in their structures, it should not be assumed that they are identical.

Placental releasing hormones are particularly interesting in their close resemblance to most or all of the hormones produced by the anterior pituitary: HPL is analogous to growth hormone and prolactin, HCG to LH, chorionic thyrotrophin (though structurally different) to TSH, and chorionic FSH and MSH to their pituitary equivalents. As regards releasing factors, there is evidence of placental biosynthesis of LH, RH, and TRH - with the likelihood that cytotrophoblast studies will reveal many more releasing hormones. Moreover, in the light of Olga Genbačev's observation that production of many of these hormones by the syncytiotrophoblast increases when the cytotrophoblast is disappearing, we should think in terms of inhibiting factors, as well as releasing ones. That may be the mode of regulation - with something like the prolactin inhibiting factor of the hypothalamus keeping a damper on the cytotrophoblast, to regulate the release of HPL.

It is interesting that the gonads and adrenals which synthesise steroids - including oestrogens and androgens as well as glycocorticoids and mineralocorticoids - all contain every one of the enzymes involved in the conversion of cholesterol; the differences lie in the quantities produced by each. By contrast, some key enzymes are missing from the human placenta. It is fully equipped for active conversion of cholesterol to progesterone, of which huge amounts are made and most reaches the fetus. But the placenta cannot by itself carry out all the steroid synthesis required in pregnancy; it therefore has to rely in part on collaboration with the fetus, which contains a transient tissue for the purpose. This is present within the adrenal gland in all species studied, not just man, but known by different names - the 'X' zone in the mouse, the fetal zone in man. The degree of collaboration is striking in human pregnancy. Large quantities of progesterone are produced by the placenta, which is rich in the most critical enzyme for all steroid hormone synthesis, 3 beta-hydroxy-steroid dehydrogenase. The transient zone in the fetal adrenal almost totally lacks this enzyme but converts ready-made placental progesterone to mineralocorticoids and glucocorticoids. Similarly, the placenta cannot itself convert the progesterone it produces into oestrogens, but the transient zone of the fetal adrenals can and does. The placenta is however, very active in oestrogen biosynthesis from a substrate provided by the same transient zone that utilises placental progesterone. The transient zone also produces large amounts of an androgen, dehydroepiandrosterone, which is rapidly aromatised to oestrone and oestradiol in the placenta.

Underlying these exchanges is the fact that the placenta, though very active in steroid synthesis, lacks three key enzymes - 17-hydroxylase, desmolase, and 16-hydroxylase - that catalyse crucial steps in the complete biosynthetic pathways for certain steroid hormones. Thus the placenta can only make oestriol, which possesses an hydroxyl group at the 16-carbon position, if the necessary 16-hydroxylation is carried out elsewhere. To make this major oestrogen, it is supplied with 16-hydroxylated precursors from the fetus. All this collaboration is so complete, especially in oestrogen biosynthesis, as to suggest that the two belong together and have somehow become separated in the process of growth and differentiation.

Finally, Dorothy Villee commented on an earlier statement that the fetus probably has little or nothing to do with initiating labour, since it is possible to do a fetectomy with the result that the placenta will remain viable for a time. There is, however, as indicated in that paper, a considerable amount of experimental evidence (mainly from sheep) that the fetus may play a part in the onset of labour. Again, the fetal adrenal is concerned in this - with an enormous increase in glucocorticoid production towards the end of gensation in man and many other species. These glucocorticoids reach the placenta and influence it, perhaps bringing about a decrease in the biosynthesis of progesterone and an increase in oestrogen production, so that the oestrogen/progesterone balance is changed. This, in turn, may influence the amount of prostaglandin present, which would affect the sensitivity of the myometrium to the hormones which usually initiate contractions, notably oxytocin. In short, the fetus may give the signal through its adrenals when it is ready to move out into an extra-uterine existence.

Commenting on the statement that the structures of placental peptide hormones differ from their pituitary counterparts in certain sequences, Hamish Munro expressed some surprise. His recent work with ACTH and beta-glycoprotein has shown these to be made in tandem by the same message, 'plus a lot of junk' discarded for secretion as peptide sequences - and precisely the same behaviour is found in placental material as in the anterior pituitary. It would be very unusual for mammalian tissues to make two different proteins in response to the same message. Moreover, the products can be precipitated both with anti-beta-glycoprotein and with anti-ACTH.

In response to questions about hormone production very early in pregnancy, Dorothy Villee said that chorionic gonadotrophin and steroids are produced through the blastocyst stage, and may be involved in the transition from morula to blastula, as well as in the implantation process. Aromatase activity is present in the trophoblast, as indeed are all the hormones that have been studied. Evidence of oestrogen biosynthesis, using labelled precursors, is found in the earliest placentas, the blood levels of oestrogen rising steadily throughout gestation as output increases. However, some hormones such as TSH are produced by placental cells in such small amounts that they probably do not influence the mother's circulating concentrations. Olga Genbačev suggests that those might play some blocker role in the fetus/placenta system. That endorphins might also influence fetal development in some such way was suggested by Hamish Munro, who pointed out that placental ACTH production is sufficient to raise the maternal level, and that this is not suppressed by dexamethasone, which confirms that the increase is unlikely to be pituitary in origin. Discussion of these controlling hormones present in low concentrations led naturally to the next paper on placental prostaglandin activity.

PROSTAGLANDINS IN THE REGULATION OF PLACENTAL FUNCTION

Olga Genbačev

The prostaglandins constitute a group of naturally occurring C-20 unsaturated hydroxy-fatty acids, the name prostaglandin being derived from the initial belief that these substances arose from the prostate. It is now the generic name for a family of closely related lipids whose basic hypothetical structure, prostanoic acid, was proposed by Bergström[1] in 1963. The nomenclature of the primary prostaglandins (E, F, D) is based on the functional groups attached to the five-membered rings of prostanoic acid. The letter designations E and F are given to the prostaglandins possessing a ketone group or hydroxyl group on C-9, and a hydroxyl group at C-11. The suffix (1 or 2) indicate the number of double bounds, while alpha and beta denote the stereochemistry of the 9-hydroxyl group. This paper will be concerned mainly with F type prostaglandins.

Prostaglandins are widely distributed throughout the animal body, and they are formed by every mammalian tissue so far investigated, though the amounts may be different. The highest concentrations of E type prostaglandins are found in human seminal plasma.[2] Elsewhere, tissue levels are rather less, being in the nanogram-microgram range per gram of tissue. Blood levels of prostaglandins in non-pregnant humans are of the order of 10 pg/ml for PGF_{2alpha} and 50 pg/ml for PGE.[3] Tissue and blood concentrations of prostaglandins rise during or approaching parturition[4-8] -

a fact that is of special relevance to this discussion.

PROSTAGLANDIN SYNTHESIS DURING PREGNANCY

The obligatory precursor of prostaglandins E and F is non-esterified or free arachidonic acid. Arachidonic acid itself is widely distributed throughout body tissues and seems to be derived almost entirely from the phosphatide fraction of the cell. Consequently, the first step in prostaglandin biosynthesis is the release of free arachidonic acid - a step controlled by the enzyme phospholipase A_2. Esterified arachidonic acid is present in high concentration in human fetal membranes.[9] Before the onset of labour, 19.3% of the fatty acid content of uterine decidua consists of esterified arachidonic acid, which is remarkably high compared with the arachidonic acid content of most other tissues in the body. The first study that confirmed the storage form of prostaglandin precursors in human fetal membranes was published by Schwartz et al[9] in 1975, these workers supporting the concept that the arachidonic acid released from the amnion diffuses to the uterine decidua where it may serve as a prostaglandin precursor. Several characteristics of the amnion suggest that it may be involved in generation of arachidonic acid, although it lacks the capacity to convert arachidonic acid to prostaglandins. The amnion is a metabolically active tissue with a high rate of glucose utilisation[10] and rapid turnover of arachidonic acid relative to palmitic acid in lecithin. The properties of fetal membrance that are pertinent to prostaglandin synthesis have been summarised by Liggins et al.[11]

The presence of phospholipases has recently been demonstrated in chorioamnion and decidua.[12,13] In many tissues the phospholipases are lysosomal enzymes whose activity depends on release from the lysosomes. This led Gustavii[14] to propose the 'lysosomal theory' of parturition, based on release of phospholipase A_2 from the lysosomes of decidual cells to hydrolise glycerophospholipids and release arachidonic acid. The evidence supporting this hypothesis has been reviewed by Liggins and can be summarised as follows: lysosomes derived from decidual cells have high fragility;[15] decidual cells obtained after caesarean section at term show marked degenerative changes and signs of lysosomal enzyme release;[11] injection of hypertonic saline into the amniotic sac induces marked degenerative changes in the decidua parietalis.[16] The control of arachidonic acid release and its further transformation to prostaglandins are poorly understood. However, Gustavii[17] has suggested progesterone as a possible factor in the regulation of lysosomal stability.

After arachidonic acid becomes available, the next step in prostaglandin biosynthesis is accomplished by a microsomal enzyme complex known as prostaglandin synthase. Elucidation of the pathway of prostaglandin biosynthesis from arachidonic acid is based on the pioneering work of Samuelsson.[18] Besides arachidonic acid, the basic requirements for prostaglandin synthesis are an enzyme complex, molecular oxygen and cofactors that can act as reducing agents.[19-21] Since the synthesis of prostaglandins seems not to be rate limited by prostaglandin synthase,[22] an increase in arachidonic acid levels promotes prostaglandin synthesis. Prostaglandins are released from the decidua and diffuse into the myometrium and amniotic fluid where a rise of concentration is observed.[6,23-25]

METABOLISM OF PROSTAGLANDINS DURING PREGNANCY

It is evident that the concentration of prostaglandins in the tissue or tissue fluids is the result of a balance between biosynthesis and degradation. The initial step in degradation of PGE and PGF is oxidation of the 15-hydroxyl group to the corresponding ketone under the influence of the enzyme 15-hydroxyprostaglandin dehydrogenase.[26,27] The enzymes regulating the degradation of prostaglandins are widely distributed throughout the pregnant uterus, and the human placenta at term is very rich in prostaglandin metabolising enzymes.[28-30] Prostaglandin dehydrogenase (PGDH) is also present in the early human placenta.[31] The highest enzyme activities are found in the fetal membranes and placenta, followed by the myometrium and decidua.[32] It is generally accepted that the high levels of PGDH in the fetal membrane and placenta are a part of the mechanism by which the fetus is protected against the potentially harmful effect of high prostaglandin concentrations. The fetus itself possesses prostaglandin metabolising enzymes and may therefore be capable of inactivating prostaglandins (Keirse - unpublished observations). According to the same author,[32] the fact that tissue of fetal origin (membranes and placenta) has substantially higher enzyme activity than that of maternal origin may indicate that prostaglandin concentrations are, to an appreciable extent, under fetal control.

This brief account of prostaglandin synthesis and catabolism in the pregnant uterus leads to the following conclusions:

Prostaglandins PGE and PGF are synthesised by uterine decidua from arachidonic acid derived from the chorionic villi

The highest activity of prostaglandin-metabolising enzymes is found in fetal membrane and placenta

Prostaglandin synthesis and metabolism both take place locally in the pregnant uterus.

All this evidence accords with the concept of prostaglandins as tissue hormones which act at, or close to, the site of their formation.[33] It is in this light that we shall consider the possible role of prostaglandin F_{2alpha} in the regulation of placental cell function.

PROSTAGLANDIN ACTION AT CELLULAR LEVEL

At cellular level prostaglandin PGF_{2alpha} acts by binding to specific receptors on the plasma membrane, to influence:

- intracellular levels of cyclic nucleotides
- DNA synthesis, and
- protein synthesis.

Prostaglandin receptors

The existence of specific prostaglandin receptors was suggested by the biological specificity of these compounds and by the inhibitory action of antagonists containing similar structural features. Evidence that such receptors are localised or fixed in the plasma membranes of diverse mammalian cell types originates from many studies on intact cells or membrane preparations from different tissues. Specific receptors for PGF_{2alpha} have been demonstrated in the cell membrane of corpora lutea,[34] and in rhesus monkey and human myometrium.[35] Binding studies reveal that PGF_{2alpha} and PGE_1 have little affinity for each other's receptors, suggesting that the conformations of the two prostaglandins differ significantly, as recently confirmed by Langs et al.[36] To our knowledge, there are no data about prostaglandin receptors in human placenta. Both binding studies with PGF_{2alpha} and PGE_1 and membrane preparations from human placentas of different gestational age (Genbačev, unpublished data) reveal the specific binding of PGF_{2alpha} to membrane from full-term placentas and no binding to the membranes from six to eight week old placentas. Further study is necessary to confirm these results.

Prostaglandin effect on intracellular cyclic nucleotide levels

Evidence is accumulating that prostaglandins and their precursors may modulate cyclic nucleotide levels in cells. Arachidonic acid stimulates cyclic-AMP accumulation in the pituitary gland.[37] Low doses (10-100 μg) of arachidonic acid stimulate guanylate cyclase activity in mammary gland homogenate,[38] but when 250 μg or more of arachidonic acid is added, the activity of guanylate cyclase is inhibited. Prostaglandins of E type influence the intracellular level of cyclic-AMP.[39-43] It has been suggested by Kuehl [44] that PGF-receptor interaction may be followed by changes in the cyclic-GMP level. This hypothesis has not yet been confirmed but remains attractive because of the accumulating data on biological regulation through the opposing influences of cyclic-GMP and cyclic-AMP.[45,46] It has recently been demonstrated [47] that prostaglandins of the F series depress adrenal cyclic-AMP with the exception of PGF_{2alpha} at a high concentration (100 μg/ml). This suggests that the change in cyclic nucleotide ratio may provide the intracellular signal, rather than alterations in the absolute levels of cyclic-AMP and GMP.

As cyclic nucleotides appear to be involved in regulating the synthesis of placental peptide hormones, particularly HCG and lactogen,[48,49] study of the relationship between prostaglandins, cyclic nucleotides and protein synthesis seem to be vital to better understanding of the regulation of placental hormone synthesis. As far as we know, there are no systematic data about the concentration of cyclic-AMP or cyclic-GMP in human placentas of different gestational age or in placental neoplasia. Our preliminary results (Genbačev and Cemerikić, unpublished) indicate that the syncytiotrophoblast content of cyclic-AMP increases from 6 to 24 weeks of pregnancy, being 21 and 36 pmol/mg protein respectively. The concentration of cyclic-GMP is about 20 times lower and does not change in the placentas of different gestational age studied. In the presence of PGF_{2alpha}, significant increase was observed in the intracellular content of cyclic-GMP.

Prostaglandin effect on DNA synthesis

There are only a few reports dealing with prostaglandin effects on RNA and DNA synthesis. It has however been demonstrated[50] that PGF_{2alpha} at a concentration of 300 ng/ml stimulates DNA synthesis and cell division in untransformed fibroblasts in tissue culture. A stimulant effect of PGF_{2alpha} on RNA biosynthesis was reported by Rillema[51] in mouse mammary gland culture. Recently, a significant increase of DNA synthesis, as determined by PGF_{2alpha} in mouse spleen cell culture was described by Egg et al.[52] There is, however, absolutely no evidence on any effect of PGF_{2alpha} on placental DNA synthesis.

Prostaglandin F_{2alpha} and protein synthesis

Only a few works deal with the effect of PGF_{2alpha} on RNA or protein synthesis, but it has been shown to stimulate the synthesis of RNA in mouse mammary gland in a prolactin-like manner, with no effect on casein synthesis.[51] And a recent report[53] showed that PGF_{2alpha} at high concentrations inhibits the formation of glycosoaminoglycans and proteins from calf rib cartilage, whereas lower concentrations were only slightly stimulating or ineffective. The effect of PGF_{2alpha} on placental protein synthesis in vitro has been studied in placentas of different gestational age.[54,55] In a concentration of 50-100 μg/ml, it inhibits total protein synthesis in mid-gestational and full-term placentas, but has no effect on protein synthesis in 6, 8, 10 and 24 week-old placentas. The strong inhibition of total protein synthesis in mid-gestational placentas induced by PGF_{2alpha} is almost entirely due to the inhibition of HPL synthesis (Figs. 1, 2 and 3).

In order to attribute some physiological role to PGF_{2alpha} in the regulation of placental protein synthesis, experiments with lower prostaglandin concentrations

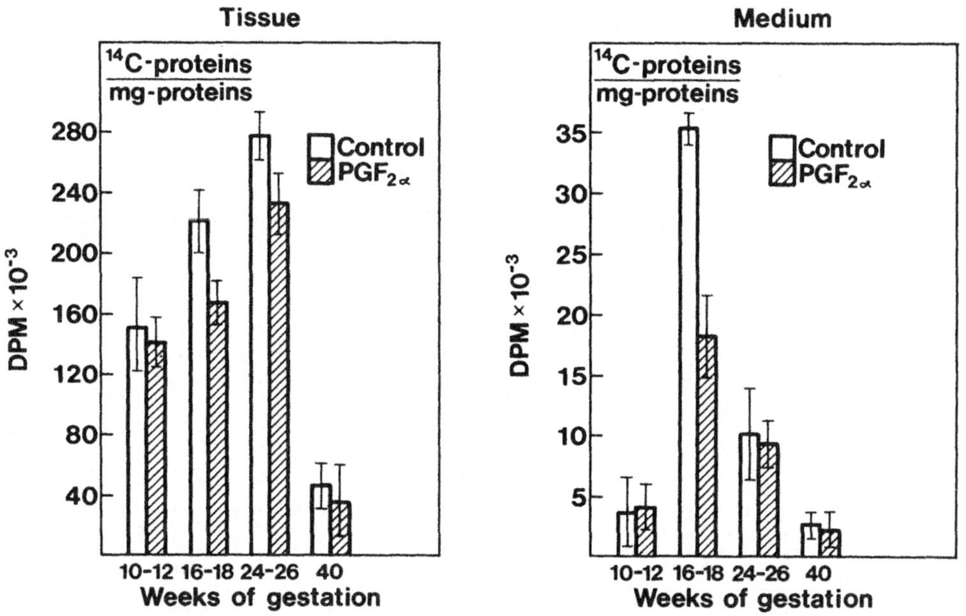

Fig. 1. The effect of PGF_{2alpha} on the incorporation rate of ^{14}C-leucine into proteins in placentas of different gestational age ($\pm$ s.e. mean).

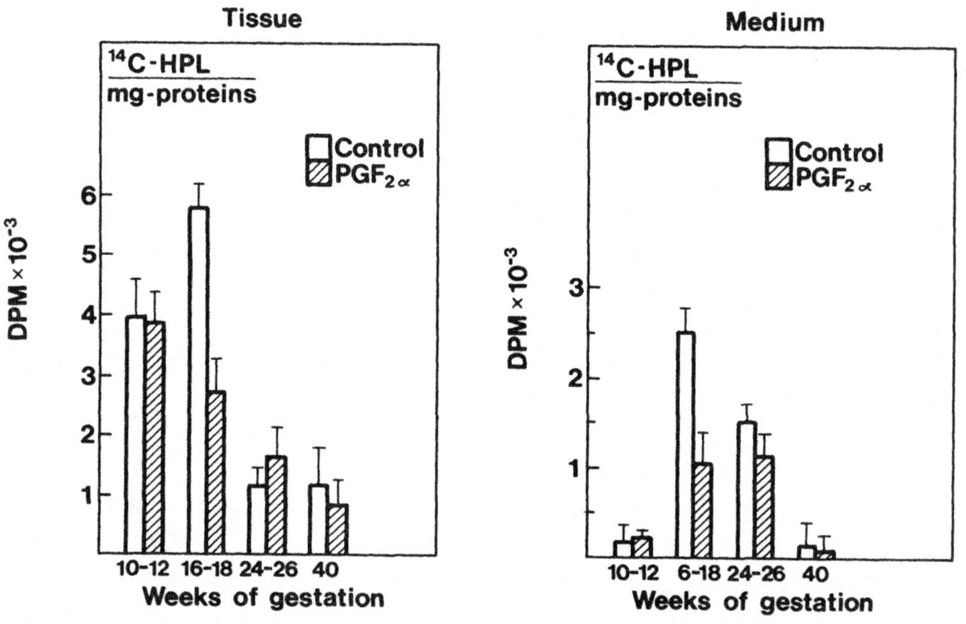

Fig. 2. The PGF_{2alpha} effect on the ^{14}C-leucine incorporation into HPL in placentas of different gestational age after 3 hours of incubation ($\pm$ s.e. mean).

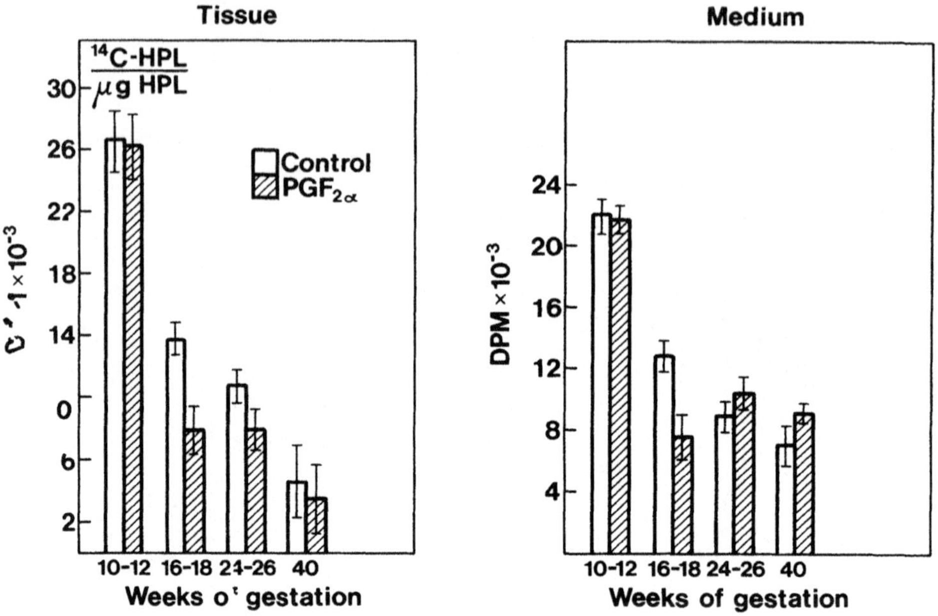

Fig. 3. Specific activity of HPL in placentas of different gestational age after 3 hours of incubation with PGF_{2alpha} ($\pm$s.e. mean).

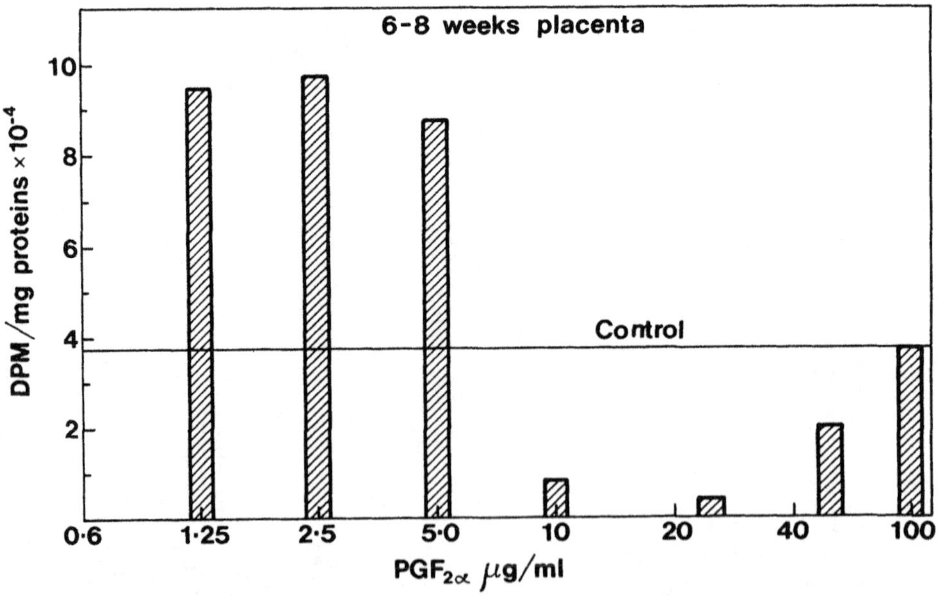

Fig. 4. Effect of different doses of PGF_{2alpha} on total protein synthesis in the first trimester placenta.

are required. Our recent observations indicate that the PGF_{2alpha} effect on placental protein synthesis depends both on the dose of prostaglandin used and on the gestational age of the placenta. In six- to eight-week-old placentas, PGF_{2alpha} at low concentration (1-5 μg/ml) stimulates placental protein synthesis and inhibits it at higher concentration (10-25 μg/ml). As noted above, the dose of 50-100 μg/ml is ineffective at that stage of gestation (Fig. 4). This finding might be explained by the existence of two types of receptor sites, occupation of one producing a positive effect and of the other a negative effect - a hypothesis put forward by Ariens et al[56] and proposed for PGF_{2alpha} action by Horrobin.[57] It postulates that the drug has higher affinity for the activating receptors than for the blocking receptors. As their concentrations rise, prostaglandins' occupancy of activating receptors is thought to reach a plateau, while the occupation of blocking receptors continues to increase until the biological response disappears.

CONCLUSIONS

We consider the PGF_{2alpha} synthesised by uterine decidua to be a local hormone that acts on the placental cells as one of the factors regulating placental protein synthesis. To induce this effect the availability of membrane bound receptor(s) seems to be important, and the existence of two classes of PGF_{2alpha} receptors is postulated.

The high concentration of prostaglandin dehydrogenase in the placenta may be part of a protective mechanism against transmembrane transport of PGF_{2alpha} since active transport has been reported for rabbit vaginae.[58]

The fetal control of PGF_{2alpha} synthesis through arachidonic acid release from chorionic villi points to the possibility of fetal control of placental protein synthesis and/or placental growth.

Further studies are required: to identify PGF_{2alpha} receptors in placentas of different gestational age, to clarify the effect of prostaglandins on cyclic-AMP and GMP levels in placental tissue, and to define the effect of different PGF_{2alpha} concentrations on protein synthesis, both in normal placental tissues and in placental tumour cells.

DISCUSSION

It is necessary to postulate two types of prostaglandin receptor to account for the placental response to PGF_{2alpha}, since it follows the bell-shaped curve common to many drugs? Posing this question, Claude Villee conceded that the two-receptor hypothesis provided a possible explanation but suggested that the lack of response to high concentrations might be explained by overloading of a step beyond the receptor, with consequent shutdown. Another possibility, mentioned by Olga Genbačev herself, is that prostaglandins may not need receptors on the placenta for their actions; there is some evidence that they can be transported across the syncytiotrophoblast membrane without the aid of receptors. Further studies are required to clarify these mechanisms and to define prostaglandin actions in the placenta - which appear to include regulation of the synthesis of HPL and of some other proteins. But does control of HPL synthesis, whether mediated by prostaglandin activity or not, rest ultimately with the mother? Olga Genbačev thought not. It seems more probably that the fetus influences the rate of synthesis of placental proteins, including HPL, indirectly through the decidual cells and the availability of phospholipase A_2.

As regards prostaglandin synthesis, Eric Newsholme described the phospholipase A_2 reaction in which esterified arachidonic acid is hydrolysed to form arachidonic acid itself as the flux-generating step. Since this provides the substrate for prostaglandin synthesis, it regulates the rate of production. Prostaglandins resemble cyclic-AMP in acting as local messengers whose biological activity must be destroyed by the utilisation reaction in which they exert their effect. With cyclic-AMP, at least two phosphodiesterases - a chymase and a deaminase - perform this inactivation, providing considerable flexibility in the system. But is there any evidence that two or more different reactions are available to inactivate prostaglandins in placental tissue? Apparently not. Studies seem to have been confined to the enzyme 15-hydroxyprostaglandin dehydrogenase, which is present in the placenta and has recently been purified and characterised. It remains an open question whether the placenta contains other prostaglandin inactivators.

Concerning the gestational age of the decidua studied, Robert Aitken drew attention to the importance of distinguishing between early and late pregnancies. In very early pregnancy, the uterus appears to make no prostaglandins at all. As early as 17 days post-ovulation, prostaglandin levels in the pregnant endometrium virtually disappear, whereas they are extremely high in the non-pregnant cycle. It has been suggested that the embryo switches off prostaglandin production by the endometrium, and that this may be a mechanism by which it prevents menstruation occuring, in addition to the corpus luteum.

Finally, discussion turned to prostaglandins and induction of labour. Commenting on the wide gulf between clinician and basic scientist, Alan Browne noted that one obstetrician might be very good at inducing labour with prostaglandin and another very bad. The one who gets good results is rather rough, sweeping the membranes and stirring up the decidua - which presumably enables the prostaglandin to exert its very localised action over a large area. And since their action is so local, higher doses of prostaglandins have no comparable effect. Referring to Dorothy Villee's earlier contribution about close interaction between the fetus and the mother in hormone production and initiation of labour, Professor Browne said he felt sure that the fetus can prevent its own entry into the world. The mechanism is not clear, but occasionally an anencephalic fetus remains in utero for a prodigiously long time - as much as 358 days alive in one case he reported, until birth when it died instantly. The absence of pituitary and adrenals was presumably responsible.

TECHNIQUES FOR STUDYING PLACENTAL METABOLISM AND TRANSFER

Maureen Young

The many techniques for studying placental metabolism and transfer are here presented in outline, with particular emphasis on in vivo techniques and reference to the transfer and metabolism of amino-acids only. An extensive review of the models used for studying placental transfer in vivo is currently in preparation.[26]

IN VITRO TECHNIQUES

Dissection, slicing and homogenising are essential when studying the component parts of the biochemical mechanisms underlying the physiological function of organs. The various techniques used for the placenta are listed in Table I, together with their sources, and the majority are very familiar to investigators. Much of the work has been done on the human placenta because of its ready availability at no cost. The recent development of a method to separate the surface microvilli of the human placenta[24] is of particular interest and the vesicles obtained have specific receptors for glucose and amino-acids;[20] the mixed membranes from homogenates also possesses specific insulin receptors.[18] The perfusion of the isolated guinea pig placenta[12] or a single lobule of the human placenta[22] must be regarded as an in

TABLE I

Placental tissue preparations for study in vitro

Isolated chorionic villi	Smith, C.H. et al[26]
Tissue slices	Longo, L.D. et al,[14] Schneider, H. and Dancis J.,[21] Enders, R.H. et al.[8]
Membranes	
- surface microvilli	Smith, N.C. et al,[24] Ruzycki, S.M. et al[20]
- intracellular	Posner, B.I.[18]
Homogenates	Hill, P.M.M. and Young, M.[9] Philipps, A.F. et al.[17]
Perfusion of both maternal and fetal circulations in isolated placenta	
- guinea pig	Leichtweiss, H.P. and Schroder, H.[12] Eaton, B.M.[6]
- lobule of human placenta	Schneider, H. et al.[22] Challier, J-C.[2]

vitro technique because the organ is perfused with artificial fluids. The guinea pig preparation is most attractive because it promises control over both the maternal and the fetal supply to the placental membrane, and the tissue is relatively undisturbed - giving it some of the advantages of the placenta perfused in situ, since substances can reach the receptors and enter and leave the placenta as they would in life. The perfused human placental cotyledon preparation allows less precise control over the two circulations, especially on the maternal side, but may still retain many of the properties characteristic of the species.

IN VIVO TECHNIQUES

It is also necessary to be able to observe transport and metabolic functions in the intact placenta with its gross and microscopical structure undisturbed. However, both the uterus and placenta present special problems for the attainment of the correct bloodflows during perfusion, because of the extreme contractility of the myometrium and the umbilical blood vessel walls. Two in vivo preparations which have partially overcome these disadvantages have been used extensively over the last 20 years. The first was developed by Barron's group[15] and is a long term preparation with indwelling catheters in the umbilical vessels and, frequently, in the maternal uterine vein of the pregnant ewe. The secret of operative success here lies in the unresponsiveness of the myometrium during hysterotomy for induction of the fetal catheters in the sheep. So far, no such preparation has been successful in primates. These preparations can be maintained for several weeks and have provided a lot of information in the unanaesthetised, unstressed feto-placental unit, with the ewe in the upright position. Comline and Silver[3] point out that attractive though the chronic preparation may be, there are no criteria to ensure that recovery is ever complete, with a return to perfectly normal intrauterine conditions. They consider that well controlled acute experiments may be more valuable than many carried out in the conscious animal.

The second preparation, developed by Dancis' group,[4] exploits the unique advantage of the placenta having two circulations; the fetal side of the placenta is perfused through the umbilical vessels, while the organ is left in situ in the uterus, nourished by maternal blood delivered at normal pressure and flow rate. The physiological, pharmacological or toxic substances to be investigated reach the receptors on either side of the placental membrane as they would in vivo; and their subsequent reactions in, and their exit from, the tissue should be relatively undisturbed. The circulation on the fetal side of the placenta is perfused, after removal of the fetus, with a relatively simple physiological solution to collect the products of placental metabolism and transfer.[19] The secret of success in cannulating the umbilical vessels is to immerse the maternal abdomen in a physiological fluid at 37°C so that there is no loss of temperature, and consequent vasoconstriction, during hysterotomy and exposure of the fetus. Such a technique was first used by Paul Zweiffel just over a hundred years ago and, later, by Joseph Barcroft in this country.

The pregnant guinea pig is a particularly suitable animal for placental perfusion studies for two reasons, First, the placenta does not separate readily from the uterine wall; although there is some retraction of the myometrium when the fetus is gently removed from the uterine cavity to introduce catheters into the umbilical vessels, and this probably accounts for some of the imperfections observed in transfer rates. Second, the structure of the placental membrane in the guinea pig is very similar to that of the human.[7] Both are haemomonochorial and have a fetal capillary wall and a layer of syncytiotrophoblast lying between the two bloodstreams, though the maternal surface of the syncytium is not so richly covered with microvilli in the guinea pig as it is in the human placenta, and the cytoplasm not so well endowed with intracellular contents. The arrangement of the two circulations is, however, very different in the two species. In the guinea pig, fetal and maternal blood both flow in separate labyrinths, and the arrangement of the major blood vessels suggests that there may be true counter-current flows between the two circulations.[10] In the human, the fetal capillaries dip in clusters into the large maternal blood sinus or intervillous space.

On the fetal side of the guinea pig placenta, there are two further advantages. First, with the removal of the fetus, the transfer of metabolites from the placenta and nutrients across it can be studied independently of fetal influences. And the use of a relatively simple physiological fluid, the second advantage, allows careful control over its composition and over the pressure at which it is perfused, and thus over the flow rate. Normally, a placenta weighing four grams is perfused at about 30-40 mm Hg (the pressure observed in the umbilical arteries in the third trimester of guinea pig gestation) which gives a flow rate of 2 ml/per minute - equivalent to 50 ml/per 100 grams of tissue per minute. Transfer rates are calculated from the umbilical venous-arterial difference and the flow rate. The whole placental tissue can be homogenised and analysed after the perfusion, and compared with control tissue. However, no one has yet described a good method of allowing for - or eliminating - the retained maternal blood and perfusion solution which must influence any estimations on placental tissue.

There are also limitations to this <u>in situ</u> preparation, as with every experimental method. The mother has to be anaesthetised (with Nembutal) and her placental circulation cannot be regarded as perfect; it cannot be controlled either, though it may be altered by drugs or by haemorrhage. Any changes which may occur in the maternal circulation during perfusion are monitored by a constant intravenous infusion of freely-diffusable antipyrine into the mother, so that the concentration ratio fetal-perfusate:maternal-plasma can be measured. This ratio is usually about 0.8, declining minimally during two hours of perfusion.[9,19] The maternal arterial blood pressure and acid/base balance are also monitored, and a fall in the antipyrine ratio is associated with a fall in maternal blood pressure or the development of acidosis. The viability of the preparation has been demonstrated by its capacity to transfer selectively the L-isomers of amino-acids[19] and the D-isomer of glucose from mother to fetus.[11] It has also been shown to transfer amino sodium[9] and potassium ions[1] at 60% and 80% respectively of the rates at which they are transported in vivo. The histological structure, observed by both light and electron microscopy, appears satisfactory after perfusion.[1] In the absence of other biochemical criteria (such as the potassium content of the tissue, the lactate:pyruvate and beta-hydroxybutyrate:acetate ratios to indicate integrity of the cytoplasmic and mitochondrial redox mechanisms, and the ATP-ADP ratios) these deficits in ion transport may be due to some impairment of bloodflow inherent in the preparation now used.

COMPARISON OF RESULTS OBTAINED IN VIVO AND IN VITRO.

The relative value of the two in vivo methods described in comparison with the in vitro can be assessed using amino-acid transport from mother to fetus by way of example. Measurement of the free amino-acids in the placenta, performed on tissue homogenates, shows that their concentration exceeds that in both maternal and fetal plasma,[9,17] the relationship between the three being shown for eight amino acids in

TABLE II

Concentration ratios of free amino-acids in guinea pig fetal and maternal plasma and placental tissue.

	Fetal:maternal	Placental levels related to:	
	Plasma ratios	Maternal plasma	Fetal plasma
Aspartate	3.9	60.6	21.5
Glutamate	4.0	74.7	22.7
Glycine	6.1	14.7	2.9
Alanine	6.0	12.5	2.4
Valine	2.8	5.5	1.5
Leucine	3.8	9.1	2.7
Lysine	4.2	7.2	2.0
Histidine	3.2	5.8	1.9

Table II. The constant relationship between the trophoblast and fetal plasma concentrations, except for the acidic amino-acids (asparate and glutamate), suggest that they all move from the placental into the fetal compartment by diffusion down a concentration gradient. By contrast, the very large gradient between the maternal plasma and trophoblast for aspartate and glutamate suggests that they are either transferred against a very large gradient indeed or synthesised de novo in placental tissue. Isotope studies in the pregnant animal with an intact fetoplacental unit show that neither glutamate nor aspartate are transferred from mother to fetus in the anaesthetised monkey[25] or the unanaesthetised rat.[5] Further, in the intact pregnant ewe,[13] the umbilical arterio-venous differences for glutamine and the majority of the amino acids are positive, demonstrating their fetal uptake (Fig.1.). Glutamic acid is the exception, with a negative difference, indicating uptake by the fetal side of the placenta. The conversion of glutamic acid to glutamine by the placenta has recently been demonstrated in preparations of isolated human placental lobule in which both circulations were perfused with artificial solutions.[2] This production of glutamine from glutamate could probably have been observed under suitable conditions in homogenates of placenta and in tissue slices, but these would not have demonstrated the direction of entry of the glutamic acid into the placenta or its relationship to fetal metabolism. Further, placental slice uptake studies would have been misleading, for Dancis' group[21] have shown that the tissue has a very

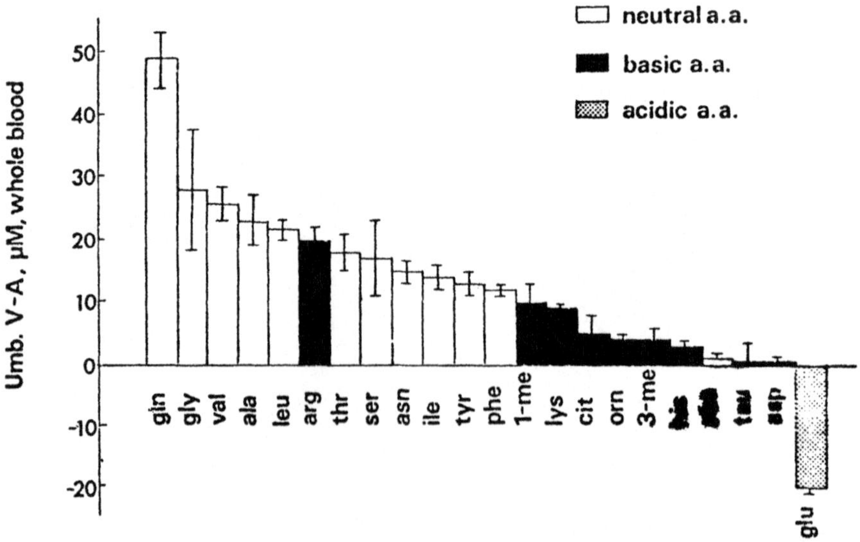

Fig. 1. Transfer of the majority of the amino-acids from the placenta to the fetal circulation, and placental uptake of glutamic acid from the fetus, in the fetal lamb.[3]

high capacity for the uptake of the two acidic amino-acids. Taken in conjunction with previous work, these observations suggest that the maternal side of the placental membrane has a low affinity but a high capacity for the uptake of acidic amino-acids, as in many other organs.[16] Other examples of the relative value of in vivo over in vitro techniques in extending our knowledge of placental function will no doubt be revealed as the former are used more extensively.

DISCUSSION

New investigative technique

A novel method of investigation involving the single passage of two tracers in the circulation of a perfused placenta was then outlined by David Yudilevich. This allows for rapid measurement of extractions, which can be very high, representing high unidirectional fluxes with, for example, as much as 82% of the input being taken up. But such high rates are revealed only if the measurements can be performed very quickly indeed, since the rate of extractions also falls very fast. The whole trick, he said, is to measure the unidirectional flux in, say, the first half minute. This gives a measurement of the carrier transport, not the net uptake, which is many times lower. The method, which has been applied to several biochemical fields in a number of different organs, is well suited to studies of placental transport, where David Yudilevich reported extractions of the order of 60 to 70% for the sugars D-flucose and D-mannose, with significantly lower extraction rates for D-fructose, and no transport of either sucrose of L-glucose. Similar studies have been done with amino-acids. In perfused guinea pig placenta, for example, it is possible to measure very significant uptakes of tryptophan.

'As leaky as the preparation may be', said Prof. Yudilevich, referring to the guinea pig placenta, 'you can carry on, over long periods, studying the unidirectionla flux by means of these very fast sampling techniques. Secondly, it is possible to do a large number of different studies in the same placenta. We are in the process of applying this to the human placenta, which is a better preparation to work on, with the aim of identifying carriers and receptors. And we have already shown that lysine is transported very significantly, on both the fetal and maternal sides, along with alanine, phenyl-alanine, tryptophan and tyrosine. Comparison with previously available methods has confirmed the striking improvement obtained with this technique. For instance, injection of glucose on the fetal side with one sample of maternal blood would have shown no stereospecificity with other methods. With the single passage technique, however, there is extremely clear differentiation between D- and L-glucose uptake, ranging from 40 to 80%. This technique is also of interest because it enables prostaglandins to be studied, and we have been able to show that about 30% of PGE_2 molecules are taken up at the fetal/maternal interface of guinea pig placenta. This should be a useful way of looking at receptor function which ties in well with Dr. Genbačev's work. It can also be extremely useful for distinguishing metabolism from transport.'

Taking up this last point, Claude Villee commented on the difficulty of answering a seemingly simple question, such as: how does substance X cross the placenta? The fact that it goes in at one side and comes out on the other does not necessarily mean that it just went across unchanged. All sorts of interesting things might have happened in between, and this new tracer technique should be of great assistance in clarifying such questions. In this context, Olga Genbačev asked which types of amino-acids would be best to use for studies of protein synthesis. Theoretically it does not matter, in Maureen Young's view, because proteins normally require them all. The ones that enter most quickly are the branch-chain neutral amino-acids, such as leucine and valine, which are incorporated in to most of the placental proteins. It should not, however be assumed that amino-acid transfer from placenta to fetus all comes from maternal blood. A study in guinea pig placenta has shown that about half the branch-chain amino-acids must have come from a highly concentrated free amino-acid pool in the placenta itself.

With regard to receptor function, Arthur Wild interpreted David Yudilevich's finding that demonstration of placental throughput depends on rapid analysis as evidence that receptors are generated very quickly on the fetal side. And he enquired whether these receptors are associated with any specific transporting organelle. In reply, Prof. Yudilevich said that the carrier is probably located in the membrane perhaps with other carriers in organelles. The important thing in his view is to try and dissociate the one from the other, because if we are eventually going to find genetic changes in these transport systems, it is vital to be sure that studies are directed to the same carrier in the same place. Page Faulk agreed that it is highly pertinent to study the involvement of the hypothesised receptor in transport mechanisms. However, the presence of a specific receptor does not necessarily imply transport of the substance it is specifically equipped to bind. In the syncytium, for example, insulin and transferrin receptors have recently been identified, yet neither insulin nor transferrin are, in fact, transported from the maternal to the fetal circulation. The purpose of such receptors remains unclear; they can hardly be there just to complicate research.

Placental energy requirements

Discussion continued with a seemingly more straightforward question: energy production for placental tissue that is actively growing, metabolising and manufacturing materials for itself and for the fetus. Yet, as Jean Ginsburg pointed out, we cannot account adequately for all the energy it needs. Some of it - though the proportion cannot be large - goes to maintaining the temperature of the fetus, which is always about $1^{\circ}C$ higher than that of the maternal blood. This has been observed in the sheep, and in man - the latter 50 or so years ago. The fact that the hand bloodflow rises progressively during human pregnancy may well be evidence of peripheral vasodilation related to the necessity for the maternal organism to dispose of excess metabolic heat generated by fetal and placental development. As regards energy sources, Eric Newsholme wondered how important fat might be, particularly the predigested fatty acid molecules known as ketone bodies, in addition to carbohydrates. Ketone body levels certainly increase markedly at parturition, and this rise is paralleled by an increase in the uterine enzymes concerned in ketone body metabolism. How important ketone bodies might be as an energy source during the whole course of pregnancy remains uncertain. Pinpointing that as a future research topic, Eric Newsholme also queried whether there might be some demand for glycolytic energy as such or whether the intermediates of glycolysis were in demand by the fetus and/or placenta for some other reason. It is at any rate noteworthy that glycolytic activity is also raised in other rapidly-growing - i.e. neoplastic - tissues.

It has been shown by several investigators that there is an inverse correlation between the maternal blood glucose and HPL concentrations - acute intravenous administration of glucose producing a fall in blood HPL. Pointing this out, Dorothy Villee drew attention to the structural similarity between HPL and growth hormone. And children deficient in growth hormone can be tested by lowering the blood glucose level: this normally increases the growth hormone level and can therefore be used to check whether they can elaborate some of the hormone. Equally, growth hormone secretion can be shut off by raising the blood sugar level. Although the placenta has usually been regarded as relatively autonomous, there might be gluco-receptors in it capable of signalling for production of MPL. And this, in its turn is a glycolytic hormone which can conserve carbohydrate in the maternal organism. There just could be a natural feedback mechanism here.

Whether the placenta really has a very high metabolic rate was queried by Maureen Young, who said that the oxygen consumption of the fetus is in reality identical with adult consumption on a weight-for-weight basis. That of the placenta is a little higher, but growth of the fetus proceeds without any great increase in overall oxygen consumption. But Hamish Munro felt that the active and inactive tissues of the placenta should be distinguished. Some tissues are very considerably energy dependent, while other fibrous structures are virtually inert. As Claude Villee pointed out, 13% of the human placenta consists of trophoblast cells - where most of the action is thought to go on. Their energy levels must obviously be very high. But just how high? - asked Hamish Munro, making a plea for better quantification not only for energy consumption but also to obtain exact data on transport mechanisms, utilisation of substrates, and outputs from the placenta. Measurement must take over from mere description in these important fields.

Noting that the meeting was intended to provide a forum for reviewing placental studies, rather than presenting detailed research findings, Peter Beaconsfield stressed the importance of discussing what is already known about placental metabolism and what needs to be known if we are to reach a better understanding of the three physiopathological fields the meeting was convened to study - cell replication, immunology and ageing. Thus far, he said there has been little if any cross-fertilisation of ideas between specialities; instead, participants have barricaded themselves in their own fields of expertise - as if fearing to venture out or risk outside contamination getting in. 'If people of our intellectual calibre and knowledge hesitate to venture outside our specific realms the entire concept of interdisciplinary meetings becomes a farce, and the term a misnomer. If we are to achieve our aim, we must be prepared to go outside our own fields. Without a willingness to indulge in some informed theorising based on the breadth of knowledge we collectively possess we shall be denying the most exciting and fundamental part of science: the evolution of fresh hypotheses and the means to test them. There is indeed a gulf between clinician and basic scientist - si science savait, si les medecins pouvaient - but as a clinician who spends part of his time familiarising himself with advances in the basic sciences and how these may be applied for the benefit of patients, I believe it can be closed. It is in this spirit that I should like briefly to draw your attention to the subject of drugs and placental metabolism.'

DRUGS AND THE PLACENTA — A PERSONAL VIEW

Peter Beaconsfield

Three questions are absolutely basic to any discussion of drugs and the placenta:

1. How do drugs affect the placenta?
2. What does the placenta do to drugs?
3. How can the placenta be used to test and evaluate chemical compounds?

Placental transfer has already been discussed at length. Many chemical compounds pass from mother to fetus, and for practical purposes we can say that all drugs cross the placenta. However, the problems that arise in the fetus are not simply due to its immature tissues being presented with a dilute dose of the drug its mother took. Metabolites also cross the placenta, and the concentrations of drug or metabolite are sometimes greater in fetal tissues than in the mother. Moreover, many drugs affect placental metabolism, and may thus induce fundamental changes affecting the fetus that are at least as, or more important than, the presence of the drug itself. Changes in physiological function can be seen by looking at metabolic pathways and intermediates with particular reference to feedback mechanisms and ramic points where metabolic flow direction is determined. If the objectives are clearly in mind, studies made at tissue level enable us to predict with a fair degree of accuracy what will take place at organ level, and at whole body level.

Ten years or so ago when I tried to introduce the concept of two-tier testing of drugs[1] - which would involve different tests for different types of drug according to their intended use, I discussed this question with Hubert Bloch of CIBA. He agreed on the value of using the placenta and said they had done some work of this kind but had avoided publicising it for fear that it might mushroom into an obligatory new protocol for testing all compounds and not simply those that might require such tests in relation to their use. His experience was that no official drug regulatory agency had ever permitted the total discarding of any test protocol, even when superceded by superior methods, and at a WHO meeting around that time he referred to the numerous toxicity tests creating a volume of work which in itself gave an apparent assurance of quality that could be quite illusory.[2] This is, paradoxically, a major risk of safety regulations. We also know that the threat of ever-increasing numbers of tests has had a suffocating effect on pharmaceutical creativity, yet there is no guarantee that this improves drug safety. In these circumstances, it seems particularly regrettable to lose a potentially useful tool such as the placenta through fears that its use might be made obligatory. As long ago as 1973, at SCIP's first meeting in Bellagio, a complete review and revision of drug testing methods was suggested - with the reasonable aim of discarding the obsolete and taking into account more specifically the nature and purpose of the chemical being studied. No more than lip service has been paid to this proposal.

That the placenta may actively modify drugs has never been systematically investigated. In 1972, by invitation, I wrote a protocol outlining such a study for a major pharmaceutical house, but nothing was ever done about it. The placenta does have microsomal enzyme systems, including some cytochrome P 450 at term,[3] so in theory at least it can produce a modifying effect on certain compounds. The metabolites thus produced could be more active and/or more toxic than the parent compound - so-called 'lethal synthesis'. Drug metabolising enzymes with oxidative, deaminating, hydroxylating and hydrolytic activity for barbiturates, amphetamine and meperidine have all been demonstrated in the placenta, and enzyme induction has also been observed after barbiturate administration.[4-7] There is a long way to go before we know the whole story.

Lastly, can we use the placenta to test and evaluate certain compounds? The answer must be 'yes', if only because it is a living mammalian system conveniently and readily available to us. An earlier paper discussed perfusion techniques, but there are a number of other methods which could be used for drug testing purposes. As the placenta is a rapidly growing tissue it would surely be a good testing ground for compounds which are being developed to slow down growth and interfere with certain aspects of metabolism - namely cytotoxic drugs, and so-called anti-metabolites. I can almost hear the old plaint about not being able to extrapolate such findings to the human condition. But why should this objection apply to the human placenta? The cellular level is the level par excellence for investigation, especially when we are talking about human cells. All complaints about the validity of extrapolation are relative. What we do need is the knowledge to decide which studies to do, on what animal or human system, and how to interpret the results. This last is usually by far the most difficult part, as it requires thought, judgement and experience, in addition to comprehensive knowledge. One of the problems today is that no one scientist can interpret all the results brought to him by the teams of specialist technicians working in this field. We therefore run three risks, all of which I can unfortunately document: first, that the interpreter will fail to notice an association between test results; second, that he will jump to a wrong conclusion from the results because of inadequate understanding; and third, that he may be tired that day and just won't look at the results properly. Investigators are, after all, part of the society in which they work.

One of the most fundamental biological laws that seems to have been forgotten lately is that the functional activity of an organ, or of the whole body, represents the total effect of many interrelated biochemical and biophysical processes. If these processes are known, and there are generally accepted norms for them, then the effect of any compound on them will serve to predict what the compound's total effects would be. However, an organ's, or the body's, compensatory mechanisms are very well developed. It is therefore quite possible for marked physico-biochemical alterations to occur as a result of innumerable processes and reactions and for a 'normal' physiological picture be preserved nevertheless, at least for some time. That is why results of hepatic and renal function tests, when these are used to assess drugs, can give an inaccurate picture of what is happening at the cellular level. The results are themselves products of tissue metabolism, and the side effects of drugs are in reality end-effects, being the manifestation of a number of disturbed biochemical and biophysical processes.

To exemplify how the placenta might be used for investigating growth-inhibiting compounds let me describe in somewhat anecdotal fashion how we first came to think about it - more than 15 years ago. Changes in pentose phosphate pathway activity affect the rate of formation of D-ribose, RNA and DNA and of protein synthesis both in non-placental tissues,[8] and in the placenta.[9] In the course of investigations into the epidemiology of cancer about 12 years ago we observed that subjects deficient in glucose-6-phosphate dehydrogenase had a reduced incidence of malignancy.[10] This observation has since been confirmed in retrospective and prospective studies.[11,12] From the results of our earlier work we could postulate a biochemical explanation for the decrease in cancer incidence, distinct from the genetic one, in these particular population groups. By using a compound that depresses pentose-phosphate shunt activity by action on an $NADPH_2$ generating system, we found that this slowed down the growth of Ehrlich's ascites cell tumours and prolonged survival time in a group of mice. In this example L-ADH was used as 'treatment', but more specific compounds are now being sought.

All abnormalities are in essence biological phenomena of multicausal origin, and the abnormalities themselves due to deviation from normal metabolism in a particular tissue. Each such deviation initiates a complex process involving a sequence of independent steps, any of which may be open to therapeutic modification. In carcinoma, they can be divided into two main stages: <u>pre-autonomous</u>, and <u>auton-</u>

omous - in respect of proliferation. Both in the field of neoplasia and in immunological processes, ageing, and the effects on tissues of drugs and other chemical compounds, the placenta represents an underestimated and underused research tool. But its use will be fully effective and the results valid only if the studies are multidisciplinary in approach. This is not an exercise for super-specialists, and that produces difficulties in itself, because in practice they dominate all research - which also creates obstacles to getting new ideas introduced and adopted. Since the mid-Victorian period, when the era of British affluence and influence was rising towards its peak with increasing reliance on science and technology, specialisation has been god - which has enabled man to travel to the moon and back, but is also one of the main reasons why cancer has not be conquered.

In a word, although the placenta suffers from the disadvantage that it consists of specialised tissues with particular functions that have to be understood in themselves, it has great advantages as an experimental animal because it is a freely available human tissue. It can be kept alive and intact long enough for its functions to be measured, and all the processes that form the themes of this meeting can be studied on it if we approach each of them with the open-minded imagination that well-instructed people should be able to exercise. The relationship between drugs and the placenta may best be considered within this broader context, not in narrow isolation.

DISCUSSION

For Dorothy Villee, two aspects of the preceding papers stood out. One was consideration of the placenta as an active interface between mother and fetus, probably treating many of the substances that reach it - drugs, hormones or whatever - as metabolic substrates, so that some of the things taken by the mother are modified en route to the fetus, while others pass through unchanged. The other interesting point she stressed was the potential value of the placenta as a human tissue for test trials of drugs, carcinogens, or other substances. In the United States there is a severe shortage of subhuman primates for laboratory work because of the cut-off of supplies from India and other past suppliers. Although the rate of breeding has been greatly increased, it cannot come anywhere near to the supply that would be needed if primate tissue were to be used for routine testing. This should stimulate work on the placenta as an alternative.

In view of the large number of women taking drugs of a particular class - the steroid hormones - Robert Aitken inquired whether a model system such as the placenta could be used to assess oestrogenicity. A lot of drugs now marketed have some associated oestrogenicity, but if a pharmaceutical company is asked about this property of one of its drugs, the response is usually to say that they injected the substance into a mouse or a rat and measured the hypertrophic response of the uterus. We know, however, that certain compounds which are highly oestrogenic in a mouse may not be so in man and that at least one has proved to be antioestrogen, an impeder of oestrogen activity. This appears to be due to species differences in the affinities of the receptor molecules. It seems probable that the placenta could be used to assess the oestrogenicity of drugs on human tissue, since it contains receptors for oestrogens (and for progesterones). A number of workers have identified oestrogen-dependent proteins in the human uterus, similar to the induced proteins in rats and mice. These are produced in large amounts, and it would be interesting to know whether the placenta produces similar proteins in response to oestrogenic compounds, and if so, whether the synthesis of these proteins could be used as a marker for the oestrogenicity of drugs. The progesterone receptor might be an alternative marker. In all species oestrogen stimulates the synthesis of progesterone receptors, which are relatively easy to assay.

That exogenous agents can induce protein synthesis in the placenta was noted by Hamish Munro. For example, iron induces ferritin synthesis - as may happen in a mother with haemolytic disease if she has extra iron in the placenta. A related question he raised is whether drugs administered chronically induce placental enzymes, increase the amount of smooth endoplasmic reticulum, increase the cytochrome P 450 concentration and so forth - since these could also provide useful markers. Peter Beaconsfield replied that the placental cytochrome concentration, including alcohol dehydrogenase, does actually rise in response to drug administration. Pointing out that probably the most used drug on earth is ferric sulphate during pregnancy, given in grams not milligrams, Page Faulk enquired whether much is known about its effects - in terms of induced ferritin synthesis in the trophoblast, for instance, or numbers of transferrin receptors in the placenta. Unfortunately not, said Peter Beaconsfield; we do not even know what effect aspirin has on the placenta.

Broadening the argument, Claude Villee emphasised the importance of studying whether drug X, say, or environmental agent Y affected the fetus. Many processes are involved. First, there is the compound's distribution in the mother, and what the mother's metabolism does to it. Then there is the question of whether the resulting compound(s) and/or the one originally administered crosses the placenta unchanged, or whether the placenta metabolises or detoxifies it - completely or in part. Finally there is the question of what the fetus does to the compounds which reach it via the placenta; in some respects the fetal liver might be a better detoxifier of a particular substance than the adult liver. On the question of

whether the placenta could be used to test drugs, Claude Villee thought it might be difficult to decide the validity of the results obtained. For example, tests might show that the placenta bound certain molecules, but it would require much more than that to conclude that drug X was less safe than drug Z. Criteria would have to be firmly established by basic studies before placental tests were introduced.
Robert Aitken agreed with this proviso, while stressing the value of being able to assess the effects of drugs on human tissue, instead of using rats or other mammals. A difference of opinion then arose between Harold Fox - who held that the placenta, being in many ways unique, would only show if a substance was toxic to placental tissue, without enabling any other conclusions to be drawn from the results - and Peter Beaconsfield who took a more sanguine view of the value of placental studies. He believes that the many metabolic processes of the placenta that are also present in normal human tissues should be studied in detail, as a first step, so that the effects of a drug or other compound to be tested could be examined with regard to each, paying particular attention to any change in the metabolic processes concerned, and the nature of their intermediates and end-products. Knowledge of a tissue's basic biochemistry should enable the effects of drugs or their metabolites on physiological processes to be predicted - and/or established by further tests. However, Claude Villee pointed out, fetal tissues must be regarded as a special case. While a drug that produces a major change in the placenta would obviously be contraindicted in pregnancy, it could not be assumed that a drug without adverse effects on the placenta would be perfectly safe for the fetus. Overall though, it seems fair to conclude, from these and other contributions to discussion, that placental studies should prove a most valuable adjunct to existing methods of drug testing - and not least as a means of learning just what compounds the fetus is exposed to in utero, and at what concentrations.

Conclusion to Section I

As in any tissue, to appreciate the function of the placenta, certain basic biochemical and physiological aspects have to be known and understood, especially for establishing normal limits. These need to include - among many other factors - blood supply, precursors, basic metabolic pathways, important intermediates and ramic points. Changes in any of these produce changes in metabolism and thus in function. Different physical and chemical assaults will produce variations in the metabolic mosaic, which must be genetically determined - and therefore variable to some degree, both within and (sometimes) beyond the normal range. These are among the fundamental considerations that underlie the major placental processes discussed in the following sections: Their understanding and thus much of their value as experimental models, defends a knowledge of basic placental biochemistry.

REFERENCES TO PAPERS IN SECTION I

PRINCIPLES OF METABOLIC REGULATION

E. A. Newsholme and B. Crabtree

1 Newsholme, E.A. and Start, C. (1973). Regulation in metabolism, Wiley, New York and London.

2 Arch, J.R.S. and Newsholme, E.A. (1976). Activities and some properties of adenylate cyclase and phosphodiesterase in muscle, liver and nervous tissues from vertebrates and invertebrates in relation to the control of the concentration of adenosine 3':5'-cyclic monophosphate. Biochem. J. 158, 603.

3 Crabtree, B. and Newsholme, E.A. (1975). Comparative aspects of fuel utilisation and metabolism by muscle. Insect Muscle Ed. Usherwood P.N.R. p.405. Academic Press, London and New York.

4 Crabtree, B. (1976). Reversible (near-equilibrium) reactions and substrate cycles. Biochem. Soc. Trans. 4, 1046.

5 Crabtree, B. and Newsholme E.A. (1978). Sensitivity of a near-equilibrium reaction in a metabolic pathway to changes in substrate concentration. Europ. J. Biochem. 89, 19.

6 Newsholme, E.A. and Crabtree, B. (1976). Substrate cycles in metabolic regulation and in heat generation. Biochem. Soc. Symp. 41, 61.

7 Sugden, P.H. and Newsholme, E.A. (1975). The effects of ammonium, inorganic phosphate and potassium ions on the activity of phosphofructokinases from muscle and nervous tissues of vertebrate and invertebrates. Biochem. J. 150, 113.

8 Newsholme, E.A. (1976). The role of fructose 6-phosphate/fructose 1, 6-diphosphate cycle in metabolic regulation and heat generation. Biochem. Soc. Trans. 4, 978.

9 Newsholme, E.A. (1977). The regulation of intracellular and extracellular fuel supply during sustained exercise, Ann. N.Y. Acad. Sci. 301, 81.

10 Newsholme, E.A. and Crabtree, B. (1973). Metabolic aspects of enzyme activity regulation. Symp. Soc. Exptl. Biol. 27, 429.

11 Crabtree, B. (1976). Theoretical considerations of the sensitivity conferred by substrate cycles in vivo. Biochem. Soc. Trans. 4, 999.

12 Newsholme, E.A. (1978). Substrate cycles: metabolic, thermic and energetic considerations, Biochem. Soc. Symp. 43, 183.

13 Newsholme, E.A. and Start, C. (1972). General aspects of the regulation of enzyme activity and the effects of hormones Handbook of Physiology: Section 7, endocrinology 1. Ed. Steiner, D.F. and Freinkel, N. pp. 369-383 American Physiological Society, Washington D.C.

14 Beis, I. and Newsholme, E.A. (1975). The contents of adenine nucleotides, phosphagens and some glycolytic intermediates in resting muscles from vertebrates and invertebrates. Biochem. J. 152, 23.

15 Newsholme, E.A. and Crabtree, B. (1970). The role of fructose 1 6-diphosphatase in the regulation of glycolysis in skeletal muscle, FEBS Letter 7, 195.

16 Clark, M.G., Bloxham, D.P., Holland, P.C. and Lardy, H.A. (1973). Estimation of the fructose disphosphatase - phosphofructokinase substrate cycle in the flight muscle of bombus affinis. Biochem. J. 134, 589.

17 Clark, D.G., Rognstad, R. and Katz, J. (1973). Isotopic evidence for futile cycles in liver cells. Biochem. Biophys. Res. Commun. 54, 1141.

18 Sutherland, E.W., Øyem I. and Butcher, R.W. (1965). The action of epinephrine and the role of adenyl cyclase system in hormone action. Rec. Progr. Hormone Res. 623.

19 Davies, J.I. and Williams, P.A. (1975). Quantitative aspects of the regulation of cellular cyclic AMP levels. 1. Structure and kinetics of a model system. J. Theor. Biol. 53, 1.

20 Perkins, J.P. (1973). Adenyl cyclase. Adv. Cyclic Nucleotide Res. 3, 1.

21 Paul, J. (1971). Transcriptional regulation in mammalian chromosones. Symp. Soc. Expt. Biol. 25, 117.

22 Wright, B.E. (1966). Multiple causes and controls in differentiation. Science, 153, 830.

23 Arch, J.R.S. and Newsholme, E.A. (1978). Activities and some properties of 5 - nucleotidase, adenosine kinase and adenosine deaminase in tissues from vertebrates and invertebrates in relation to the control of the concentration and the physiological role of adenosine. Biochem. J. 174, 965.

24 Arch, J.R.S. and Newsholme, E.A. (1978). The control of the metabolism and the hormonal role of adenosine. Essays in Biochem. 14, 82.

25 Medvedev, Zh. A. (1967). Molecular aspects of ageing. Symp. Soc. Expt. Biol. 21, 1.

26 Hermansen, L. Personal communication.

27 Opie, L.H. and Owen, P. (1975). Effects of increased mechanical work by isolated perfused rat heart during production or uptake of ketone bodies, Biochem. J. 148, 403.

28 Houghton, C.R.S. (1971). Studies on the metabolism of exercise with special reference to perfused isolated skeletal muscle. D.Phil. thesis Oxford.

29 Rowan, A.N. and Newsholme, E.A. (1978). Changes in the contents of adenine nucleotides and intermediates of glycolysis and the citric acid cycle in flight muscle of the locust upon flight and their relationship to the control of the cycle. Biochem. J. 176 (In press).

PLACENTAL CARBOHYDRATE, PROTEIN AND FAT METABOLISM

Peter Beaconsfield and Jean Ginsburg

1 Moya, F. and Thorndike, V. (1962) Passage of drugs across the placenta. Am. J. Obstet. Gynec. 84, 1778.

2 Moya, F. and Smith, B.A. (1965) Uptake distribution and placental transport of drugs and anaesthetics. Anesthesiology 26, 465.

3 Villee, C.A. (1965) Placental transfer of drugs. Ann. N.Y. Acad. Sci. 123, 237.

4 Wild, A.E. (1974) Protein transport across the placenta. Symposia Soc. Exptal. Biology XXVIII, 521.

5 Ginsburg, J. (1971) Placental drug transfer. Ann. Rev. Pharmacol 11, 387.

6 Dawes, G.S. (1969) Foetal blood gas homeostasis, p. 162 in Foetal Autonomy, Ciba Foundation Symposia, Edited Wolstenholme, G.W. and O'Connor, M. Churchill, London.

7 Kermit, K.E., Blakey, J., Yoshida, K. and Romito J.A. (1971) Demonstration of viability of perfused human term placenta. Obstet. and Gynec. 37, 183,

8 Widdas, W.F. (1952) Inability of diffusion to account for placental glucose transfer in the sheep and consideration of the kinetics of a possible carrier transfer, J. Physiol. 118, 23.

9 Karvonen, M.J. and Raichä, N. (1954) Permeability of placenta of guinea pig to glucose and fructose. Acta Physiol. Scandinav. 31, 194.

10 Chinard, F.P., Danislino, V., Hartmann, W.L., Huggett, A.St. G., Paul, W. and Reynolds, J.R.M. (1956) Transmission of hexoses across placenta in human and rhesus monkey (Macaca mulatta). J. Physiol. 132, 289.

11 Carstensen, M., Leichweiss, H.P., Molsen, G. and Schroder, H. (1977) Evidence for a specific transport of D-hexoses across the human term placenta in vitro, Arch. Gynaekol. 222, 187.

12 Lumley J.M. and Wood, C. (1967) Influence of hypoxia on glucose transport across the human placenta, Nature 216, 403.

13 Schröder, H., Leichtweiss, H.P. and Madee, W. (1975) The transport of D-glucose, L-glucose and D-mannose across the isolated guinea pig placenta. Pfluegers Arch. 356, 267.

14 Ely, P.A. (1966) The placental transfer of hexoses and polyols in the guinea-pig, as shown by umbilical perfusion of the placenta. J. Physiol. 184, 255.

15 Rosso, P. (1975) Changes in the transfer of nutrients across the placenta during normal gestation in the rat. Am. J. Obstet. Gynecol. 122, 761.

16 Villee, C.A. (1953) The metabolism of human placenta in vitro. J. Biol. Chem. 205, 113.

17 Ginsburg, J. and Jeacock, M.K. (1968) Effect of epinephrine on placental carbohydrate metabolism. Am. J. Obstet. Gynecol. 100, 357.

18 Sakurai, T., Takagi, H. and Hosoya, N. (1969) Metabolic pathways of glucose in human placenta: changes with gestation and with added 17-estradiol. Am. J. Obstet. Gynecol. 105, 1044.

19 Cori, C.F. and Cori, G.T. (1925) The carbohydrate metabolism of tumors. II Changes in the sugar, lactic acid, and CO_2-combining power of blood passing through a tumor. J. Biol. Chem. 65, 397.

20 Warburg, O. (1931) The Metabolism of Tumors. Constable, London.

21 Bierich, R. and Rosenbehm, A. (1933) Uber den milchsauregehalt von normalen unt von krebsgeweben, Hoppe-Zeyler's Z. Physiol. Chem. 214, 271.

22 Pasteur, L. (1861) Expériences et vues nouvelles sur la nature des fermentations. C.R. Acad. Sci. 52, 1260.

23 Krebs, H.A. (1972) The Pasteur effect and the relations between respiration and fermentation. Essays in Biochemistry. 8, 1.

24 Parry, M.J. and Walker, D.G. (1966) Purification and properties of adenosine-5-triphosphate-D-glucose-6-phosphotransferase from rat liver, Biochem. J. 99, 266.

25 Walker, D.G., Lea, M.A., Rossiter, G.and Addison, M.E.B. (1967) Glucose metabolism in the placenta, Arch. Biochem. and Biophys. 120, 646.

26 Roux, J.F. and Villee, C.A. (1960) Effects of anoxia on the metabolism of the human placenta, Am. J. Obstet. & Gynecol. 80, 224.

27 Pocchiari, F. (1968) Initial stages in the conversion of glucose in glycogen, p. 129 in Proc. 4th meeting Europ. Bioch. Soc. Academic Press, New York.

28 Beaconsfield, P. (1969) On the need of a two tier system for evaluating drugs intended for long term administration. Ann. Istituto Sup. di Sanità 5, 536.

29 Kamel, R. and Schwarz Fischer, F. (1975) Hexokinase isozymes in human neoplastic and fetal tissues; the existence of hexokinase II in malignant tumors and in placenta. Humangenetic. 30, 181.

30 Newsholme, E.A. and Start, C. (1973) Regulation in Metabolism. J. Wiley & Sons, London.

31 Fridhandler, L. (1961) Pathways of glucose metabolism in fertilised rabbit ova at various pre-implantation stages. Exp. Cell Res. 22, 303.

32 Edwards, R.G. (1977) Early human development: from the oocyte to implantation. Chapter 15 in Scientific Foundations of Obstetrics and Gynaecology. Edited E.E. Philipp, J. Barnes and M. Newton. William Heinemann, London.

33 Beaconsfield, P., Ginsburg, J. and Kosinski, Z.(1965) Glucose metabolism via the pentose phosphate pathway relative to cell replication and immunological response. Nature 205, 50.

34 Beaconsfield, P. and Reading, H.W. (1964) Pathways of glucose metabolism and nucleic acid synthesis. Nature, 202. 464.

35 Sweeney, M.J., Ashmore, J., Morris, H.P. and Weber, G. (1963) Comparative biochemistry of hepatomas. IV Isotope studies of glucose and fructose metablism in liver tumours of different growth rates. Cancer Res. 23, 995.

36 Ginsburg, J. and Jeacock, M.K.(1964) Effect of adrenaline on human placental lactate production in vitro. Am. J. Obstet. and Gynecol. 90, 794.

37 Burd, L.I., Jones, M.D., Simmons, M.A.,Makowski, E.L., Meschia, G. and Battagla, F.C. (1975) Placental production and foetal utilisation of lactate and pyruvate. Nature 254, 710.

38 Schreiner, W. and Villee, C.A. (1961) Oxidative phosphorylation in mitochondria from human placentas. Am. J. Obstet. & Gynecol. 91, 961.

39 Bernard, C. (1859) Sur une nouvelle fonction du placenta. J. de la Physiologie de l'homme et les animaux 2, 31.

40 Ross, S.A. and Hytten, F.E. (1976) Placental glycogen. Brit. J. Obstet. Gynaec.83, 43.

41 Burg, E., Hertig, A.T., McKay, D.G. and Adams, E.C. (1962) Histochemical aspects of hydatidiform mole and choriocarcinoma, Obstet. Gynecol. 19, 156.

42 Cédard, L., Alsat, E., Urtasum, M.J. and Varangot, J. (1970) Studies on the mode of action of luteinizing hormone and chorionic gonadotrophin on estrogenic biosynthesis and glycogenolysis by human placenta perfused in vitro. Steroids 16, 361.

43 Demers, L.M., Gabbe, S.G., Villee, C.A. and Greep, R.C. (1973) Human chorionic gonadotrophin-mediated glycogenolysis in human placental villi: a role of prostaglandins. Biochim. et Biophys. Acta 313, 202.

44 Longo, L.D., Yuen, P. and Gusseck, D.J. (1973) Anaerobic, glycogen dependent transport of amino acids by the placenta, Nature 243, 531.

45 Gabbe, S.G., Demers, L.M., Greep, R.O., Villee, C.A. (1972) The effects of hypoxia on placental glycogen metabolism. Am. J. Obstet. Gynec. 114, 540.

46 Demers, L.M. Gabbe , S.G., Villee, C.A. and Greep, R.C. (1972) The effects of insulin on human placental glycogenesis. Endocrinology 91, 270.

47 Posner, B.I. (1974) Insulin receptors in human and animal placental tissue. Diabetes 23, 209.

48 Podskalny, J.M.,Chou, J.Y. and Rechler, M.M. (1975) Insulin receptors in a new human placenta cell line: demonstration of negative cooperativity, Arch. Biochem. Biophys. 170, 504.

49 Takano, K., Hall, K.,Fryklund, L., Holmgren, A., Sievertsson, H. and Uthne, K. (1975) The binding of insulin and somatomedin A to human placental membrane, Acta Endocrinol. 80, 14.

50 Villee, C.A. (1953) Regulation of blood glucose in the human fetus, J. Appl. Physiol 5, 437.

51 Holmberg, N.G., Kaplan, M.J., Karvonen, M.J., Lind, J. and Malm, M. (1956) Permeability of human placenta to glucose, fructose and xylose. Acta Physiol. Scand. 36, 291.

52 Alexander, D.P., Huggett, A. St. G., Nixon, D.A. and Widdas, W.F. (1955) The placental transfer of sugars in the sheep: studies with radioactive sugar. J. Physiol. 129, 352.

53 Bacon, J.S.D. and Bell, D.J. (1948) Fructose and glucose in the blood of the fetal sheep. Biochem. J. 42, 397.

54 Huggett, A. St. G. (1954) The transport of lipids and carbohydrates across the placenta. Cold Spring Harbor Symp. Quant. Biol. 19, 82.

55 Hagerman, D.D. and Villee, C.A. (1952) The transport of fructose by the human placenta, J. Clin. Invest. 131, 911.

56 Zakim, D. (1973) Influence of fructose on hepatic synthesis of lipids. p.161 in Effects of carbohydrates on lipid metabolism. Ed. I. Macdonald. Karger, Basle.

57 Coltart, T.M. Bateman, C. (1975) Carbohydrate-induced lipogenesis in the human placenta of normal and diabetic pregnancies. Brit.J.Obstet.Gynaec. 82, 471.

58 Yoshioka, T. and Roux, J.F. (1972) In vitro metabolism of palmitic acid in human fetal tissue. Pediat. Research 6, 675.

59 Roux, J.F. and Myers, R.E. (1974) In vitro metabolism of palmitic acid and glucose in the developing tissues of the rhesus monkey, Am. J. Obstet. & Gynec. 118, 385.

60 Sutherland, E.W. and Wosilait, W.D. (1955) Inactivation and activation of liver phosphorylase. Nature 175, 169.

61 Krebs, E.G. and Fischer, E.H. (1956) The phosphorylase (b to a) converting enzyme of rabbit skeletal muscle. Biochim. Biophys. Acta 20, 150.

62 Cohen, P.D., Antonin, J.F., Nimmo, H.S. Yeaman, S.J. (1976) Protein phosphorylation and hormone action, p.281 in, Polypeptides: Molecular and Cellular Aspects: CIBA Found. Symp. Churchill London.

63 Kram, R., Moens, W. and Vokaer, A. (1975) Control of cellular growth and differentiation by cyclic nucleotides, p.53 in, Reproductive Endocrinology, Ed. Vokaer, A. and de Bock, G. Pergamon Press.

64 Goldberg, N.D., Haddox, M.K., Nicol, S.E., Acott, T.S., Glass, D.B. and Zeitig, C.E. (1976) Cyclic GMP and cyclic AMP in biological regulation. p.99 in Control Mechanisms in Cancer, Ed. Criss, W.E., Ono, T. and Sabine, J.R. Raven Press, New York.

65 Satoh, K. and Ryan, K.J. (1971) Adenyl cyclase in the human placenta. Biochim. Biophys. Acta 244, 618.

66 Ferre, F. and Cédard, L. (1971) Etude du méchanisme de la regulation hormonale dans le placenta humain: 1. mise en évidence d'une activité adenyl cyclasique dans les homogenats de placenta à terme. Biochim. Biophys. Acta 237, 316.

67 Ferre, F., Breuiller, M. and Cédard, L. (1972) Demonstration of 3'5'-cyclic AMP phosphodiesterase activity in the human placenta at term. C.R. Acad. Sci. 274, 3313.

68 Ferre, F., Breuiller, M. and Cédard, L. (1975) Human placental CAMP phosphodiesterase activity, kinetic properties and sensitivity to some drugs and hormones. FEBS Lett. 52, 295.

69 Gelot, M.A., Paysant, P. and Nabet, P. (1973) Demonstration and study of physico-chemical characteristics of a placental protein binding cyclic AMP. C.R. Soc. Biol. 167, 1439.

70 Anguy, A., Alsat, E. and Cédard, L. (1976) Phosphorylase activity of human placenta perfused in vitro: effect of gonadotrophins, dibutyryl cyclic AMP and prostaglandins. C.R. Acad. Sci. 281, 897.

71 Handwerger, S., Barrett, J., Tyrey, L. and Schemberg, D. (1973) Differential effect of cyclic adenosine monophosphate on the secretion of human placental lactogen and human chorionic gonadotrophin. J. Clin. Endocrinol. Metab. 36, 1268.

72 Lewlliers, J., Alsat, E., Laudat, P. and Cédard, L. (1974) Hormone-stimulated CAMP production in human placenta perfused in vitro. FEBS Lett. 47, 146.

73 Hussa, R.O., Story, M.T. and Pattillo, R.A. (1974) Cyclic adenosine monophosphate stimulates secretion of human chorionic gonadotrophin and estrogens by human trophoblast in vitro. J. Clin. Endocrinol. Metab. 38, 338.

74 Matsuda, T., Nakano, Y., Nishikawa, Y. and Yamaguchi, R. (1977) Feto-maternal amino acid patterns and cyclic AMP in the human placenta with abnormal pregnancies, particularly with SFD, Tohoku J. Exp. Med., 121, 253.

75 Voorhees, J.J. and Duell, E.A. (1975) Imbalanced cyclic AMP-cyclic GMP levels in psoriasis. Adv. Cyclic Nucleotide Res. 5, 735

76 Nishiyama, K., Katakami, H., Yamamura, H., Takai, Y., Shimomura, R. and Nishizuka, Y. (1975) Functional specificity of guanose 3' : 5' monophosphate-dependent and adenosine 3' : 5' monophosphate-dependent protein kinases from Silkworm. J. Biol. Chem. 250, 1297

77 Newsholme, E.A. (1977) The regulation of intracellular and extracellular fuel supply during sustained exercise. Ann. N.Y. Acad. Sci. 301, 81.

78 Nelson, G.H., Zuspan, F.P. and Mulligan, L.T. (1966) Defects of lipid metabolism in toxemia of pregnancy, Am. J. Obstet. Gynec. 94, 310.

79 Younoszai, M.K. and Haworth, J.C. (1968) Chemical composition of the placenta in normal preterm, term and intra-uterine growth retarded infants. Am. J. Obstet. Gynec. 103, 262.

80 Robertson, A.F. and Sprecher, H. (1968) A review of human placental lipid metabolism and transport. Acta Paediatr. Scand. Supplement 183.

81 Vikrot, O. (1964) Quantitative determination of plasma phospholipids in pregnancy and non pregnant women with special reference to lysolecithin. Acta Med. Scand. 175, 443.

82 Popjak, G. and Beekmans, M. (1950) Are phospholipids transmitted through the placenta? Biochem J. 104, 99.

83 Biezenski, J.J. (1969) Role of placenta in fetal lipid metabolism. 1. Injection of phospholipids double labelled with C^4 glycerol and P^{32} into pregnant rabbits. Am. J. Obstet. Gynec. 104, 1177.

84 Biezenski, J.J., Carrozza, J. and Li, J. (1971) Role of Placenta in fetal lipid metabolism. 3. Formation of rabbit plasma phospholipids. Biochim. Biophys. Acta 239, 92.

85 Mallov, S. and Alousi, A.A. (1965) Lipoprotein lipase activity of rat and human placenta. Proc. Soc. Exptl. Biol. Med. 119, 301.

86 Koren, Z. and Shafrir, E. (1964) Placental transfer of free fatty acids in the pregnant rat. Proc. Soc. Exptl. Med. 116, 411.

87 Van Duyne, C.M., Parker, H.R., Havel, R.J. and Holm, L.W. (1960) Free fatty acid metabolism in fetal and newborn sheep. Am. J. Physiol. 199, 987.

88 Hershfield, M.S. and Nemeth, A.M. (1968) Placental transport of free palmitic and linoleic acids in the guinea pig. J. Lipid Res. 9, 460.

89 Kayden, H.J., Dancis, J. and Money, W.L. (1969) Transfer of lipids across the guinea pig placenta. Am. J. Obstet. Gynec. 104, 564.

90 Elphick, M.C., Hudson, D.G. and Hull, D. (1975) Transfer of fatty acids across the rabbit placenta. J. Physiol. 252, 29.

91 Portman, O.W., Behrman, R.E. and Soltys, P. (1969) Transfer of free fatty acids across the primate placenta. Am. J. Physiol. 216, 143.

92 Szabo, A.J., Grimaldi, R.D. and Jug, W.F. (1969) Palmitate transport across perfused human placenta. Metab. Clin. Exptl. 18, 406.

93 Dancis, J., Jansen, V. and Levitz, M. (1976) Transfer across perfused human placenta. IV. Effect of protein binding on free fatty acids. Pediatr. Res. 10, 5.

94 Zuspan, F.P., Whaley, W.H., Nelson, G.H. and Ahlquist, R. (1966) Placental transfer of epinephrine. 1. Maternal-fetal metabolic alterations of glucose and non-esterified fatty acids. Am. J. Obstet. Gynec. 95, 284.

95 Edson, J.L., Hudson D.G. and Hull, D. (1975) Evidence of increased fatty acid transfer across the placenta during a maternal fast in rabbits. Biol. Neonate 27, 50.

96 Edson, J.L. and Hull, D. (1977) The effect of maternal starvation on the metabolic response to cold of the newborn rabbit. Pediatr. Res. 11, 793.

97 Hummel, L., Schwartze, A., Shirrmeister, W. and Wagner, H. (1976) Maternal plasma triglycerides as a source of fetal fatty acids, Acta Biol. Med. Ger. 35, 1635.

98 Hummel, L., Zimmermann, T., Shirrmeister, W. and Wagner, H. (1976) Synthesis, turnover and compartment analysis of the free fatty acids in the placenta of rats. Acta Biol. Med. Ger. 35, 1311.

99 Hosoya, N., Hagerman, D.D. and Villee, C.A. (1960) Stimulation of fatty acid synthesis by oestradiol in vitro. Biochem. J. 76, 297.

100 Roux, J.F., Yoshioka, T. and Myers, R.E. (1974) Conversion of palmitate to respiratory carbon dioxide by foetal tissues of man and monkey. Nature. 227, 936.

101 Szabo, A.J., de Lellis, R. and Grimaldi, R.D. (1963) Triglyceride synthesis by the human placenta. 1. Incorporation of labelled palmitate into placental triglycerides. Am. J. Obstet. Gynec. 115, 257.

102 Hummel, L., Schirrmeister, W., Zimmermann, T. and Wagner, H. (1974) Quantitative studies on the metabolism of placental triglycerides and phospholipids in the rat. Acta Biol. Med. Ger. 32, 311.

103 Kleine, U. (1967) Studies on the lipid metabolism of villi of mature human placentas. Clin. Chim. Acta 17, 95.

104 Szabo, A.J., Grimaldi, R.D. and de Lellis, R. (1963) Triglyceride synthesis by the human placenta. 11. The effect of cyanide and fluoride on the incorporation of labelled palmitate into placental triglycerides. Am. J. Obstet. Gynec. 115, 257.

105 Karp, W., Sprecher, H. and Robertson, A. (1973) Human placental phospholipid synthesis. Biol. Neonate 22, 398.

106 Roux, J.F. and Green, R. (1968) Lipid metabolism by the human placenta. Obstet. Gynec. 29, 446.

107 Winkler, L. (1963) Uber die Lipide der Ratteplacenta und deren quantitative Veränderungen im Laufe der Trächtigkeit soure einige Fragen des Phosphatidumsatzes in der Placenta Physiol. Chem. 76, 199.

108 Villee, C.A. and Hagerman, D.D. (1961) Studies of pyridine nucleotide metabolism in placenta. J. Gen. and Comp. Endocrinol. 1, 371.

109 Barnabei, O. and Ninni, A. (1963) Possible role of a placental lipid fraction in the transport of (1-^{14}C) glycine from maternal to fetal blood. Biochim. Biophys. Acta 70, 586.

110 Nelson, G.H. (1966) Lipid metabolism in toxemia of pregnancy. Clin. Obstet. Gynecol. 9, 882.

111 Chevallier, F. (1964) Transferts et synthèse du cholestérol chez le rat au cours de sa croissance. Biochim. Biophys. Acta 84, 316.

112 Connor, W.E. and Lin, D.S. (1967) Placental transfer of cholesterol-4-^{14}C into rabbit and guinea pig fetus. J. Lipid. Res. 8, 558.

113 Kramsch, D.M. and Hollander, W. (1969) The transplacental passage of cholesterol, protein and sulfate from maternal plasma into fetal arteries. Fed. Proc. 28, 516.

114 Van Leusden, H. and Villee, V.A. (1965) The de novo synthesis of sterols and steroids from acetate by preparations of human term placenta. Steroids 6, 31.

115 Villee, C.A., Van Leusden, H. and Zelewski, L. (1966) The regulation of the biosynthesis of sterols and steroids in the placenta. Adv. Enzyme Reg. 4, 161.

116 Villee, C.A. (1968) The placenta and fetal tissues. A cooperative enterprise for the synthesis of steroids. Israel J. Med. Sci. 4, 270.

117 Robertson, A.F., Sprecher, H. and Dobbs, C. (1969) Metabolism of cholesterol esters in the human placenta. Biol. Neonate 14, 32.

118 Di Luzzio, N.R. (1972) Employment of lipids in the measurement and modification of cellular, humoral and immune responses. Adv. Lipid Res. 10, 43.

119 Mertin, J. (1976) Effect of polyunsaturated fatty acids on skin allograft survival and primary and secondary cytotoxic response in mice. Transplantation 21, 1.

120 Mihns, A.A., Gibson, R.G. and Hirschowitz, B.I. (1975) Suppression of lymphocyte transformation by 16 (16) dimethyl-prostaglandin E_2 and unsaturated fatty acids. Proc. Soc. Exp. Biol. Med. 149, 1026.

121 Roman-Franco, A.A. and Santiago-Delpin, E.A. (1977) The immunoregulatory role of cholesterol and other lipids: a hypothesis. Medical Hypotheses 3, 235.

122 Chatterjee M. and Munro, H.N. (1977) Structure and biosynthesis of human placental peptide hormones. Vitamins & Hormones 35, 149.

123 Hubert, C., Balinga, B.S., Villee, C.A. and Munro, H.N. (1974) Protein synthesis in cell-free systems prepared from human placenta: II p.45. Enzyme inefficiency due to defects in t-RNA charging with resulting loss of elongation factor - 1. Biochim. Biophys. Acta 374, 359.

124 Chatterjee, M., Baliga, B.S. and Munro, H.N. (1976) Synthesis of human placental lactogen and human chorionic gonadotropin by polyribosomes and messenger RNAs from early and term human placentas. J. Biol. Chem. 251, 2945.

125 Campbell, P.N. (1978) Personal communication.

126 Whipple, G.H., Hill, R.B., Terry, R., Lucas, F.V. and Yuili, C.L. (1955) The placenta and protein metabolism: transfer studies using carbon^{14}-labelled proteins in dogs. J. Exptl. Med. 101, 617.

127 Sybulski, S. and Tremblay, P.C. (1967) Uptake and incorporation into protein of radioactive glycine by human placentas in vitro. Am. J. Obstet. Gynec. 97, 1111.

128 Beaconsfield, P. Unpublished observations.

129 Campbell, P.N. (1958) Protein synthesis with special reference to growth processes both normal and abnormal. Adv. Cancer Research. V, 98.

130 Christensen, P.J. and Streicher, J.A. (1948) Association between rapid growth and elevated cell concentrations of amino acids. 1. In foetal tissues. J. Biol. Chem. 175, 95.

131 Crumpler, H.R., Dent, C.E. and Linden O. (1950) The amino acid pattern in human foetal and maternal plasma at delivery. Biochem J. 47, 223.

132 Litonjua, A.D., Caulas, M., Soliman, J. and Paulino, D.O. (1967) Uptake of alpha-aminoisobutyric acid in placental slices at term. Am. J. Obstet. Gynec. 99, 242.

133 Enders, R.H., Judd, R.M., Donohue, T.M. and Smith, C.H. (1976) Placental amino acid uptake III. Transport systems for neutral amino acids. Am.J. Physiol. 230, 706.

134 Cédard, L. (1972) Placental perfusion in vitro. Acta Endocrinol. (Suppl.) 158, 331

135 Dancis, J., Olsan, G., and Folkart, G. (1955) Transport of histidine and xylose across the placenta and into the red blood cells and amniotic fluid. Am. J. Physiol. 194, 44.

136 Young, I.M. (1969) Three topics in placental transport. in Foetus and Placenta. Edited, A. Klopper and Diczfalusy, E. Blackwell Scientific Publications, Oxford.

137 Page, E.W., Glendenning, M.B., Margolis, A.J. and Harper, H.A. (1957) Transfer of D- & L-histidine across the human placenta. Am. J. Obstet. Gynec. 73, 589.

138 Glendenning, M.B., Margolis, A.J. and Page, E.W. (1961) Amino acid concentration in foetal and maternal plasma. Am. J. Obstet. Gynec. 81, 591.

139 Szabo, A.J. and Grimaldi, R.D. (1970) The metabolism of the placenta. Adv. Metab. Disord. 4, 185.

140 Schneider, H. and Dancis, J. (1974) Amino acid transport in human placental slices. Am. J. Obstet. Gynec. 120, 1092.

141 Miller, R.K. and Berndt, W.C. (1974) Characterization of neutral amino acid accumulation by human term placental slices. Am. J. Physiol. 227, 1236.

142 Southgate, D.A. (1971) The accumulation of amino acids in the products of conception of the rat and in the young animal after birth. Biol. Neonate 19, 272.

143 Kelleher, P.C., Kenyon, C.D. and Villee, C.A. (1963) Serum protein synthesis by the fetal rat. Science 139, 839.

144 Dancis, J., Money, W.L., Springer, D. and Levitz, M. (1968) Transport of amino acids by placenta. Am. J. Obstet. Gynec. 101, 820.

145 Dancis, J., Baverman, M. and Lind, J. (1957) Plasma protein synthesis in the human fetus and placenta. J. Clin. Invest. 36, 398.

146 Freda, V.J. (1962) Placental transfer of antibodies in man. Am. J. Obstet. Gynec. 84, 1756.

147 Joel, F.B., Hagerman, D.D. and Villee, C.A. (1961) Effects of estradiol added in vitro on the metabolism of human placenta. J. Biol. Chem. 236, 3151.

148 Goldberg, M.L. and Atchley, W.A. (1966) The effect of hormones on DNA. Proc. Nat. Acad. Sci.U.S. 55, 989.

149 Gnaprakasam, M.S. and Talwar, G.P. (1975) Influence of human chorionic gonadotrophin on placental metabolism. in Regulation of growth and differentiated function in eukaryote cells. Edited Talwar, G.P. New York, Raven Press.

150 Bohn, H. (1976) Isolation and characterization of placental specific proteins SP_1 and PP.5. p117 in Protides of the Biological Fluide. Ed. Peeters, H., Brügge, Belgium.

151 Horne, C.H., Towler, C.M., Pugh-Humphreys, R.G., Thomson, A.W. and Bohn, H. (1976) Pregnancy specific beta-1-glycoprotein - a product of the syncytiotrophoblast. Experientia 32, 1197.

152 Stimson, W.H. (1976) Studies on the immunosuppressive properties of a pregnancy associated alpha-macro-globulin. Clin. Exp. Immunol. 25, 199.

153 Petropoulos, E.A. (1973) Maternal and fetal factors affecting the growth and function of the rat placenta. Acta Endocrinologica 73 Supplement. 176.

154 Vincent, R.A., Huang, P.C. and Parmley, T.H. (1976) Proliferative capacity of cell cultures derived from the human placenta. In Vitro 12, 649.

155 Winnick, M., Coscia, A. and Noble, A. (1967) Cellular growth in human placenta. Pediatrics 39, 248.

156 Tedde, G. and Tedde, P.A. (1979) Mitotic index of the Langhans' cells in the normal human placenta from the early stages of pregnancy to the term. Acta Anat. 100, 114.

157 Jollie, W.P. (1964) Radioautographic observations on variations in desoxyribonucleic acid synthesis in rat placenta with increasing gestational age. Am. J. Anat. 114, 161.

158 Weinberg, P.C., Cameron, I.L., Parmley, T., Jeter, J.R. and Pauerstein,C.J. Gestational age and placental cellular replication. Obstet. Gynecol. 36, 692.

159 Dobbing, J. (1978) Personal communication

160 Butterstein, J.M.B. and Leathem, J.H. (1974) Placental growth modification during pregnancy in the rat. Endocrinology 95, 645.

161 Beydoun, S.N., Abdul-Karim, R.W. and Hairland, M.E. (1974) The regulatory effect of estrogens on fetal growth. III Placental deoxyribonucleic acid, ribonucleic acid and proteins. Am. J. Obstet. Gynecol. 120, 918.

162 Croskerry, P.G. and Dobbing, J. (1978) Placental inhibition of foetal growth enhancement in the rat. Nature 273, 147.

163 Kurz, L. (1971) Propagation and hormone production by human normal and malignant trophoblast in rats. I. Normal trophoblast from term human placentas in Millipore diffusion chambers. Am. J. Obstet. Gynecol. 109, 1049.

164 Kurz, L. (1971) Propagation and hormone production by human normal and malignant trophoblast in rats. II. Choriocarcinoma in Millipore diffusion chambers in rats. Am. J. Obstet. Gynecol. 109, 1058.

165 Hytten, F.E. and Leitch, I. (1971) The Physiology of Human Pregnancy. Oxford, Blackwell.

166 Rosso, P. (1975) Maternal malnutrition and placental transfer of alpha-aminoisobutyric acid in the rat. Science 187, 648.

167 Rosso, P. (1977) Maternal-fetal exchange during protein malnutrition in the rat. Placental transfer of alpha-amino isobutyric acid. J. Nutr. 107, 2002.

168 Hastings-Roberts, M.M. and Zeman, F.J. (1977) Effects of protein deficiency, pair-feeding, or diet supplementation on maternal, fetal and placental growth in rats. J. Nutr. 107, 973.

169 Zamenhof, S., Hall, S.M., Grand, L., Van Martheus, E. and Donahue, M.J.(1974) Deprivation of amino-acids and pre-natal brain development in rats. J. Nutr. 104, 1002.

170 Nelson, M.M. and Evans, H.M. (1953) Relation of dietary protein levels to reproduction in rat. J. Nutr. 51, 71.

171 Kinzey, W.G. and Srebnik, H.H. (1963) Maintenance of pregnancy with pituitary hormones in protein-deficient rats. Anat. Record. 145, 249.

172 Hazelwood, R.L. and Nelson, M.M. (1965) Steroid maintenance of pregnancy in rats in the absence of dietary protein. Endocrinology. 77, 999.

173 Kalivas, D.T. and Nelson, M.M. (1966) Maintenance of pregnancy by reserpine in the absence of dietary protein. Endocrinology. 79, 460.

174 Naismith, D.J. and Morgan, B.I. (1976) The biphasic nature of protein metabolism during pregnancy in the rat. Br. J. Nutr. 36, 563.

175 Winick, M. (1970) Cellular growth in intrauterine malnutrition. Pediatric Clinics N. Am. 17, 69.

176 Winick, M. (1971) Cellular changes during placental and fetal growth. Am. J. Obstet. Gynec. 109, 166.

177 Velasco, E.G., Rosso, P., Brasel, J., and Winick, M. (1975) Activity of alkaline RNase in placentas of malnourished women. Am. J. Obstet. Gynec. 123, 637.

178 Hellman, L.M., Harris, B.A. and Andrews, M.C. (1950) Studies of the metabolism of the human placenta.II Oxygen consumption and anaerobic glycolysis in relation to ageing and severe toxaemia. Bull.Johns Hopkins Hosp. 87, 203.

179 Holliday, R. and Tarrant, G.M. (1972) Altered enzymes in ageing human fibroblasts. Nature 238, 26.

180 Ginsburg, J. and Jeacock, M.K. (1967) Placental lactate production in toxaemia of Pregnancy. Am. J. Obstet. Gynec. 98, 239.

181 Konttinen, A., Pyorala, T. and Carpen, E. (1964) Serum lipid pattern in normal Pregnancy and Pre-eclampsia. J. Obst. Gynaec. Brit. Cwlth. 71, 453.

182 Nelson, G.H. (1971) Placental phospholipid patterns in normal and eclamptic pregnancies. Am. J. Obstet. Gynec. 110, 352.

183 Speroff, L. (1973) An Essay: Prostaglandins and toxaemia of pregnancy. Prostaglandins 3, 721.

184 Demers, L.M. and Gabbe, S.G. (1976) Placental prostaglandin levels in pre-eclampsia. Am. J. Obstet. Gynec. 126, 137.

185 Alam, N. A., Clary, P. and Russell, P. T. (1973). Depressed placental prostaglandin metabolism in toxaemia of pregnancy. Prostaglandins 4, 363.

186 Butterfield, L. J. and O'Brien, D. H., (1963). The effect of maternal toxaemia and diabetes on transplacental gradients and free amino acid. Arch. Dis. Child 38, 326.

187 Rahman, S. A., Hingorani, V., Malkani, P. K., and Laumas, K. R. (1973). In vitro biosynthesis of proteins in human placentae from normal and toxaemic pregnancies. Acta Endocrinol. 73, 567.

188 Heijkenskhold, F. and Geimzell, C. A. (1957). Glycogen content in the placenta of diabetic mothers. Acta Paediatr, 46, 74.

189 Ginsburg, J. and Jeacock, M. K. (1966). Some aspects of placental carbohydrate metabolism in human diabetes. J. Obstet. Gynaec. Brit. Cwlth. 73, 452.

190 Gabbe, S. G., Demers, L. M., Greep, R. O., and Villee, C. A. (1972). Placental glycogen metabolism in diabetes mellitus. Diabetes 21, 1185.

191 Olsen, R. E., (1962). Physiology of cardiac muscle p.199 in Handbook of Physiology - Circulation Vol. 1. Ed. Hamilton, W. F., and Dow, P. Washington.

192 Szabo, A. J. and Szabo, O. (1974). Placental free-fatty-acid transfer and fetal adipose tissue development: an explanation of fetal adiposity in infants of diabetic mothers. Lancet ii 498.

193 Sybulski, S. and Tremblay, P. C. (1969). Placental glycogen content and utilisation in intra-uterine fetal malnutrition. Am. J. Obstet. Gynec. 103, 257.

194 Oh, W., D'Amodio, M., Yap, L. L. and Hohenauer, L. (1970). Carbohydrate metabolism in experimental intra-uterine growth retardation in rats. Am. J. Obstet. Gynec. 108, 415.

195 Patillo, R. A., Hussa, R. O. and Garancis, J. C. (1971). Glycogen metabolism in human hormone producing trophoblastic cells in continuous culture. 1. regulation of glycogen metabolism by glucose. In Vitro 7, 59.

196 Hers, H. G., and de Wuls, H. (1967). The regulation of glycogen synthesis in the Liver. Fed. Eur. Biochem. Soc. Proc. 4th Meeting, 65.

197 Buschiazzo, H., Exton, J. H. and Park, C. R. (1970). Effects of glucose on glycogen synthetase, phosphorylase and glycogen deposition in the perfused rat liver. Proc. Nat. Acad. Sci. 65, 383.

198 Alpers, J. B., Wu, R. and Racher, E. (1963). Regulatory mechanisms in carbohydrate metabolism. VI Glycogen metabolism in HeLa cells. J. Biol. Chem. 238, 2274.

199 Patillo, R. A., Hussa, R. D., Terragno, W. A., Storey, M. T., and Mattingly, R. F. (1973). Absence of prostaglandin synthesis in the malignant human trophoblast in culture. Am. J. Obstet. Gynec. 115, 91.

200 Carminati, P., Luzzani, F. and Lerner, L. J. (1974). Chances in the metabolism of PGE1 and PGF2 alpha in rat placenta during pregnancy. Prostaglandins 8, 205.

201 Hussa, R. O., Storey, M. T., Pattillo, R. A., and Kemp, R. G. (1977) Effect of cyclic 3 : S - AMP derivatives, prostaglandins and related agents on human chorionic gonadotrophin secretion in human malignant trophoblast in culture. In Vitro 13, 443.

202 Pattillo, R. A., Gey, G. O., Dells, E., Huang, W. Y., Hause, L., Garancis, J., Knoth, M., Amatruda, J., Bertino, J., Griesen, M. G., and Mattingly, R. S. (1971). The hormine synthesizing trophoblast cell in vitro: A model for cancer research and placental hormone synthesis. Ann. N.Y. Acad. Sci. 1972, 288.

NUCLEIC ACIDS AND PLACENTAL DEVELOPMENT

Hamish Munro

1 Laga, E. M., Driscoll, S. G. & Munro, H. N. (1972). Comparison of placentas from two socioeconomic groups. 1. Morphometry. Pediatrics, 50, 24.

2 Mozayani, S.,Baliga, B. S. & Munro, H. N. (1978b). Unpublished results.

3 Winick, M. & Noble, A. (1966). Quantitative changes in ribonucleic acids and protein during normal growth of rat placenta. Nature, 212, 34.

4 Velasco, E. G. & Brasel, J. A. (1975). DNA polymerase activity in normal and malnourished rat placentas. Journal of Pediatrics, 86. 274.

5 Beaconsfield, P., Ginsburg, J., & Jeacock, M. K. (1964). Glucose metabolism via the pentose phosphate pathway relative to nucleic acid and protein synthesis in the human placenta. Develop. Med. and Child Neurol. 6, 469.

6 Winick, M.,Coscia, A. & Noble, A. (1967). Cellular growth in human placenta. 1. Normal placental growth. Pediatrics. 39, 248.

7 Butterstein, G. M. & Leathem, J. H. (1974). Placental growth modification during pregnancy in the rat. Endocrinology, 96, 645.

8 Novak, T. S. & Munro, H. N., (1977). Effects of protein-calorie malnutrition on biochemical aspects of brain development. In: Nutrition and the brain, Vol. 2, edited by R. J. Wurtman and J. Wurtman. New York, Raven Press, p.193.

9 McCance, R. A. & Widdowson, E. M. (1964). Protein metabolism and requirements in the newborn. In: Mammalian Protein metabolism, Vol. 2, edited by H. N. Munro and J. B. Allison. New York and London, Academic Press. p.225.

10 Munro, H. N. (1969). In Mammalian Protein Metabolism, Vol.3, p.133 (ed. H.N. Munro). Academic Press, New York.

11 Rosso, P. (1975). Placental nucleic acids and protein metabolism during prolonged gestation. Pediatric Research, 9, 279.

12 Mozayani, S.,Baliga, B. S. & Munro, H. N. (1978a). Unpublished results.

13 Chatterjee, M., Baliga, B. S. & Munro, H. N. (1976). Synthesis of human placental lactogen and human chorionic gonadotrophin by polyribosomes and messenger RNA's from early and full term placentas. Journal of Biological Chemistry, 251, 2945.

14 Chatterjee, M. & Munro, H. N. (1977). Structure and biosynthesis of human placental peptide hormones. Vitamins and Hormones, 35, 149.

15 Chatterjee, M. & Munro, H. N. (1977). Changing ratio of human chorionic gonadotropin subunits synthesized by early and full-term placental polyribosomes. Biochemical and Biophysical Research Communications, 77, 426.

16 Drake, R., Kusamran, T., Mozayani, S., Baliga, B. S. & Munro, H. N. (1978). Unpublished data.

17 Kusamran, T., Drake, R., Baliga, B. S. & Munro, H. N. (1978). Unpublished data.

18 Gibbons, J. M., Mitnick, M. & Chieffo, V. (1975). In vitro biosynthesis of TSH- and LH-releasing factors by the human placenta. American Journal of Obstetrics and Gynecology, 121, 127.

19 Brody, S. (1952). Interrelations between nucleic acids and growth of the human placenta. Experimental Cell Research, 3, 702.

20 Brody, S. (1953). Quantitative studies on nucleic acids and nuclease activities during development of human placenta. Acta Obstetricia et Gynecologica Scandinavica, 32, Supplement 6,1.

21 Laga, E. M., Driscoll, S. G., & Munro, H. N. (1973). Quantitative studies of human placenta. II. Biochemical characteristics. Biology of the Neonate, 23 260.

22 Mori, M. (1965). Study of protein biosynthesis in fetus and placenta. I. Incorporation of C-14-amino acids into the human placenta. American Journal of Obstetrics and Gynecology, 93, 1164.

23 Stark, G. & Klinkhart, H. (1956). Nucleinsäuren und Wachstum der Placenta. (Nucleic acids and growth of the placenta.) Klinische Wochenschrift, 34, 1251.

24 Munro, H. N., Lau, A., Roy, R., Sarkar, S. & Baliga, B. S. (1978). Unpublished results.

ENDOCRINE FUNCTION OF THE PLACENTA

Dorothy Villee

1 Davies I.J. and Ryan K.J. (1972) Comparative endocrinology of gestation. Vitamins and Hormones 30. 223.

2 Aschheim, S. and Zondek B. (1927) Ei und Hormon. Hypophysenvorder-lappenhormon und Ovarialhormon im Harn von Schwangeren. Klin. Wschr. 6: 1321.

3 Josimovich, J.V. and MacLaren J.A. (1962) Presence in the human placental and term serum of a highly lactogenic substance immunologically related to pituitary growth hormone. Endocrinology 71: 209.

4 Hennen G.P. (1965) Detection and study of a human chorionic thyroid-stimulating factor. Arch. int. Physiol. Biochim. 73: 689.

5 Genazzani, A.R., Hurlimann J., Fioretti, P., and Felber J.P. (1974) In vitro synthesis of an ACTH-like hormone and human chorionic somatomamotrophin by placental and amniotic cells. Experientia 30: 430.

6 Vandeputte M. and Sobis H. (1972) Histocompatibility antigens on mouse blastocysts and ectoplacental cones. Transplantation 14: 331.

7 Amoroso E.C., Perry F.R.S. and Perry J.S. (1975) The existence during gestation of an immunological buffer zone at the interface between maternal and fetal tissues. Phil.Trans.Roy.Soc. Lond. B 271: 343.

8 Martin B.J., Spicer S.S., and Smythe N.M. (1974) Cytochemical studies of the syncytiotrophoblast of human early and term placenta. Anat. Rec. 178: 769.

9 Wiley, L.D. (1974) Presence of a gonadotrophin on the surface of preimplanted mouse embryos. Nature 252: 715.

10 Haour F. and Saxena B.B. (1974) Detection of a gonadotropin in rabbit blastocyst before implantation. Science 185: 444.

11 Adcock E.W. et al. (1973) Human chorionic gonadotropin: Its possible role in maternal lymphocyte suppression. Science 181: 845.

12 Finn R. et al.(1976) The placenta as an immunological barrier. Brit. Med. J. 2: 527.

13 Dickman W.J. and Cauchi M.N. (1978) Lymphocyte induced stimulation of human chorionic gonadotrophin production by trophoblastic cells in vitro. Nature 271: 377.

14 Perry J.S., Heap R.B. and Amoroso E.C. (1973) Steroid hormone production by pig blastocysts. Nature 245: 45.

15 Dickmann Z. and Dey S.K. (1974) Steroidogenesis in the preimplantation rat embryo and its possible influence on morula-blastocyst transformation and implantation. J. Reprod. Fert. 37: 91.

16 Dickmann Z., Dey S.K. and Gupta J.S. (1975) Steroidogenesis in rabbit preimplantation embryos. Proc. Nat . Acad. Sci. 72: 298.

17 Huff, R.L. and Eik-Nes K.B. (1966) Metabolism in vitro of acetate and certain steroids by 6-day old rabbit blastocysts. J. Reprod. Fert. 11: 57.

18 Seamark, R.F. and Lutwak-Mann C. (1972) Progestins in rabbit blastocysts. J. Reprod. Fert. 29: 147.

19 Villee, C.A. (1977) Synthesis of proteins in the placenta. Gynecol. Invest. 8: 145.

20 Beas, F. et al. (1975) A human placental hormone (UTPH) with uterine growth and DNA promoting effects. Horm. Metab. Res. 7: 515.

21 Chatterjee, M. and Munro H.N. (1977) Structure and biosynthesis of human placental peptide hormones. Vit. Horm. 35: 149.

22 Ross, G.T. (1977) Clinical relevance of research on the structure of human chorionic gonadotropin. Am. J. Obstet. Gynec.129: 795.

23 Naughton, M.A. et al.(1975) Localization of the β chain of human chorionic gonadotropin on human tumor cells and placental cells. Cancer Res. 35: 1887.

24 Mori, K.F. (1969) Antigenic structure of human gonadotropins. Contribution of carbohydrate moiety to the antigenic structure of pituitary follicle-stimulating hormone. Endocrinology 85: 330.

25 Braunstein, G.D. et al.(1971) The effects of desialylation on the biologic and immunologic activity of human pituitary luteinizing hormone. Biochem. biophys. Res. Commun. 42: 962.

26 Bossaert, Y. et al.(1965) Demonstration of hCG in human placenta during gestation by immunofluorescence. Revue fr. Etud. clin. biol. 10: 919.

27 Dreskin, R.B., Spicer, S.S. and Greene W.B. (1970) Ultrastructural localization of chorionic gonadotrophin in human term placenta. J. Histochem. Cytochem. 18: 862.

28 Ikonikoff, L.K. de and Cédard L. (1973) Localisation of human chorionic gonadotrophin and somatomammotrophic hormone by the peroxydase immunohisto-enzymologic method in villi and amniotic epithelium of human placenta from six weeks to term. Am. J. Obstet. Gynec. 116: 1124.

29 Gau, G. and Chard, T.(1976) Location of the protein hormones of the placenta by the immunoperoxidase technique. Brit.J. Obstet. Gyn. 83: 876.

30 Catt, K.L., Dufau, M.L. and Vaitukaitis J.L. (1975) Appearance of hCG in pregnancy plasma following the initiation of implantation of the blastocyst. J. Clin. Endocrinol. Metab. 40: 537.

31 Braunstein, G.D., Grodin, J.M. Vaitukaitis, J. and Ross G.T. (1973) Secretory rates of human chorionic gonadotropin by normal trophoblast. Am. J. Obstet. Gynec115: 447.

32 Boroditsky, R.S., Reyes, F.E., Winter, J.S.D., and Faiman C. (1975) Serum human chorionic gonadotropin and progesterone patterns in the last trimester of pregnancy: Relationship to fetal sex. Am. J. Obstet. Gynec121: 238.

33 Thiery, M., Dhout, M. and Vanderkerckhove D. (1976) Serum hCG and hPL in twin pregnancies. Acta Obstet. Gynecol. Scand. 56: 495.

34 Ashitaka, Y. et al.(1974) Serum and chorionic tissue concentrations of human chorionic gonadotropin and its subunits during pregnancy. Endocrinol. Japon. 21: 547.

35 Vaitukaites, J.L. (1974) Changing placental concentrations of human chorionic gonadotropin and its subunits during gestation. J. Clin. Endocrinol. Metab. 38: 755.

36 Chatterjee, M. and Munro H.N. (1977) Changing ratio of human chorionic gonadotropin subunits synthesized by early and full-term placental polyribosomes. Biochem. Biophys. Res. Comm. 77: 426.

37 Handwerger, S., Barrett, J., Tyrey, L. and Schomberg, D. (1973) Differential effect of cyclic adenosine monophosphate on the secretion of human placental lactogen and human chorionic gonadotropin. J. Clin. Endocrinol. Metab. 36: 1268.

38 Hussa, R.O., Story, M.T., and Pattillo R.A. (1974) Cyclic adenosine monophosphate stimulates secretion of human chorionic gonadotropin and estrogens by human trophoblast in vitro. J. Clin. Endocrinol. Metab. 38: 338.

39 Story, M.T., Hussa, R.O., and Pattillo R.A. (1974) Independent dibutyryl cyclic adenosine monophosphate stimulation of human chorionic gonadotropin and estrogen secretion by malignant trophoblast in vitro. J. Clin. Endocrinol. Metab. 39: 877.

40 Chou, J.Y., Wang, S.S. and Robinson J.C. (1978) Regulation of the synthesis of human chorionic gonadotrophin by 5-bromo-2'-deoxyuridine and dibutyryl cyclic AMP in trophoblastic and nontrophoblastic tumor cells. J. Clin. Endocrinol. Metab. 47: 46.

41 Gibbons, J.M., Mitnick, M., and Chieffo V. (1975) In vitro biosynthesis of TSU- and LH-releasing factors by the human placenta. Am. J. Obstet. Gynec. 121: 127.

42 Cédard, L., Alsat, E., Urtasun, M.J. and Varangot, J. (1970) Studies on the mode of action of luteinizing hormone and chorionic gonadotropin on estrogenic biosynthesis and glycogenolysis by human placenta perfused in vitro. Steroids 16: 361.

43 Levilliers, J., Alsat E., Laudat, Ph. and Cédard, L. (1974) Hormone-stimulated cAMP production in human placenta perfused in vitro. FEBS Letters 47: 146.

44 Channing, C.P. (1970) Influences of the in vivo and in vitro hormonal environment upon luteinization of granulosa cells in tissue culture. Recent Prog. Hormone Res. 26: 589.

45 Villee, D.B. (1967) Development of endocrine function in the human placenta and fetus. New Engl. J. Med. 281: 533.

46 Blank, M.S., Chan, J.S.D. and Friesen H.G. (1977) Placental lactogens, new developments. J. Steroid Biochem. 8: 403.

47 Grumbach, M.M. and Kaplan, S.L. (1964) On the placental origin and purification of chorionic growth hormone-prolactin and its immunoassay in pregnancy. Trans. N.Y. Acad. Sci. 27: 167.

48 Friesen, H., Suwa, S., and Pare, P. (1969) Synthesis and secretion of placental lactogen and other proteins by the placenta. Recent Prog. Hormone Res. 25: 161.

49 Hubert, C. and Cédard, L. (1975) Isolation and in vitro translation of human placental lactogen messenger RNA from human term placenta. Nucleic acids Res. 2: 1903.

50 Boime, I., and Boguslawski, S. (1974) Synthesis of human placental lactogen by ribosomes derived from human placenta. Proc. Nat. Acad. Sci. 71: 322. 1322.

51 Chatterjee, M., Baliga, B.S., and Munro H.N. (1976) Synthesis of human placental lactogen and human chorionic gonadotropin by polyribosomes and messenger RNAs from early and full term placentas. J. Biol. Chem. 251: 2945.

52 Hubert, C., Mondon, F. and Cédard L. (1977) Specific binding of purified human chorionic somatomammotrophin antibody to polyribosomes from term placenta. Biochimie 59: 1977.

53 Belleville, F., Peltier, A., Paysant, P. and Nabet,P. (1975) Isohormones: Molecular forms of the human chorionic somatomammotropic hormone. Eur. J. Biochem. 51: 429.

54 Chatterjee, M., Laga, E.M., Merrill, C.C. and Munro, H.N. (1977) Microheterogeneity of human placental lactogen showing different patterns in individuals. Biochim. Biophys. Acta 493: 332.

55 Cox, G.S., Weintraub, B.D., Rosen, S.W. and Maxwell,E.S. (1976) Properties of biologically active messenger RNA from human placenta. J. Biol. Chem. 251: 1723.

56 Szczesna, E. and Boime I. (1976) mRNA-dependent synthesis of authentic precursor to human placental lactogen. Proc. Nat.Acad.Sci.73: 1179.

57 Niall, H.D. et al.(1971) Sequences of pituitary and placental lactogenic and growth hormones: Evoluation from a primordial peptide by gene reduplication. Proc. Nat. Acad. Sci. 68: 866.

58 Shine, J. et al.(1977) Construction and analysis of recombinant DNA for human chorionic somatomammotropin. Nature 270: 494.

59 Patrito, L.C., Flury, A., Rosato, J. and Martin, A. (1973) Biosynthesis in vitro of chorionic gonadotrophin from human placenta. Hoppe-Seyler's Z. Physiol. Chem. 354: 1129.

60 Maruo, T., Ashitaka, Y., Mochizuki, M. and Tojo, S. (1974) Chorionic gonadotropin synthesized in cultivated trophoblast. Endocrinol. Japon. 21: 499.

61 Gaspard U., and Franchimont, P. (1972). Variations secretoires vers hormones polypeptidiques placentaires humains en culture de tissue. C.R.Acad.Sci.(Paris) 275, 1661.

62 Choy, V.J. and Watkins, W.B. (1976). Effect of ionic environment on the release of human placental lactogen in vitro. J. Endocrin. 69, 349.

63 Prieto, J.C., Cifuentes, I. and Serrano-Rios, M. (1976). HCS regulation during pregnancy. Obstet. Gynec. 48, 297.

64 Gaspard, U, Sandront, H. and Luychx, A. (1974) Glucose-insulin interaction and the modulation of human placental lactogen (hPL) secretion during pregnancy. J. Obstet. Gynaec. Brit.Commonw. 81: 201.

65 Burt, R.L., Leake, N.H. and Rhyne, A.L. (1970) Human placental lactogen and insulin-blood glucose homeostasis. Obstet. Gynec. 36: 233.

66 Gaspard, U., Sandront, H. and Lambotte R. (1973) Control by glucose of maternal serum levels of chorionic somatomammotrophin (hCS) during pregnancy. Acta paediat Belg. 27: 218.

67 Josimovich, J.B. and Archer D.F. (1977) The role of lactogenic hormones in the pregnant woman and the fetus. Am. J. Obstet. Gynec. 129, 777.

68 Josimovich, J.B. and Brande, B.L. (1964) Chemical properties and biological effects of human placental lactogen (hPL). Trans N.Y. Acad. Sci. 27: 161.

69 Ashton, I.K. and Francis, M.J.O. (1978) Response of chondrocytes isolated from human fetal cartilage. J. Endocrinology 76: 473.

70 Gusdon, J.P., Caudle, M.R., and Herbst, G.A. (1975) Localization of anti-hPL in fetal, placental and maternal renal tissues. Gynecol. Invest. 6: 321.

71 Williams, C., and Coltart, T.M. (1978) Adipose tissue metabolism in pregnancy: The lipolytic effect of human placental lactogen. Brit. J. Obst. Gyn. 85: 43.

72 Talamantes, F., Jr. (1975) Comparative study of the occurrence of placental prolactin among mammals. Gen. Comp. End. 27: 115.

73 Hennen, G.P. (1965) Detection and study of a human chorionic thyroid-stimulating factor. Arch. Int. Physiol. Biochim. 73: 689.

74 Hershman, J.M. and Starnes, W.R. (1969) Extraction and characterization of a thyrotropic material from the human placenta. J. Clin. Invest. 48: 923.

75 Nisula, B.C., Morgan, F.J. and Canfield, R.E. (1974) Evidence that chorionic gonadotropin has intrinsic thyrotropic activity. Biochem. Biophys. Res. Commun. 59: 86.

76 Shepard, T.H. (1967) Onset of function in the human fetal thyroid: biochemical and radioautographic studies from organ culture. J. Clin. Endocrinol. Metab. 27: 945.

77 Tojo, S., Ashitaka, Y., Maruo, T. and Nishimoto, H. (1975) Some biological properties of human chorion follicle stimulating hormone. Endocrinology 22: 585.

78 Maruo, T. (1976) In vitro biosynthesis of human chorionic follicle stimulating hormone. Endocrinology 23: 65.

79 Gennazzani, A.R., et al. (1975) Detection and partial purification of corticotrophin-like placental hormone. The human chorionic corticotrophin (hCG) Clin. Endocr. 4: 1.

80 Diczfalusy, E. (1964) Endocrine functions of the human foetoplacental unit. Fed. Proc. 23: 791.

81 Schubert, K. and Schade, K. (1977) Placental steroid hormones. J. Steroid Biochem. 8: 359.

82 Cassmer. O. (1959) Hormone production of the isolated human placenta. Acta endocr. Suppl. 45.

83 Ryan, K.J. (1962) Hormones and the placenta. Am. J. Obstet. Gynec. 84: 1695.

84 Lauritzen, Ch. (1973) Endokrinologie der normalen Schwangerschaft. Med. Klin. 68: 897.

85 Chan, S.W.C. and Leathem, J.H. (1975) Placental steroidogenesis in the rat: Progesterone production by tissue of the basal zone. Endocrinology 96: 298.

86 Tam, W.H. (1977) Steroid synthesis in vitro by the placenta of the guinea pig and progesterone concentrations in systemic and uterine plasma. J. Endocrinol. 73: 483.

87 Marchut, M. (1976) Progesterone formation and metabolism by rabbit placenta in vitro. Experientia 32: 1211.

88 Edwards, D.P. et al. (1976) Human placental 3β-hydroxysteroid dehydrogenase: 9 -isomerase. J. Biol. Chem. 251: 1632.

89 Ferre, F., Breuiller, M. and Cédard, L. (1975) Human placental Δ5- 3β -hydroxysteroid dehydrogenase activity (Δ5-3β HSDH): Intracellular distribution, kinetic properties, retroinhibition and influence of membrane delipidation. Steroids 26: 551.

90 Weidenfeld, J., Ben-Uzilio, R. and Ne'eman, Y. (1975) Cofactor requirements of microsomal 3β-hydroxysteroid oxidoreductase, 5-eneisomerase from human placenta. J. Steroid Biochem. 6: 1243.

91 Falkay, G. (1978) Correlation between the concentrations of prostaglandin dehydrogenase and progesterone in the early human placenta. J. Endocrinol. 76: 173.

92 Klimek, J. et al. (1976) Regulation of progesterone biosynthesis in human placental mitochondria by Krebs cycle metabolites. Acta Biochim. Pol. 23: 185.

93 Milewich, L. et al. (1978) Initiation of human parturition. IX. Progesterone metabolism by placentas of early and late human gestation. Obstet and Gynec. 51: 278.

94 Hagemenas, F.C., Baughman, W.L. and Kittinger, G.W. (1975) The effect of fetal hypophysectomy on placental biosynthesis of progesterone in rhesus. Endocrinology 96: 1059.

95 Chan, S.W.C. and Leathem, J.H. (1977) Comparison of normal and giant placenta. Endocrinology 100: 1418.

96 Braunstein, G.C., et al. (1976) Prenatal diagnosis of placental steroid sulfatase deficiency. Am. J. Obstet. Gynec126: 176.

97 Bolte, E. et al. (1964) Studies on the aromatisation of neutral steroids in pregnant women. I. Aromatisation of C-19 steroids by placentas perfused in situ. Acta Endocrin. 45: 535.

98 Varangot, J., Cédard, L., and Yannotti, S. (1965) Perfusion of the human placenta in vitro. Am. J. Obstet. Gynec 92: 534.

99 Wolf, A.S. et al. (1978) Steroid metabolism in the perfused human placenta. Acta Endocrinol. 87: 181.

100 Dziadkowiec, I., Czarnik, Z. and Rembiesa, R. (1977) Metabolism of 4-14C-Dehydroepiandrosterone and 4-14C-4-androstene-3, 17-dione by isolated cells of early human placenta. Endocrinologia Experimentalis 11: 19.

101 Engel, L.L. and Orr, J.C. (1974) The flux of intermediates and products in aromatisation of C19 steroids by human placental microsomes. Eur. J. Biochem. 48: 35.

102 Siiteri, P.K. and Thompson, E.A. (1975) Studies of human placental aromatase. J. Steroid Biochem. 6: 317.

103 Reed, K.C. and Ohno, S. (1976) Kinetic properties of human placental aromatase. J. Biol. Chem. 251: 1625.

104 Kelly, W.G., Judd, D. and Stolee, A. (1977) Aromatization of Δ4-androstene-3, 17-dione, 19-hydroxy-4-androstene-3, 17-dione, and 19-oxo-4androstene-3, 17-dione at a common catalytic site in human placental microsomes. Biochem. 16: 140.

105 Thompson, E.A., Jr. and Siiteri, P.K. (1974) The involvement of human placental microsomal cytochrome P-450 in aromatization. J. Biol. Chem. 249: 5373.

106 Cédard, L., Alsat, E., Ego, C. and Varangot, J. (1968) Influence of luteinizing hormone on the aromatization of testosterone by human placenta perfused in vitro. Steroids 11: 179.

107 Tominaga, T. and Troen, P. (1967) Stimulation of aromatization by human placental lactogen. J. Clin. Invest. 46: 1124.

108 Page, E., Villee, C.A. and Villee, D.B. (1976) Human Reproduction: The Core Content of Obstetrics, Gynecology and Perinatal Medicine, W.B. Saunders Co. Philadelphia.

109 Liggins, G.C. et al. (1973) The mechanism of initiation of parturition in the ewe. Recent Prog. Hormone Res. 29,111.

ROLE OF PROSTAGLANDINS

Olga Genbačev

1 Bergström, S., Ruhage, R., Samuelsson, B. and Söval, J., (1963). Prostaglandins and related factors. 15. The structures of prostaglandin E_1, F_1 and $F_{1\alpha}$. J. Biol. Chem. 238.

2 Bergström, S., Carloson, L.A. and Weekes, J.R. (1968). The prostaglandins a family of biologically active lipids. Pharmacol. Rev. 20, 148.

3 Dray, F. and Vharbonnel, B. (1974). Radioimmunoassay of $PGF_{2\alpha}$ in human plasma: very low levels. Prostaglandins. 5, 173.

4 Karim, S.M.M. (1968). Appearance of prostaglandins $F_{2\alpha}$ in human blood during labour. Brit. Med. J. 4, 618.

5 Karim, S.M.M. (1972). Physiological role of prostaglandins in the control of parturition and menstruation. J. Reprod. Fertil. Suppl. 16, 195.

6 Karim, S.M.M. and Devlin, J. (1967). Prostaglandin content of amniotic fluid during pregnancy and labour. J. Obstet. Gynaecol. Brit. Cwlth. 74, 230.

7 Williams, K.J. (1973). Prostaglandin synthesis by the pregnant rat uterus at term and its possible relevance in parturition. Brit. J. Pharmacol. 47,628.

8 Twomey, S.L., Benett, G.E. and Drewes, P.A. (1975). Serum prostaglandin $F_{2\alpha}$ levels during normal pregnancy. Clin. Biochem. 8, 60.

9 Schwartz, B.E., Schultz, F.M., MacDonald, P.C. and Johnston, J.M. (1975). Initiation of human parturition. III Fetal membrane content of prostaglandin E_2 and F precursor. Obstet-Gynecol. 46, 564.

10 Baltzan, M.A., Andres, P. and Cader, G. (1962). Heterogeneity of forearm metabolism with special reference to free fatty acids. J. Clin. Invest, 41, 116.

11 Liggins, G.C., Forester, C.S., Grieves, S.A. and Schwartz, A.L. (1977). Control of parturition in man. Biol. Reprod. 16, 39.

12 Grieves, S.A. and Liggins, G.C. (1976). Phospholipase A activity in human and ovine uterine tissue. Prostaglandins. 12, 229.

13 Schultz, F.M., Schwartz, B.E., MacDonald, P.C. and Johnson, J.M. (1975). Initiation of human parturition. II Identification of phospholipase A_2 in fetal choriamnion and uterine decidua. Am. J. Obstet. Gynecol. 123,650.

14 Gustavii, B. (1972). Labour: a delayed menstruation? Lancet, ii, 1149.

15 Brunk, U. and Gustavii, B. (1973). Lability of human decidual cells. In vitro effects of autolysis and osmotic stress. Am. J. Obstet. Gynec. 115, 811.

16 Vassiliakos, P., Wyss, R. and Stastny, J. (1974). ecidual changes during hypertonic saline-induced abortion. Am. J. Obstet. Gynecol. 119, 889.

17 Gustavii, B. (1975). Release of lysosomal acid phosphatase into the cytoplasm of decidual cellsbefore the onset of labour in humans. Brit. J. Obstet. Gynecol. 82, 177.

18 Samuelsson, B. (1965). On the incorporation of oxygen in the conversion of 8, 11, 14-eicosatrieonic acid to prostaglandin E_1. J. Amer. Chem. Soc. 87, 3011.

19 Wlodawer, P. and Samuelsson, B. (1973). On the organisation and mechanism of prostaglandin synthase. J. Biol. Chem. 248, 5673.

20 Hinman, J.W. (1972). Prostaglandins. Ann. Rev. Biochem. 41, 161.

21 Sih, C.J. and Takeguchi, C.A. (1973). Biosynthesis of the prostaglandins, Ed. Ramwell, I.P. Plenum Press, New York. p.83.

22 Pace-Asciak, C. and Wolfe, L.S. (1970). Biosynthesis of prostaglandins E_2 and $F_{2\alpha}$ from tritium-labelled arachidonic acid by rat stomach homogenates. Biochem. Biophys. Acta 218, 539.

23 Karim, S.M.M. (1966). Identification of prostaglandins in human aminotic fluid. J. Obst. Gynecol. Brit. Cwlth. 73, 903.

24 Salmon, J.A. and Amy, J,J, (1973). Levels of prostaglandin F in amniotic fluid during pregnancy and labour. Prostaglandins 4, 523.

25 Keirse, M.J.N.C., Flint, A.P.F. and Turnbull, A.C. (1974). F Prostaglandins in amniotic fluid during pregnancy and labour. J. Obstet.Gynaecol. Brit. Cwlth. 81, 131.

26 Anggard, E. and Samuelsson, B. (1964). Prostaglandins and related factors. J. Biol. Chem. 239, 4097.

27 Hamberg, M. and Samuelsson, B. (1967). On the mechanism of the biosynthesis of prostaglandin E_1 and F_1. J. Biol. Chem. 242, 5336.

28 Jarabak, J. (1972). Human placental 15-hydroxyprostaglandin dehydrogenase. Proc. Nat. Acad. Sci., 69, 533.

29 Thaler-Dao, H., Saintot, M., Bandin, G., Descomps, B. and Vrastes de Paulet, A. (1974). Purification of the human placental 15-dehydroxyprostaglandin dehydrogenase: properties of the purified enzyme. FEBS Letters 48, 204.

30 Schlegel, W., Demera, L.M., Hildebrant-Stark, H.E., Behrman, H.R. and Greep, R.O. (1974). Partial purification of human placenta 15-hydroxyprostaglandin dehydrogenase; kinetic properties. Prostaglandins 5, 417.

31 Falkey, G. and Sas, M. (1978). Correlation between the concentrations of prostaglandin dehydrogenases and progesterone in the early human placenta. J. Endocr. 76, 173.

32 Keirse, M.J.N.C. and Turnbull, A.C. (1975). Metabolism of prostaglandins within the pregnant uterus. Brit. J. Obstet. Gynaecol. 82, 887.

33 Wiqvist, N., Bygdeman, M. Green, K. and Landstrom, V. (1975). Endogenous prostaglandins and the initiation of labour. Acta Obstet. Gynecol. Scad. Suppl.37,7.

34 Rao, Ch.V. (1975). The presence of discrete receptors from prostaglandin F_2 in the cell membranes of bovine corpora lutea. Biochem. Biophys. Res. Comm. 64, 416.

35 Wakeling, A.E. and Wyngarden, L.J. (1974). Prostaglandin receptors in the human, monkey and hamster uterus. Endocrinology, 5, 55.

36 Langs, D.A., Erman, M. and Detitta, G.T. (1977). Conformations of prostaglandins $F_{2\alpha}$ and recognition of prostaglandins by their receptors. Science 197, 1003.

37 Bergeron, L. and Barden, N. (1975). Stimulation of cyclic AMP accumulation by arachidonic and 8, 11, 14-eicosatrieonic acids in rat anterior pituitary gland. Mol. Cell. Endocrinol. 2, 253.

38 Rillema, J.A. (1978). Activation of guanylate cyclase by arachidonic acid in mammary gland homogenate from mice. Prostaglandins 15, 857.

39 Shaw, J.E., Jessup, S.J. and Ramwell, P.W. (1972). Prostaglandin-adenyl cyclase relationship. Adv. Cyclic Nucleotide Res. Raven Press, New York.

40 Ratner, A.M.C., Wilson, L., Srivastava, N. and Peake, G.T. (1974). Stimulatory effects of prostaglandin E_1 on rat anterior pituitary cyclic AMP and luteinizing hormone release. Prostaglandins 5, 165.

41 MacLeod,R.M. and Lehmeyer, J.E. (1976). Release of pituitary growth hormone by prostaglandins and dibutyryl adenosine cyclic 3':5'-monophosphate in the absence of protein synthesis. Proc. Nat. Acad. Sci. 67, 1172.

42 Kuehl, F.A., Cirillo, V.J., Ham, E.A. and Humes, J.L. (1972). The regulatory role of prostaglandins on the cyclic 3':5'-AMP system. in: Advances in the Biosciences Ed. Raspe, G., No.9 p.155, Pergamon Press, Vieweg.

43 Borgeat, P., Labrie, L. and Garneau, P. (1975). Characteristics of action of prostaglandins on cyclic AMP accumulation in rat anterior pituitary gland. Can. J. Biochem. Vol. 53, 455.

44 Kuehl, F.A. (1974). Prostaglandins, cyclic nucleotides and cell function. Prostaglandins, 5, 325.

45 Goldberg, N., Haddox, M.K., Nicol, S.E., Glass, D.B., Sanford, C.H., Kuehl, F.A. and Estenson, R. (1975). Biological regulation through opposing influences of cyclic GMP and cyclic AMP: the Ying Yang hypothesis. Adv. Cycl. Nucl. Res. 5, 307, Ed. Drummond, G.J., Greengard, P. and Robinson, G.A. Raven Press, New York.

46 Newrath, H. (1976). Cyclic AMP and cyclic GMP may play opposing roles in influencing force of contraction in mammalian myocardium. Nature 262, 509.

47 Honn, K.V. and Chavin, W. (1978). Temporal effect of prostaglandins E and F on human adrenal c-AMP and cortisol output. Life Sci. 22, 543.

48 Handwerger, S.J., Barrett, L., Tyrey, and Schomberg, D. (1973). Differential effect of human placental lactogen and human chorionic gonadotrophin. J. Clin. Endocrinol. Metab. 36, 1268.

49 Chov, Janice Yang, Shaw-Shyan Wang and Robinson, J.C. (1978). Regulation of the synthesis of human chorionic gonadotropin by 5-bromo-2'-deoxyuridine and dibutyryl cyclic AMP in trophoblastic and nontrophoblastic tumour cells. J. Clin. Endocrinol. Metab. 47, 46.

50 Asva de,L.J., Clingan, D. and Rudland, P.S. (1975). Imitation of cell proliferation in cultured mouse fibroblasts by prostaglandin $F_{2\alpha}$. Proc. Nat. Acad. Sci. 72, 2724.

51 Rillema, J.A. (1976). Effects of prostaglandins on RNA and casein synthesis in mammary gland explants of mice. Endocrinology, 99,490.

52 Egg, D., Altmann, H., Günther, R., Klein, W. and Kocsis, F. (1978). The influence of some prostaglandins on DNA synthesis and DNA excision repair in mouse spleen cells in vitro. Prostaglandins, 15, 437.

53 Kleine, T.O. and Jugmann, U. (1977). Inhibitory and stimulating effects of prostaglandins A, E, F on the in vitro biosynthesis of glycosaminoglycans and protein from calf rib cartilage. Pharmacol. Res. Com. 9, 823.

54 Genbačev, O., Kraincanić, M., Sulvoić, V., Kostić, G. and Aleksić, M. (1975). In vivo and in vitro effect of $PGF_{2\alpha}$ on placental protein and HPL synthesis. in: Physical and chemical bases of biological information transfer, p.147, Ed. Vassileva-Popova, J., Plenum Press, New York

55 Genbačev, O., Kraincanić, M., Ratković, M. and Sulović, V. (1977). Effect of prostaglandin $PGF_{2\alpha}$ on the synthesis of placental proteins and human placental lactogen (HPL). Prostaglandins, 13, 723.

56 Ariens, E.J., Simonis, A.M. and van Rossum, J.M. (1964). Drug-receptor interactions: interactions of one or more drugs with different receptor system. in Molecular Pharmacology I Ed. Ariens, E.J., Academic Press, New York.

57 Horrobin, D.F. (1977). Interactions between prostaglandins and calcium: The importance of bell-shaped dose response curve. Prostaglandins 14, 667.

58 Bito, L.Z. (1975). Saturable, energy dependent transmembrane transport of prostaglandins against concentration gradients. Nature, 265, 134.

TECHNIQUES USED IN STUDY OF PLACENTAL METABOLISM

Maureen Young

1 Bradbury, M., Firth, A.J., Hedley, R. (personal communication).

2 Chailier, J-C. (1978) Analyse expérimentale des échanges materno-foetaux dans le placenta humain perfusé 'in vitro'. Relation avec le metabolisme placentaire. D.Sc thesis Université Pierre et Marie Curie, Paris.

3 Comline, R.S. and Silver, M. (1973) Recent observations on the undisturbed fetus 'in utero' in its delivery . Recent Adv. in Physiol. 9, 406 Ed. Linden, J., Churchill Livingstone, Edinburgh.

4 Dancis, J. and Money, W.L. (1960) Transfer of sodium and iodoantipyrine across guinea pig placenta with an 'in situ' perfusion technique. Am. J. Obstet. Gynec., 80, 215.

5 Dierks-Ventling, C., Cone, A.L. and Wapnir, R.A. (1971) Placental transfer of amino acids in the rat. I. L -Glutamic acid and L-Glutamine. Biol. Neonate, 17, 361.

6 Eaton, B.M , Leichtweiss, H.-P., Short, A.H. and Yudilevich, D.L. (1978) Transport of hexoses across the trophoblast in the dually perfused isolated placenta of the guinea-pig. J. Physiol. (in press)

7 Enders, A.C. (1965) A comparative study of the fine structure of the trophoblast in several hemochorial placentas. Am. J. Anat., 116, 29.

8 Enders, R.H., Judd, R.M., Donohue, T.M. and Smith, C.H. (1976) Placental amino acid uptake. III. Transport systems for neutral amino acids. Am. J. Physiol, 230, 706.

9 Hill, P.M.M. and Young, M. (1973) Net placental transfer of free amino acids against varying concentrations. J. Physiol., 235, 409.

10 Kaufmann, P. and Davidoff, M. (1977) The guinea-pig placenta. In Advances in Anatomy Embryology and Cell Biology , vol. 53, p.7, Springer-Verlag, Berlin: Heidelberg: New York.

11 Krauer, F., Joyce, J. and Young, M. (1973) The influence of high maternal plasma glucose levels and maternal blood flow on the placental transfer of glucose in the guinea pig. Diabetologia. 9, 453.

12 Leichtweiss, H -P, Schröder, H. (1971) Untersuchung über den Glukosetransport durch die isolierte, beidseits künstlich perfundierte Meershweinchenplacenta. Pflügers Arch., 325, 139.

13 Lemons, J.A., Adcock, E.W., Jones, D.M., Naughton, M.A., Meschia, G. and Battaglia, F.C. (1976) Umbilical uptake of amino acids in the unstressed fetal lamb. J. Clin. Invest., 58, 1428.

14 Longo, L.D., Yuen, P. and Gusseck, D.J. (1973) Anaerobic, glycogen-dependent transport of amino acids by the placenta. Nature. 243, 531.

15 Meschia, G., Cotter, J.R., Breathnach, C.S. and Barron, D.H. (1965) The haemoglobin, oxygen, carbon dioxide and hydrogen ion concentrations in the umbilical bloods of sheep and goats as sampled by indwelling plastic catheters. Q. J . exp.Physiol., 50, 185.

16 Oldendorf, W.H. and Szabo, J. (1976) Amino acid assignment to one of three blood-brain barrier amino acid carriers. Am. J. Physiol., 230, 94.

17 Phillips, A.F., Holzman, I.R., Teng, C. and Battaglia, F.C. (1978) Tissue concentrations of free amino acids in term human placentas. Am. J. Obstet. Gynec., 131, 881.

18 Posner, B.I. (1974) Insulin receptors in human and animal placental tissue. Diabetes. 23, 209.

19 Reynolds, M.L. and Young, M. (1971) The transfer of free amino nitrogen across the placental membrane in the guinea-pig. J. Physiol., 214, 583.

20 Ruzycki, S.M., Kelley, L.K. and Smith, C.H. (1977). Placental amino acid uptake. IV. Transport by microvillous membrane vesicles. Am. J. Physiol., 234, p.C27.

21 Schneider, H. and Dancis, J. (1974) Amino acid transport in human placental slices. Am. J. Obstet. Gynec., 120, 1092.

22 Schneider, H., Panigel, M. and Dancis J. (1972) Transfer across the perfused human placenta of antipyrine, sodium, and leucine. Am. J. Obstet. Gynec. 114, 822.

23 Smith, C.H., Adcock, E.W., Teasdale, F., Meschia, G. and Battaglia, F.C. (1973) Placental amino acid uptake: tissue preparation, kinetics, and preincubation effect. Am. J. Physiol., 224, 558.

24 Smith, N.C., Brush, M.G. and Luckett, S. (1974) Preparation of human placental villous surface membrane. Nature. 252, 302.

25 Stegink, L.D., Pitkin, R.M., Reynolds, W.A., Filer, L.J., Boaz, D.P. and Brummel, M.C. (1975) Placental transfer of glutamate and its metabolites in the primate. Am. J. Obstet. Gynec., 122, 70.

26 Young, M. (1979). Small animal models. In Animal Models in Fetal Medicine , Ed. Nathanielsz, P.W., (in preparation).

DRUGS AND THE PLACENTA

Peter Beaconsfield

1 Beaconsfield, P. (1969). On the need for a two-tier system for evaluating drugs intended for long-term administration. Ann. Istituto Sup. di Sanità, 5, 536.

2 Paget, G.E. and Bloch, H. (1968). Responsibilities of the pharmaceutical industry in the assessment of drug safety and efficacy. In CIOMS Round Table : Evaluation of Drugs : Whose Responsibility? W.H.O., Geneva, p.47.

3 Meigs, R.A. and Ryan, K.J. (1968). Cytochrome P - 450 and steroid biosynthesis in the human placenta. Biochem. Biophys. Acta, 165, 476.

4 Van Petten, G.R., Hirsch, G.H. and Cherrington, D.A. (1968). Drug metabolising activity of the human placenta. Can. J. Biochem., 46, 1057.

5 Kyegombe, D., Franklin, C. and Turner, P. (1973). Drug metabolising enzymes in the human placenta, their induction and repression. Lancet i, 405.

6 Juchau, M.R., Niswander, K.R.and Yaffe, M.J. (1968). Drug metabolising systems in homogenates of human mature placenta. Am. J. Obstet. Gynec. 100, 318.

7 Juchau, M.R. (1972). Mechanisms of drug biotransformation reactions in the placenta. Fed. Proc. 31, 38.

8 Beaconsfield, P. and Rainsbury, R. (1964). Réduction de la synthèse des acides nucléiques et des protéines dans les tumeurs malignes par inhibition de la voie métabolique des pentoses phosphates. C.R. Acad. Sci. 259, 2729.

9 Beaconsfield, P., Ginsburg, J. and Kosinski, Z. (1965). Glucose metabolism via the pentose phosphate pathway relative to cell replication and immunological response. Nature, 205, 50.

10 Beaconsfield, P., Rainsbury, R. and Kalton, G. (1965). Glucose-6-dehydrogenase deficiency and the incidence of cancer. Oncologia, 19,11.

11 Naik, S.N. and Anderson, D.E. (1970). G-6-PD deficiency and cancer. Lancet i, 1060.

12 Addis, S. (1971). Distribuzione della deficienza in glucosio-6-fosfato deidrogenasi tra pazienti ricoveratic nell' ospedale civile di Sassari, Appl. bio-med. Calcolo elettrinico, No.4, 230. Università di Milano.

SECTION II

CELL REPLICATION

NEOPLASIA – GROWTH OR MALIGNANCY?

Editors' note: Since the word neoplasm means 'new foundation' or 'new growth', it could equally well be applied to the conceptus as to malignant tumours. But where does the borderline lie? According to Dorland's Medical Dictionary, malignant neoplasms are characterised by 'a greater degree of anaplasia' than benign tumours and have 'the properties of invasion and metastasis' - which seems clear enough. But the embryo outstrips most malignant tumours in its normal rate of growth, and the normal trophoblast not only invades maternal tissue but also 'metastasises', to a limited extent, into the mother's lungs. The parallels between cell replication *in utero* and in malignant tumours are closer in these respects than we commonly recognise.

What of the old distinction that normal cells stop growing where as malignant ones fail to? That truism is no longer entirely true. Both normal and malignant cells of certain types can be grown indefinitely in culture. Moreover, there are no known specific differences that distinguish malignant cells from normal ones. We don't even know what governs the maturity of a healthy cell - or how to detect the moment when it falters in its functions and needs to be replaced, by normal replication. Perhaps malignancy is best described as the inability of one cell type, in a multicellular organism, to stop replicating. Dorland's definition of neoplasia comes close to this: 'the progressive multiplication of cells under conditions that would not elicit, or would cause cessation of, multiplication of normal cells'.

'... under conditions that ...' - those seem to be the crucial words which set this definition above most others. But what conditions? External to the cell, as the words seem to imply without quite saying so, or within its own constitution? Or perhaps the conditions that result from an interplay between the two? These were the questions that underlay much of the discussion on cell replication, which opened with Richard Gardner's exposition on its control - quoting examples from embryonic and placental development. Faults in control must, it seems fair to assume, underlie malignant change. And whatever 'conditions' bring them about, those faults must presumably be located in the DNA of malignant cells or very closely associated with it.

In discussion, Peter Beaconsfield stressed the need to change our orientation to cancer so that this question can be investigated. Instead of endlessly analysing data in the Micawberish hope that something unusual or specific would eventually turn up, we should - in his view - be following up likely leads. Research is not, after all, a game of pure chance. Investigation of 'highly-instructed intelligent guesses' should surely prove more rewarding than an uncritical blanket approach. What's more, the necessary knowledge and facilities for analysis of DNA function are now becoming available, as R.J.C. Harris pointed out in a forward-looking contribution to discussion.

It is by such means that it should be possible to identify what Peter Beaconsfield believes to be the irrevocable step from normal cell replication to cancer - a genetic mutation occurring in the course of 'unzipping' DNA for cell repair or replacement. Research into the so-called pre-DNA phase of the cell cycle may enable such a mutation (or mutations) to be identified - with the prospect that this might open the door to prevention and/or correction of the fault, and thus of cancer itself. Success cannot of course be guaranteed, but research into this 'intelligent guess' should certainly provide cancer research with the sense of direction and purpose it has long lacked.

But we have jumped the gun in outlining the session on cell replication. The discussion points noted above followed a masterly review of the characteristics of malignant cells and of the cell cycle in tumours, together with methods for their investigation, by Philip Dendy. And before that Robert Aitken described the origin and formation of the placenta, followed by Christopher Elston's review of choriocarcinoma and related growth anomalies. It was against the background of this factual guide to what is and is not known in these important fields that discussion of future cancer research developed. That the placenta may well play a major part in that research speaks for itself.

SECTION II

CELL REPLICATION

Chairman: Peter Beaconsfield

The contrast between the first session and this one will be marked - not surprisingly, perhaps, because biochemistry lends itself to orderly discussion based on clear-cut classification, but cell replication does not. It is a disorderly subject on which our thoughts are often disorderly too, making it difficult to organise and interpret the results of the extensive research that has been done in the field. Even the words 'cell replication' mean different things to different people, and enlarging the title of this session to cover cell behaviour as well as replication has helped only marginally. I wish I could say that we were going to discuss growth and replication from the blastocyst and implantation stage, through the replication and invasiveness of the trophoblast, to the final cessation of growth - and to compare and contrast all this with growth in tumours.

Unfortunately, such a simplistic approach is not possible. I suspected as much when writing the participants' briefs, and my suspicion has been amply confirmed by reading their reviews. Nevertheless, much of the material to be presented not only describes the complex patterns of normal and abnormal placental growth, but also sets the scene for our subsequent discussion by drawing comparisons with growth in tumours. At least the aims of this session can be simply stated - in the form of questions: What do we really want to know about cancer? Where should we look to find some of the answers? And of what value could the placenta be as a model for some of the studies required?

CONTROL OF CELL REPLICATION – LESSONS FROM EMBRYONIC AND PLACENTAL DEVELOPMENT

Richard L. Gardner

This paper concentrates on two main issues:

1. Control of the cell cycle, and
2. Cell programming, including differential gene activity.

In studying cell replication, it would be a great help if we could dissociate the various phases of the cell cycle to see how each operates and how they are linked together and coordinated. In micro-organisms, an extensively used approach to this problem has been to generate various mutants for studying particular functions of the cell cycle, but in higher organisms an embryo with a cell-cycle mutant would not develop. We are left with two alternatives. One is to work on somatic cells in culture and generate mutants of the cell cycle, but virtually all the obtainable permanent cell lines are grossly aneuploid, which means starting with a system which is very ill-defined. That difficulty can be overcome by the second alternative, a system in which there are tissue deficiencies in certain aspects of cell-cycle function. One example comes from the mouse blastocyst. At 3½ days, it has a monolayer of trophectoderm cells forming the outer layer of the embryo, and there is good evidence, from transplanting genetically-marked cells, that this outer layer generates all the later trophoblast tissues of the placenta and the fetus. At 4½ days the so-called mural trophectoderm cells that surround the cavity of the embryo, but do not form a layer over the inner cell-mass, stop dividing; over a period of days they then transform into mononuclear giant cells. The available biochemical evidence suggests that they do so by repeated endoreduplication of the entire genome, not by amplification of part of it. In other words, this is a system in which cycles of DNA replication occur without cytokinesis.

Trophectoderm studies

It is noteworthy that trophectoderm isolated microsurgically at 3½ days, i.e. before the first giant cells are produced, continues to develop in a predictable way in culture (as it does in utero or at an ectopic site) - transforming into a series of mononuclear giant cells, without any further increase in cell number. But if, instead of culturing that trophectoderm (or transplanting it directly into the uterus of another site) it is put back into a genetically-marked unrelated inner cell-mass, then reimplantation of the reconstructed embryo - comprising mural trophoblast surrounding a genetically-dissimilar inner cell-mass - results in generation of an entirely normal conceptus. Analysis of the trophoblast derivatives shows that they have proliferated quite normally and that they all possess the same genetic markers as the original mural trophectoderm. In short, what has been done is to prevent giant cell transformation by recombining the tissue with an inner cell-mass, and thus enabling the trophoblast cells to continue proliferating normally. That can be done from the blastocyst stage right up to the last stage in development (9½ days) at which it is possible to isolate a pure trophectoderm production - so-called extra embryonic ectoderm.

The trophectoderm is a tissue composed exclusively of diploid cells with an extrodinarily high mitotic index, yet once it is removed from the context of the embryo, all mitotic activity ceases within 24 hours. Then, as noted above, all the existing cells start to endoreduplicate, producing a population of mononuclear giant cells. The immediate implication of this, at least in the mouse, is that proliferation of trophoblast depends in some way upon interaction with the inner cell-mass and its derivatives. If the embryo/fetus fails to continue developing and growing, all the trophoblast cells in effect become terminal cells, because they can no longer divide. Although nothing is known about the details of trophoblast/inner cell-mass interaction, these findings suggest that trophoblast or trophectoderm cells have an uncoupling between DNA synthesis, nuclear division and cytokinesis - which can be overcome by interaction with a different type of cell or cells present in the inner cell-mass. As a system for research into control of cell replication this is of considerable value. It provides a means of studying the mechanisms by which DNA-replication is coupled with other events in the cell cycle. It also enables some answers to be given to the important question of relevance to other species, since the mouse findings reported have been provisionally confirmed by similar results obtained by performing the same experiments in guinea pig embryos. Man may well be different, however, because the primate trophoblast can undergo uncontrolled proliferation to become a choriocarcinoma. Spontaneous neoplasms of the trophoblast are virtually unheard of in other mammals, but this does not necessarily mean that normal human or primate trophoblast possesses its own proliferative potential. An abnormal trigger produced by other cells (or even by an anomalous trophobalst element), in much the same way as the inner cell-mass normally acts in mice, could conceivable set off a neoplastic change in normal primate trophoblast.

Differential gene activity

Studies of developmental biology are based on two fundamental assumptions. The first says that differentiation is a question not of differences in gene content between cells, but of differences in gene activity. In other words, all cells in a given tissue or organism contain the same genetic information, and differentiation is a question of the switching on and off of certain blocks of genes in different cells. The second assumption is that restrictions in the genetic programmes of cells, observed in the course of differentiation, involve stable activation or repression of blocks of genes (since tissues would otherwise vary in their features). As a model for studying control of gene activity, a system which has attracted much interest is based on X-chromosome inactivation. In female uterian mammals, only one of the two X-chromosomes is active in each cell of an adult female, and inactivation of the other X is believed to occur early in development. If a particular cell happens to have switched off the paternally inherited X, all its clonal descendents will have the same X inactive. There is considerable evidence to show that this repression is very stable. It is peculiar that it involves all the genes on one particular chromosome, and is therefore not a tissue-specific form of differential gene activity but chromosome-specific. But how can one be sure that the initial suppression is a random process, affecting either the paternal or the maternal X-chromosome in a particular stem cell, and that this same X will then be stably repressed in all its daughter cells? In seeking answers to these questions, much attention is currently focused on precisely when X-chromosome inactivation occurs in early development and what mechanisms are involved.

By transplanting a single cell carrying different coat-colour markers on each of its two X-chromosomes into early embryos of a third, unrelated mouse genotype, we have tried to determine the time of inactivation. If injection of such a cell results in a chimaeric animal with only one donor coat colour, plus the host coat colour, then one of its X chromosomes must have been switched off before or immediately after it was transplanted. But if the host animal shows both donor colours, in addition to its own, X inactivation must have occurred after the transplanted cell had propagated clonally in the host embryo. The result we have obtained is that X inactivation in the primitive ectoderm of the mouse - which is capable of generating the entire fetus - occurs around the time of implantation. That initial inactivation of one or other X-chromosome may not be a random event is suggested by recent work with the primitive endoderm that forms the yolk-sac and with tissue of trophectoderm origin, using polymorphism for the X chromosome or iso-enzymes of X-linked genes. Virtually all, if not all, the cells of primitive endoderm or trophectoderm derivation show inactivation of the paternally inherited X-chromosome. The evidence for this interesting selectivity is now quite secure.

One possible mechanism would be a double step - consisting of random X inactivation, followed by selective cell survival, such as might be a means of ensuring that embryonic cells would survive implantation only if they had the same X active as the mother's own cells. This notion has proved to be incorrect. If a heterozygote embryo is implanted into a mother that is homozygous for the paternal allele of the particular gene being studied, it is still the paternal allele that gets switched off. Another interesting hypothesis, recently put forward to explain the selective inactivation of the paternal X chromosome, is that it may be initiated during spermatogenesis. Maybe what we are observing is residual imprinting of an X-chromosome that was already modified earlier. In those embryonic tissues which differentiate precociously, after only a few rounds of DNA replication, the paternal X-chromosome remains different from the maternal X and may be switched off preferentially. On the other hand, in the derivatives of the primitive ectoderm, which differentiates relatively late in development, that imprinting might have been erased by a larger number of rounds of DNA replication. This is, at present, just a hypothesis. But it serves to remind us that if we can find out what is different about the paternal X-chromosome, it should shed light on this particular mechanism of gene repression - and perhaps on other aspects of differential gene activity.

Finally, may I plead that the placenta should not be referred to as 'a tissue'. Its heterogeneity is of the very essence. Trophectoderm, primitive endoderm, and primitive ectoderm must be distinguished just as clearly in all work on the placenta as they are in its development. There is evidence from transplanting single, genetically-marked cells that these three cell lineages diverge even before implantation. They are distinct cell types that cannot be intercoverted by experimental manipulation. All three are represented in close proximity in the mature placenta, as a secondary coming together, yet each retains its distinct identity in terms of structure, function and genetic activity. Whether we are discussing biochemistry, cell replication, immunology, ageing or indeed any other features of the placenta, it is vital to specify which of its constituent tissues we mean.*

For discussion of this paper, see end of section

*see also Gardner, R.L. (1977). Developmental potency of normal and neoplastic cells of early mouse embryo. Excerpta Medica International Congress Series 432, Birth Defects. Ed. Littlefield, J.W. & de Grouchy, J., Excerpta Medica, Amsterdam.

ORIGIN AND FORMATION OF THE PLACENTA

Robert J. Aitken (Speaker),
Rebecca Beaconsfield and Jean Ginsburg

We all start from one cell - the fertilised ovum - and our first cell division begins within a very few hours of the union of ovum and sperm in the ampulla of the oviduct. The stimulus for this initial division is fertilisation itself, although the molecular basis of the trigger mechanism is not known. The finding that an unfertilised ovum can divide after electric or other stimulation[1-3] is irrelevant to this discussion. The rate of tubal activity and hence of ovum transport are influenced by hormonal and other factors, but the initial cleavage of the zygote is not. No further stimulation is required for cell division as the fertilised ovum moves down the oviduct into the uterus, and cell cleavage continues as a series of mitotic divisions and incomplete cell cycles.[4] The fertilised ovum and cancer cells are the only ones which continue to divide without the stimulation of tissue demands for cellular replacement or regeneration.

INITIAL DIVISION

Up to about the eight-cell stage the individual blastomeres are distinct and undergo regular cleavage appearing to be similar in gross morphology. Thereafter, cell outlines become less clear; desmosomes differentiate between adjacent outer cells, later forming junctions which produce the barrier protecting the internal milieu of the embryo.[5] These junctional changes in the outer cell layer may possibly be the first indication of the formation of the trophoblast.[6] The cells which will become the placenta and those which will become the fetus are differentiated early at the blastocyst stage of around 120 cells. *In vitro*, the earliest time at which this has been observed in the human embryo is 5 days after fertilisation.[7] The blastocyst consists of a single layer of cells, the trophoblast - surrounding a fluid-filled cavity - the blastocoele - which contains a mass of cells at one end - the inner cell mass (ICM). The ICM is the forerunner of the embryo and the trophoblast cells round the blastocyst subsequently contribute to formation of the placenta.[8] Alone, the ICM cannot implant in the uterus, but full trophoblastic proliferation in the mouse does not seem to take place without it. On the other hand, the mouse uterus will produce decidua whether the intact blastocyst is implanted or merely some of its mural cells.

BLASTOCYST FORMATION

Validity of placental model

Before considering how the blastocyst is formed and implants, and how the trophoblast differentiates to form the major part of the placenta, the purpose of this communication needs stating. Our object is to try to evaluate whether the placenta is a valid experimental model for the study of cell replication, and whether any aspects of trophoblast or placenta activity can be compared with malignant cell replication on the one hand and with normal replication on the other. As many embryological changes are only incidental to this purpose they are simply outlined here, with emphasis on those aspects which relate to our objective.

Biochemical changes

DNA reduplication starts within a few hours of fertilisation[9,10] and RNA synthesis from the two-cell stage[11] at the latest. The enzymes for this nucleic acid synthesis are probably all present in the egg before fettilisation. The stage is set; but what is it about fertilisation that gets the players into motion? Once cell division has started and certainly by the two-cell stage, virtually all the mechanisms required for normal cell metabolism and replication are available. Synthesis of all types of RNA increases considerably with the first few cleavages so that the amount of RNA per cell also rises rapidly. At this stage cleavage can be prevented by administration of a transcriptional inhibitor such as actinomycin-D which suppresses RNA synthesis in the first part of the cell cycle.[11] Protein synthesis increases enormously as cleavage continues and embryonic cellular differentiation begins. The protein synthesised in the first few hours after fertilisation may depend on preformed RNA present in the oocyte - and therefore maternal in origin. With the early formation of embryonoid RNA, new embryonic protein is rapidly synthesised and by the eight-cell stage at the latest over 1 000 new proteins are present.[12-14] These represent virtually all the proteins which will eventually be found in the blastocyst, and from the eight cell stage onwards; although the total amount of protein increases as the cell unmber rises its variety does not.

Precursors for nucleic acid synthesis - i.e. glucose (which is then metabolised to d-ribose via the pentose shunt), nucleosides, purines, and pyrimidine bases - are initially provided from the oocyte itself. But after the first cleavage, cellular incorporation of nucleosides, purines, and pyrimidines from the external milieu increases rapidly and differentially.[12] Glucose uptake increases markedly with the first few cell divisions and continues at an elevated rate thereafter.[15] Amino-acid uptake also increases rapidly soon after fertilisation.[12] Many of the biochemical changes parallel those observed in carcinoma and other proliferating tissues, including the early placenta itself. Can we use these parallels to learn anything about cancer? Are there any important differences?

The energy requirements for protein synthesis and cellular differentiation are met in the first instance by endogenous sources from within the ovum. With the onset of cleavage, oxygen consumption increases together with glucose uptake.[15] Glucose is converted into glycogen in the cell where it can be used for the cleaving zygote, which has an extremely high demand for ATP.[16] Glycolysis rates in the dividing ovum are also high. All this parallels the metabolic pattern in the cancer cell and other rapidly growing tissues, including the early placenta - as discussed in the previous paper. It is therefore of interest that activity of lactate dehydrogenase, which metabolises lactic acid, is extremely high in the ovum - representing as much as 5% of all the protein in the mouse oocyte.[17] Pentose phosphate pathway activity is greater in the dividing ovum and pre-implantation blastocyst than in more differentiated embryonic tissues.[18] This resembles the situation in other proliferating tissues, but what is the initiating stimulus for the variation in metabolic activity essential for cell replication? And what is the distinctive signal that produces the metabolic alteration in abnormal cellular activity? The enzyme systems for steroidogenesis are present after the early stages of division in several species, but whether the cleaving ovum or balstocyst produces peptide hormones is still disputed.[19,20]

Structural development of blastocyst

The blastocyst is a highly-differentiated polarised structure, whose formation is not dependent on any specific maternal influences, since fertilisation and replication up to this stage have been achieved in vitro.[20] Formation of the blastocyst is the first stage of embryonic morphogenesis and involves two separate processes - differentiation of the ICM and trophectoderm cells[18] and formation of the blastocyst cavity or blastocoele.[21,22] Two theories have been proposed to explain the first process. It was originally suggested that polarity occurs very early in development and that two cell lines are formed from specific parts of the cytoplasm of the fertilised ovum distributed among the blastomeres, but this is no longer accepted.[23] There is no evidence of polarity in the fertilised ovum, and isolated blastomeres from the four- or eight-cell stage can form trophectoderm.[24,25] According to the more recent inside/outside hypothesis, differentiation into ICM and trophoblast starts when there are sufficient blastomeres to form two cell layers at the eight- to 16-cell stage, so that the outer layer forms the placenta and the inner one the embryo.[24] This theory is supported by animal studies with aggregation chimaeras. In these experiments pairs of mouse embryos, in which one member has been labelled with ^{3}H-thymidine, were aggregated and allowed to develop to the blastocyst stage. The results suggested that no sorting of cells had occured during the process of development and that the component blastomeres had differentiated according to their position.[26]

Similarly with aggregation chimaeras formed by arranging genetically or radioactively labelled blastomeres round the otuside of unlabelled four- to 16 cell embryos, labelled cells are found in a majority of cases in the extra-embryonic trophectoderm layer or its derivatives. With the converse experiment - labelled eight-cell stage embryos surrounded by unlabelled embryos - the labelled cells are invariably though not exclusively found in the ICM of the blastocysts.[27] Separation of ICM and trophectoderm cells from expanded 3½-day mouse blastocysts (by micro-[28-32] and immuno-surgical[33-35] methods) shows that the two cell populations have limited developmental potential by the late blastocyst stage. We know that blastomeres are totipotent at the eight-cell stage,[24] so when does determination first occur during early embryogenesis? The 'inside-cells' from mouse embryos undergoing transition from morula to blastocyst have been isolated by an immuno-surgical technique and their development fate analysed in vitro.[35] The results show that at least some inside cells do not lose their capacity to form trophectoderm, and do not become fully committed ICM cells until after the initiation of blastocoele formation.

The first stage in formation of the blastocoele seems to be the appearance of tight junctions between adjacent 'outside' blastomeres.[36] These junctions are thought to form a structural barrier which permits fluid retention within the cavity and so facilitates blastocyst expansion. The mechanism of fluid entry into the blastocoele is thought to involve active transport of solutes[21,38-40] initially and subsequently the passive entry of water.[21,22] What triggers the altered solute and fluid movement?

PRE-IMPLANTATION BLASTOCYST GROWTH AND THE EMBRYONIC DIAPAUSE

Species differ considerably in the time interval between formation of the blastocyst and its implantation and also in the extent of growth during this period.[41] The human embryo implants relatively early, between the sixth and seventh day after fertilisation, and the blastocyst grows little after the fifth day.[42] In contrast, other species, such as the ungulates which implant later, grow considerably before implantation, and in the pig the blastocyst can be as long as 1 mm by the 13th day after fertilisation.[43] Certain species exhibit embryonic diapause-delayed implantation with the blastocyst undergoing a quiescent dormant phase.[44-47] This delay can be facultative, occurring only if the mother is lactating heavily,[44,48-52] or an obligative regular feature of pregnancy.[44,53-58] The quiescent phase of an obligate diapause generally lasts for a fixed period; its length appears to be controlled by environmental stimuli such as light and temperature[44,53-58] and can be as long as nine months.[59]

During diapause the length of the cell cycle in embryos is progressively increased and cellular metabolism is depressed.[60,61] We do not know what causes diapause, how cell replication is slowed or what stimulates resumption of growth before implantation. It would plainly be of immense value in studying abnormal cellular proliferation if we knew something about the biophysical and biochemical mechanisms responsible for this phenomenon. In all species investigated, embryonic quiescence has been found linked temporally with absence of uterine secretions and resumption of embryonic growth with their reappearance.[62-68] The uterine secretions contain a mixture of proteins, amino-acids, inorganic ions and carbohydrates[44,63-4,66,68] but no specific growth stimulating factors have been isolated from them.

Is there any relation between blastocyst growth and uterine secretory activity in species which do not undergo delayed implantation? In animals which undergo marked blastocyst growth and expansion before implantation, there is indeed a coincidental increase in endometrial secretory activity,[69,70] but once again no specific growth stimulating factors have been isolated from the secretions. The fact that implantation of an embryo nurtured <u>in vitro</u> can result in a normal fetus and that an ectopic pregnancy may go to term also argues against a specific product of uterine secretion being essential for local embryonic cellular growth. The reverse may be more likely for it seems that uterine secretory activity may be stimulated by the implanting blastocyst.[71-73]

Is this due to a stimulant factor from the trophoblast and if so, what is its nature? In the rabbit, pre-implantation expansion of the blastocyst is associated with the appearance of a protein, so called uteroglobulin[69,70,74-78] whose synthesis is modulated by progesterone.[82,83] Uteroglobulin was initially thought to stimulate blastocyst development,[84] but its function is now considered to be that of a progesterone binding protein.[80-82, 85,86] In the rabbit uteroglobulin seems to be a protease inhibitor[87-89] and is also present in other tissues such as the lung,[90,91] seminal vesicle[92] and oesophagus.[93] It has been suggested that uterglobulin might counteract the activity of proteolytic enzymes produced by the trophoblast.[94]

There is only slender evidence for the presence of uteroglobulin in the reproductive tract of man[95] and other species,[96] but it would be worth investigating whether there are other substances capable of counteracting the activity of lytic factors liberated by the trophoblast and which could be responsible for limiting trophoblast invasion.

IMPLANTATION OF THE BLASTOCYST

Implantation of the blastocyst to the uterus is conventionally divided into three phases - apposition, adhesion and invasion. This division may facilitate morphological description, but there is normally no functional break in the process. Our particular interest lies in the parallels between the behaviour of the trophoblast at this stage and that observed in tumour cells. Studies of malignant tissue show altered cellular adhesive properties - reduced mutual adhesiveness of tumour cells[97-100] and increased adhesion of malignant cells to their substrate[101] - which are thought to be key factors in the initiation of invasion. The trophoblast of the implanting blastocyst appears to possess these properties during its invasive phase and apposition and adhesion between trophoblast and endometrial cells mirror the increased adhesion between malignant cells and their substrates.

Apposition

The first phase of implantation, apposition, involves orientation of the ICM of the blastocyst towards the mucosa of the uterus. During this stage, the microvilli on the surface of trophectoderm cells and uterine epithelium interdigitate and are only separated by a narrow gap not exceeding 250Å.[41] The mechanism by which the blastocyst becomes located at the definitive site of implantation in the human and is held in apposition to the uterine epithelium is unknown. Studies in animals suggest that resorptive activity or endocytosis exhibited by the endometrial epithelia during the luteal phase leads to closure of the uterine lumen around the blastocyst.[102]

Adhesion

Once the trophoblast and luminal epithelium have become apposed, the gap between these cell layers narrows further by adhesion.[103] During this phase, the regular microvilli on the apical borders of the uterine and trophoblast cells disappear, and the two cell surfaces follow a common, irregular course. We do not know exactly what happens in the human during this phase, because penetration of the uterine epithelium has already occurred in the earliest human embryo examined in situ.[104] Areas of initmate contact bwtween the trophoblast and uterine glandular epithelium are seen on examination of later stages in human implantation.[105-6] These closely resemble attachment sites in rodents, where adhesion of the blastocyst is accompanied by mutual adhesion between the opposing walls of the uterine lumen. The molecular basis of this adhesion is unknown. Could it involve changes in glycoproteins and other constituents of the membrane, as in carcinoma? Maternal steroid hormones are considered essential in preparing the uterine epithelium for implantation, and exogenous steroids can prevent or interfere with implantation.[107] It is interesting that trophoblast invasion of stromal tissues in animals seems more rapid when implantation takes place ectopically, and that specific steroids do not seem to be needed for such implantation.[108]

Invasion

Trophoblast invasion of the uterine epithelium with subsequent implantation obviously resembles malignancy but, as discussed above, similarities are also apparent in earlier phases and these presumably set the stage for invasion. What is the physico-chemical basis of the invasion process? In tumours, a number of factors are presumed responsible, including increased adhesion to substrate, decreased mutual adhesion, inhibition of growth of normal cells in the region of invasion, abnormal cell movement (particularly decreased contact inhibition) and liberation of lytic substances. However, none of these, with the exception of decreased contact inhibition of movement, is specific for carcinoma.

Does the physico-chemical basis of trophoblast invasion differ from that in malignant tumours? The enzyme that acts as plasminogen activator is secreted by trophoblast during invasion of the uterus,[109] and this is also released by cancer cells when they invade.[110] In the mouse, blastocyst invasion seems to be facilitated by the autolytic degeneration of luminal epithelial cells in advance of the invading trophoblast,[111,112] presumably as the result of proteases or other lytic substances produced by the trophoblast. This again mirrors what happens in cancer. What are the trophoblastic factors that initiate this process? Are similar factors involved in tumour invasion? Is the stimulus imminent implantation or invasion, or is some other feedback mechanism involved? Does the trophoblast exhibit contact inhibition movement, or lack this property like cancer cells? Again, there are many questions yet to be answered.

Limitation of trophoblast invasion

The degree of endometrial penetration by the trophoblast during the invasive phase varies in different species - being virtually absent in the pig[113] and marked in the human. But even the former can be highly invasive when implanted in ectopic sites such as the ureter.[114] Is it the uterus that limits trophoblast invasiveness and if so, how? If we knew what normally curtails trophoblast growth, would this help us to understand the local spread of cancer? In normal pregnancy both trophoblast invasiveness and decidual formation are strictly defined and limited. There is no trophoblastic migration in the human beyond the inner myometrium. Why? What is the signal for this and who gives it? Is it predetermined in the placenta? Feedback from the developing fetus seems unlikely because placental growth in animals continues to term after fetectomy without becoming invasive.[115] In the macaque monkey, the extent of trophoblast invasion may be limited by proliferation of the uterine epithelial cells in the immediate vicinity of the blastocyst to form an epithelial plaque. This extends beneath the implantation site and temporarily cuts off the advancing trophoblast from the endometrial stroma.[116] But plaque formation as a component of the uterine mechanisms for limiting the extent of trophoblast invasion is not universal in primates. The baboon blastocyst also implants superficially but without plaque formation.[117] There is no epithelial plaque in the human.

FORMATION OF THE PLACENTA

The heterogeneous tissue complex which constitutes the human placenta is produced by the trophoblast invasion and differentiation combined with a maternal uterine decidual reaction. The human placenta may therefore be defined as 'those tissues which intervene between the maternal and fetal circulations and which limit or facilitate the movement of endogenous or exogenous material between mother and fetus'.[118] The haemochorial type of placenta found in the human reflects the most invasive type of trophoblast and the most pronounced decidual response.[113,119] At the same time it provides the closest possible relation between mother and fetus for nutrient and other exchange, since the trophoblast is in direct contact with maternal blood. The human blastocyst penetrates deep into the endometrial stroma, and is eventually separated from the uterine lumen by regeneration of the luminal epithelium over the invasion site. In summary, the distinguishing features of this phase of implantation in the human are:

1. Marked decidual response
2. Formation of irregular projections of the cytotrophoblastic shell extending deep into the endometrium
3. Trophoblastic penetration of the myometrium, and
4. Late invasion of the spiral arterioles by trophoblast cells.[41,113,119]

Differentiation of trophoblast after implantation

During the early stages of trophoblast invasion, the tissue differentiates to form two cell layers, a peripheral syncytiotrophoblast,[120] and an inner cytotrophoblast, which starts proliferating to form the forerunners of primary villi. The syncytium then undergoes vacuolation to form a system of lacunar spaces, which connect with the maternal sinusoids and fill with blood.[113,121] In this way, the placenta is supplied with maternal arterial blood directly from the uterine vessels. How do the foreigners - placenta and fetus - elicit this response in the maternal host? The process has some similarities to the provisions of a blood supply by the host to a tumour, but there are major morphological differences, possibly related to the different natures of the 'grafts'.

The final stage of implantation - differentiation of the chorionic villi - involves two processes. Active proliferation of the cytotrophoblast carries the tips of the primary villi through the syncytial layer and into the decidualised endometrial stroma. At the same time the cytotrophoblast cell columns spread laterally in the peripheral syncytium and endometrium, and join together to form a shell around the conceptus. Although initial formation of the cytotrophoblastic shell is associated with proliferation of the cytotrophoblast and rapid expansion of the implantation area,[120,121] completion of the shell limits the area of trophoblast invasion. By eight weeks, trophoblast proliferation in the human is virtually confined to the tips of the anchoring villi in contact with the basal decidua. Why does trophoblast proliferation stop in this way?

Maternal uterine decidual response

Decidual transformation of the endometrial stroma, which is such a prominent feature of early human pregnancy, can be simulated in ectopic sites other than the prepared uterus, with a response sufficient to form a placenta capable of sustaining fetal growth to term. How does the placenta evoke such a response in other tissues and how does it ensure that it continues for the required period of normal gestation? The type of uterine reaction in different species seems to correlate with trophoblast invasiveness, the former being most marked when the latter is most invasive, as in the human. Twenty-five years ago, Amoroso[113] suggested that the possible functions of the decidua were limitation of trophoblast invasion, formation of a cleavage zone at the time of parturition, endocrine secretion and nutrition of the embryo. This holds true today, and we can only add a possible immunological role - an inhibiting effect of the decidua on immune responses as a result of blocking afferent lymphatics to the regional nodes.[122]

Invasion and inflammatory response

There is no classic inflammatory response to the blastocyst implanting in the uterus and only minimal lymphocytic infiltration. Perivascular leucocyte infiltration has been observed with the initial wave of trophoblast migration[123,124] but not subsequently. Similarly, when a carcinoma implants there is no local inflammatory reaction. Which structure is responsible for this - the donor placenta or the recipient uterus? It is unlikely to be the latter, since pregnancy can flourish outside the uterus. As to the placenta, a substance can be extracted from teratocarcinomata which inhibits inflammatory responses in mice,[125] and it has been suggested that a similar mechanism might be responsible for the absence of an inflammatory reaction in the pregnant uterus. What is the nature of the compound extracted from the teratocarcinoma and what initiates its formation? Is there a similar substance in the placenta? Histaminase is present in high concentration in both placentae[126,127] and tumours,[128,129] with multiple common isoenzymes.[130] The levels in the placenta are higher than in any other tissue.[127] It seems plausible that histaminase could limit the inflammatory responses to histamine released during the invasive phase of placental and neoplastic growth.

Modification of maternal vessels and intravascular migration of trophoblast

The uterine arteries undergo major structural alterations during formation of the placenta after implantation. A characteristic feature of the early placenta, as distinct from stromal invasion, is the presence of trophoblast cells within the maternal arteries supplying the decidua. This occurs in the human and in many other species and is thought to result from retrograde migration of trophoblast cells into the maternal spiral arteries supplying the decidua.[131-134] The intra-arterial invasion starts with plugging of the distal tips of the uterine decidual spiral arteries by trophoblastic tissue, continuous either with the cytotrophoblast shell or with the proliferating tips of the anchoring villi.[131-133] Later trophoblast seems to migrate deep into the spiral arteries, but the intra-arterial migration stops at the medial terminal arteries.[134,135] Why?

Trophoblast cells also become incorporated in the arterial wall, which loses its normal histological characteristics to become a tube of fibrinoid material with a wider diameter than the original vessel and trophoblastic cells embedded in the wall.[132,135] In animals, changes are observed in the vessel walls even before trophoblast migration.[132] What is the stimulus for this early change? The structural changes disrupt the autonomic supply to the vessels, with the result that the placental vascular bed does not actively participate in reflex homoeostatic adjustments of the maternal vasculature. The placental vasculature forms a low resistance system, supplied directly from the systemic circulation so that flow through the placenta depends on the prevailing systemic pressure. Hence, despite the absence of autonomic vasomotor supply, changes in placental bed haemodynamics occur as a passive secondary response to changes in systemic pressure, and/or to chemical stimuli.

Why do the blood vessels of the host invade a tumour to provide it with a circulation? And how is the flow through these vessels regulated - if it is? The retrograde intravascular migration of trophoblastic cells might explain local spread of trophoblast. Could a similar mechanism account for adjacent neoplastic spread with intervening normal tissue? It would certainly not account for 'Blood-borne metastatic spread', as usually conceived, but what does this really mean? What is spread? - the cancer cell itself, part of the cell or its DNA? Here, once again, there are more questions than answers. But, on reflection, there is no satisfactory evidence of blood-borne metastatic spread except to the lungs.

REPAIR OF PLACENTAL BED AFTER PARTURITION

Tissue reconstruction, without scarring, takes place in the uterus after the placenta has been shed at term. How is this achieved? Clarification of the mechanism responsible for healing of the placental bed and replacement of its vasculature without fibrosis would revolutionise clinical management of wound healing and skin grafts. Cound the absence of scar tissue be due to the action of a placental hormone - peptide or steroid? Immunosuppressive properties which could influence survival of the placental graft have been claimed for human chorionic gonadotrophin (HCG)[136,137] for some of the fetal[138,139] or placental proteins[140] (which are also re-expressed in tumour tissue) and also for some of the so-called pregnancy-specific proteins.[141-143] Could any of these be involved in the prevention of uterine fibrosis after delivery of the placenta?

The enormous research effort devoted to studying the use as tumour markers of the many compounds common to placenta or fetal tissues and cancers has shown only that the differences are quantitative not qualitive. The different placental alkaline phosphatase isoenzymes in bronchial carcinoma for example are also found in normal bronchial mucosa,[144] suggesting that they may be a feature of normal replication. The question that should be asked is not which particular placental isoenzymes are present in tumours, or whether they are identical in all respects to the placental variety, but what is their function in the tumour and why is there also so much in placental or fetal tissues? That the various alkaline phosphatases appear in the placenta at different stages of development must result from altered cellular demand. What creates this demand? Is it related to normal cell growth or to protection against rejection?

CONCLUSION

This summary of placental growth has shown that, in its early stages, the behaviour of the placenta has more similarities to cancer than differences, especially in the early stages of its development. Taking the similarities first,

1. No stimulus is required for cell division in the placenta, which replicates autonomously beyond the needs of tissue replacement

2. The placenta invades at the site of implantation and infiltrates locally

3. The placenta produces lytic substances during implantation and invasion, placental cells showing increased adhesiveness to their substrate and decreased adhesiveness between themselves

4. The placenta is tolerated by the maternal host, possibly due to an alteration in immune responsiveness. There is no sustained inflammatory response to implantation of the blastocyst or to trophoblastic invasion
5. The placenta induces an adaptive circulatory response in the maternal host, although the morphology of the circulation to the placenta differs from that associated with tumours
6. Biochemical similarities can be demonstrated, for example the production of isoenzymes and many peptide hormones.

As for the differences,

1. Placental growth is limited in extent and duration even in an ectopic site outside the uterus
2. The placenta does not metastasise in the true sense of the term
3. The placenta is shed after a defined period in balance with the maternal host

These differences in no way detract from the use of the placenta as a model for studying abnormal cell replication, but enable us to ask what the differences depend on. Are they a feature of the placenta or of the maternal host? The placenta has brakes imposed on its growth; who applies them - the host, the placenta or both? And where are these brakes? Answers to these and the many other questions posed in this review should shed considerable light on the mechanisms by which tumours spread - as well as enabling us to learn more about placental development.

For discussion of this paper, see end of section

CHORIOCARCINOMA AND RELATED GROWTH ANOMALIES

Christopher W. Elston

Because of its origin from the trophoblast, gestational choriocarcinoma occupies a unique position in the field of human oncology - as the only example of a naturally occurring neoplastic allograft. Furthermore, this tumour, which only a few years ago was one of the most malignant of all neoplasms, has now proved to be gratifyingly susceptible to treatment by cytoctoxic agents. It has a well-recognised geographical distribution, and a link between normal and abnormal trophoblast is provided by the fact that it is preceded by a hydatidiform mole in at least 50% of cases, a sufficiently close association to regard molar change in the placenta as a pre-malignant condition. Such data, taken at face value, suggest that choriocarcinoma might provide a useful model for the study of normal and abnormal cell replication. Our current concept of neoplastic growth is based on comparative studies of human and experimental tumours in which structure and function is related to clinical behaviour. We thus distinguish benign tumours such as thyroid adenomas - which closely resemble normal tissue, remain confined to the organ of origin, and do not cause the death of the patient - from malignant tumours such as carcinoma of the breast - which differ from normal structures, may disseminate to other sites and are frequently fatal. Malignant tumours may be further subdivided according to their degree of malignancy, assessed both structurally and clinically. In this review a similar approach is applied to choriocarcinoma in order to examine its suitability as a tumour model.

CLINICAL BEHAVIOUR

It is notoriously difficult to give a definition of clinical malignancy which is applicable in all circumstances; in practice, death is the criterion usually employed. In this respect untreated choriocarcinoma must be regarded as a highly malignant neoplasm, almost invariably killing the patient, and even when surgery and radiotherapy were the standard treatment the mortality was over 80%, most patients dying within a year of diagnosis.[1,2] This gloomy picture has been transformed by the introduction of cytotoxic drugs, and following Hertz's initial hopeful reports[3,4] chemotherapy has become the treatment of choice.[5-8] So successful is chemotherapy that the crude mortality has been reduced to less than 20%, and a permanent cure can reasonably be expected in the presence of widespread metastatic disease. This dramatic reversal in mortality is without parallel in the field of human oncology. In no other solid tumour has such a reduction in mortality been achieved,[9] and it is still a general rule that highly malignant, widely metastatic tumours remain incurable. It is beyond the scope of this review to discuss this aspect further, but it must be concluded that in its clinical behaviour choriocarcinoma is quite unlike any other human tumour.

STRUCTURE AND FUNCTION

The morphological characteristics of a tumour which are most helpful in arriving at a pathological assessment of malignancy are its degree of cytological differentiation, and its invasiveness, linked with its ability to form metastases.

Cytological differentiation

Normal trophoblast develops from the outer cell layer of the blastocyst, and by the seventh day has usually differentiated into two layers, an inner layer of mononuclear cytotrophoblast cells and an outer layer of multinucleated syncytiotrophoblast. There is now good evidence from studies of DNA synthesis[10,11] and from electron microscopy[12,13] that the syncytiotrophoblast is formed by fusion of cytotrophoblast cells, and is itself incapable of division. Intermediate trophoblast cells have also been identified ultrastructurally.[14] As implantation proceeds lacunae are formed within the trophoblastic cell mass, to become the precursors of the intervillous spaces, and these gradually become filled with maternal blood. Between the 14th and 20th days, trabecular columns of proliferating cytotrophoblast covered by syncytiotrophoblast become radially arranged and partially separate the lacunae. These are not true chorionic villi, but have been termed primary villous stems.[15] The microscopical structure of choriocarcinoma[1,16-21] has been shown to consist of central cores of cytotrophoblast cells surrounded by peripheral rims of syncytiotrophoblast. The syncytiotrophoblast is usually arranged around lacunae containing maternal red cells. A variable number of intermediate trophoblast cells is seen. Although this relationship between the cytotrophoblast and syncytiotrophoblast is not always as regular as that normally seen,[20] it is remarkable how closely the overall microscopic structure of choriocarcinoma recapitulates that of the trophoblast of the early implanting blastocyst.[18,21-23] Indeed, the similarity may be so great that care needs to be taken in the interpretation of endometrial curettings, to avoid misdiagnosing an early conceptus as choriocarcinoma.[20-24]

While the basic bilaminar pattern is virtually always present in gestational choriocarcinoma, variations are seen within individual tumours, and from case to case. In some tumours cytotrophoblast predominates, and in others the syncytiotrophoblast is in excess. Since the syncytiotrophoblast is known to be derived from the cytotrophoblast (see above), it is theoretically possible that measurement of the proportions of the two elements in a tumour could be used to estimate its degree of differentiation - the greater the amount of cytotrophoblast the greater the degree of malignancy. This argument was advanced by Sutherland[25] to explain the rapidly fatal course in a patient whose tumour was composed almost entirely of cytotrophoblast. Examination of this hypothesis by estimating the relative proportions of the two cell types, using a point counting method, has revealed no relationship between the cytotrophoblast-syncytiotrophoblast ratio and patient survival.[23] Differentiation can also be assessed by cytological examination of nuclear appearances. Most of the early reports noted the regularity of nuclear features,[1,16,17,26] but others have commented on the degree of nuclear atypicality in choriocarcinoma.[19,20,27] It is true that a variable amount of nuclear pleomorphism occurs in choriocarcinoma - many of the nuclei being large and vesicular, with prominent nucleoli. However, careful study of the trophoblast in the early implanting blastocyst shows a similar variation in nuclear size, with multiple nucleoli, and I am unconvinced that the nuclei of choriocarcinoma cells differ to any great extent from normal as seen by light microscopy. My own observations showed no correlation between nuclear changes and prognosis, nor was the mitotic rate useful as an index of malignancy. As seen by light microscopy, choriocarcinoma therefore appears to be more remarkable for the similarity of its trophoblast to the normal than for any specific differences, its structure being more akin to a benign than a malignant neoplasm. Additionally, unlike tumours such as carcinoma of the breast in which a definite correlation can be shown between cytological differentiation and prognosis,[28,29] no relationship can be found between the structure of a choriocarcinoma and the patient's response to treatment.

This leads to consideration of the status of invasive and non-invasive molar trophoblast. Hydatidiform mole is included in the spectrum of trophoblastic neoplasia, not because it is considered to be a neoplasm in itself, but rather because of its close association with choriocarcinoma. Next in this spectrum is the intriguing lesion described as invasive hydatidiform mole - an entity characterised by local invasion of the uterus and related structures by chorionic villi which have undergone molar change accompanied by a variable degree of trophoblastic proliferation. In addition, metastases may occur and these have been shown to contain molar villi.[30,31] Invasive mole thus possesses two of the conventional markers of malignancy, local invasion and metastasis. Following his experience with the treatment of trophoblastic disease in Singapore, Tow[32] proposed that invasive mole be renamed 'villous choriocarcinoma', and that choriocarcinoma be called 'avillous choriocarcinoma'. He argued that the former was merely an early stage of the avillous form. This view has received some support,[33] and it is tempting to suggest a continuous spectrum of malignancy, from hydatidiform mole through invasive mole to choriocarcinoma. The presence of chorionic villi would then be regarded as a marker of good differentiation. This concept would have more validity if the mesenchymal component of the villi were indeed derived from the cytotrophoblast,[34] but it seems more likely to develop from the extra-embryonic mesoderm.[35] Although invasive mole has a documented mortality,[36,37] death due to histologically proven villous metastases has only rarely been recorded[38,39] - and most of the deaths appear to be due more to local catastrophic events, such as haemorrhage or perforation, than to true metastatic trophoblastic disease. In the specialised unit at Charing Cross Hospital there have been no deaths in a large series of patients[23] (Bagshawe, 1976, personal communication). There is little evidence to suggest that a patient with invasive mole is more likely to develop choriocarcinoma,[20] indeed the opposite may be true,[40] but our present evidence is too conflicting for precise assessment of this question. It certainly does not appear to have the relationship with choriocarcinoma that say, a transitional cell papilloma of the bladder has with an invasive bladder carcinoma. Invasive mole has clinical features which suggest relatively benign behaviour, yet it is capable of metastasis. Perhaps it is best regarded as a form of limited trophoblastic proliferation that follows a less aggressive pathway than choriocarcinoma - a biologically separate but related entity.[20,21]

There have been numerous electron-microscopic studies of the normal placenta at different stages of its development,[41-49] and Fox[35] has recently provided a general review. Not surprisingly fewer studies have been carried out in choriocarcinoma owing to the difficulty in obtaining suitable material.[50-53] In general, the ultrastructure of choriocarcinoma is remarkably similar to that of normal early placental trophoblast, but the two cell types are clearly identifiable, and intermediate cells can also be recognised. Most accounts note nuclear differences, the nuclei of choriocarcinoma being larger than normal, with greater infolding of the nuclear membrane. Cytotrophoblastic mitochondria are more prominent and enlarged in choriocarcinoma, while the endoplasmic reticulum in the syncytiotrophoblast is slightly increased. The findings with cell lines of transplanted human choriocarcinoma in experimental animals have been very similar to those described above.[52-54] As yet there have been too few ultrastructural studies in choriocarcinoma to draw firm conclusions, but apart from the nuclear abnormalities, relatively few significant variations from the normal have been described.

Invasiveness of normal and abnormal trophoblast

One of the most fascinating aspects of placental physiology is the process of implantation and the establishment of the uteroplacental vasculature.[55,56] Briefly the lacunae which develop in the early proliferating trophoblastic cell mass become confluent to form the precursors of the intervillous space, possibly as a result of engulfment within the syncytiotrophoblast of endometrial capillaries.[57] Later, the spiral arteries of the decidua basalis become invaded by cytotrophoblast cells, which partly replace the vascular endothelium and infiltrate into the walls to become intramural. At the same time the decidua is diffusely infiltrated by trophoblast cells. This completes the first phase of haemochorial placentation, but between the 16th and 20th weeks a second wave of endovascular trophoblast moves down the spiral arteries to reach the myometrial segments and even the terminal segments of the parent radial arteries.[58] Trophoblast cells also migrate into the adjacent myometrium to complete the fully developed picture of 'placental site reaction'.[59] Invasiveness is, therefore, a normal and essential physiological property of the trophoblast. Although widespread myometrial invasion is a conspicuous feature in choriocarcinoma, surprisingly little muscle destruction and necrosis is seen, and where malignant trophoblast is in contact with myometrium preservation of the latter is usually excellent. Injection studies have shown that the extensive local invasion in choriocarcinoma is really vascular permeation of dilated uterine venous sinuses rather than true invasion.[23] Choriocarcinoma is quite unlike other solid human tumours in one fundamental anatomical aspect - its lack of an integral stromal vasculature. It relies for its nutrition entirely on invasion of maternal blood vessels, very like the trophoblast of the early implanting blastocyst. Examination of the edge of a nodule of choriocarcinoma in the uterus always shows permeation of maternal vessels, and malignant trophoblast can frequently be seen infiltrating and replacing the vascular endothelium in a manner reminiscent of normal trophoblast. Tumour cells then proliferate within the sinuses and embolise towards the uterine venous plexus.

Another type of trophoblastic lesion also shows invasive properties. This is the curious form of exaggerated placental site reaction first described by Marchand[60] as 'atypical choriocarcinoma' and later called 'syncytial endometritis' by Ewing,[17] in which there is wide-spread permeation of the uterine musculature by trophoblast cells, without tissue destruction, The invading cells may extend a long way from the original placental site, and Elston[61] has referred to one case in which they had spread throughout the myometrium and into one ovary. Clinically, the lesion does not behave in a neoplastic way and is rarely, if ever, fatal. Most authorities now consider it to be an abnormal persistence of placental site cells[19,21,62-64] but its true nature remains uncertain.

The similarity in the invasive properties of normal and abnormal trophoblast can be further emphasised by considerating their metastatic potential. Metastatic spread is of course a diagnostic feature of choriocarcinoma and - not surprisingly in view of its blood vessel invasion - almost always haematogenous (lymph node metastases are extremely rare in choriocarcinoma). Local metastasis to the vagina and vulva is common, but the lungs and brain are most frequently involved. However, malignant trophoblast is not the only cause of such metastatic lesions. Deportation of trophoblastic fragments to the lungs has long been recognised in eclamptic and other maternal deaths,[65-67] and it probably takes place to some extent in normal pregnancy.[68] The phenomenon can, therefore, be regarded as a physiological function of normal trophoblast, related to its invasiveness. Metastatic lesions are also well recognised in molar pregnancies, where the clinical course resembles benign rather than malignant deportation.[21] While choriocarcinoma displays a similar metastatic pattern to many other tumours, such as breast and renal carcinomas, its innate invasiveness and deportation closely parallels that of normal trophoblast and benign trophoblastic lesions. This distinguishes it from other human tumours, in which invasion can be taken as prima facie evidence of malignancy.

CYTOGENETIC ASPECTS

Some of the greatest differences between normal and abnormal trophoblast have been revealed by cytogenetic studies. The sex chromatin distribution in the trophoblastic and stromal cells of hydatidiform moles shows consistent predominance of female genetic sex - the female to male ratio varying from 3:1 to 18:1.[21,69-74] Similarly 14 out of 18 choriocarcinomas were found to be chromatin positive in one study,[73] while the world literature shows that 81% of 163 trophoblastic lesions, including 48 choriocarcinomas, were genetically female.

The results of chromosome analysis have been variable and inconsistent. One study reported aneuploidy in three hydatidiform moles,[75] with a predominant chromosome number of 38, while others have shown that the cells of a hydatidiform mole are usually euploid.[72,76,77] A progressive increase in abnormalities from hydatidiform mole through invasive mole to choriocarcinoma has been described, the two choriocarcinomas showing aneuploidy with counts of between 86 and 90 in one and 48 and 49 in the other.[78] Triploidy has been reported in abortuses showing marked hydropic change,[79-81] and trisomy 2 in a case of hydatidiform mole.[82] The borderline between hydropic abortion and true hydatidiform mole is blurred, and the significance of these reports difficult to assess. No rational explanation has yet been given for the undoubted female sex predominance in hydatidiform mole. There is a possible connection between the triploidy commonly found in abortuses showing hydropic change and the lesser degree in hydatidiform mole.[81] Most hydatidiform moles have normal chromosomal patterns, and two groups have claimed an increase in chromosomal abnormality with increased malignancy.[78,83] Further studies are clearly needed in this area, and it would be of particular interest to assess hydatidiform moles prospectively to see whether malignant trophoblastic proliferation develops from those with normal or abnormal chromosomes.

BIOCHEMICAL ASPECTS

The placenta, in addition to its role in the transfer of oxygen and nutrients to the fetus, is an endocrine organ of considerable complexity.[84-86] Briefly, the trophoblast synthesises both steroidal and polypeptide hormones. The oestrogenic steroidal hormones are oestriol, oestradiol and oestrone, produced from preformed substrate derived from the fetal and maternal adrenals. Progesterone is also synthesised, the substrate being maternal cholesterol. A variety of polypeptide hormones is produced, including human chorionic gonadotrophin (HCG), human chorionic somatomammotrophin (HCS), human chorionic prolactin, human placental lactogen (HPL) and human chorionic thyrotrophin (HCT). These hormones are produced without significant use of substrate preformed elsewhere.

Hormonal activity has been consistently recorded in trophoblastic neoplasia, oestrogen excretion from choriocarcinoma being demonstrated by several groups.[87-90] Progesterone has been found in choriocarcinomatous tissue in concentrations similar to those in normal placenta,[91] and the serum progesterone levels are raised in most patients with metastatic trophoblastic disease.[92] By far the most important hormonal activity demonstrated in choriocarcinoma has been secretion of HCG. This was originally demonstrated by biological methods,[30,93-95] but the greatest advance came with the development of a highly sensitive radioimmunoassay by Bagshawe and his colleagues.[96-97] This method has enabled synthesis of HCG to be detected in 500 cases of active malignant trophoblastic disease,[7] a finding that has proved to be a most valuable 'marker' for the presence of continuing tumour activity. A further advance has been the development of a radioimmunoassay for the distinctive beta subunit of HCG[98] – which, by discriminating between HCG and LH, further improves specificity and sensitivity in monitoring therapy. Bagshawe[7] has concluded that choriocarcinoma resembles early pregnancy trophoblast in its secretion of HCG, whilst HPL production, characteristic of late pregnancy, is low or absent. As with its structure, so with its functional production of both steroidal and polypeptide hormones, choriocarcinoma has properties closely resembling those of normal trophoblast. This is another respect in which choriocarcinoma differs from other malignant neoplasms that rarely retain the normal functional capacity of the tissue of origin to any significant extent.

IMMUNOLOGICAL ASPECTS

Many explanations have been proposed for the fact that the fetus survives rejection in the gestational period despite its tissues containing paternal antigens.

Although most of the evidence points to the trophoblast as the site of an immunologically protective mechanism, its precise nature remains in doubt. It is possible that fetal antigens are not expressed on the surface of the trophoblastic cell, that they are masked by a protective covering, or that the trophoblast acts as a neutral filter, limiting the access of maternal cells and immunoglobulins to the fetus.[99] Since choriocarcinoma arises from the trophoblast, it too must be regarded as an allograft, indeed as a unique neoplastic allograft. The morphological expression of the allograft reaction is well documented[100-102] and the cellular infiltrates are composed of lymphocytes, macrophages and plasma cells. It has been stated that no such inflammatory reaction is seen in the normal placental bed,[34] but although this is probably true during the first two weeks of nidation, a variable lymphocytic response can be found during the rest of human pregnancy.[20] We have found similar infiltrates in relation to choriocarcinoma in about 90% of cases, and they are particularly intense in 40%.[23,61,103,104] These findings have been confirmed by others[20,105] although one paper reported a cellular reaction in less than half the cases studied.[106] We have further shown that the intensity of the reaction is related to prognosis, the response to treatment being much more favourable in the presence of a marked reaction.[23,61,103,104] It is possible that the infiltrates represent an attempt at tumour rejection on an immunological basis,[23,104] and this receives circumstantial support from the fact that gestational choriocarcinoma can be cured by chemotherapy, whilst teratomatous choriocarcinoma, which has an identical morphological appearance, cannot.[107,108]

Disappointingly there is as yet little confirmatory evidence for this theory.[109] Most current research has been related to studies of individual specific, rather than tissue or tumour related, antigens. Despite numerous studies of HLA data[110-4] no consistent pattern has emerged, and the risk of a woman developing trophoblastic disease does not appear to be influenced by the HLA antigens of her mate.[109] In contrast the ABO blood groups appear to have an important effect. An increased frequency of blood group A has been shown in patients with choriocarcinoma,[115] and the risk for women of blood group A is increased if the husband is group O rather than group A.[116] The risk of a blood group O woman developing choriocarcinoma also depends on the group of the husband, greater risk being associated with group A husbands.[117] Our current knowledge of the immunological aspects of both the materno-fetal relationship and choriocarcinoma is intriguing but incomplete. There is increasing evidence to suggest that immunogenetic mechanisms play a part in the genesis of gestational choriocarcinoma, but more detailed studies are clearly needed.

RELATIONSHIP WITH PREVIOUS PREGNANCY

From the large numbers of epidemiological studies carried out, it is clear that choriocarcinoma may follow any of the various types of pregnancy - normal, abortion, hydatidiform mole or ectopic. In addition, a small number of cases has been reported in which the tumour has no direct relationship with any pregnancy, and this has given rise to speculation that the trophoblast of the early ovum could itself be malignant, constituting a choriocarcinoma 'ab initio'. It is difficult to see how such a contention can be confirmed or disproved, and it seems at least as likely that the tumour could have arisen from an unnoticed spontaneous abortion. Most of the epidemiological evidence is circumstantial and there are very few cases in which a definite origin in placental tissue can be traced. This is not altogether surprising, since the onset of clinical symptoms from the choriocarcinoma usually occurs several weeks or even months after the preceding pregnancy has terminated. The sequential relationship between hydatidiform mole and choriocarcinoma is so well documented that there can be little doubt that hydatidiform change in the placenta is a significant factor in the aetiology of malignant trophoblastic disease. In the United States and Europe hydatidiform mole precedes choriocarcinoma in about 50% of cases, whilst in developing countries the figure is nearer 80%.[21] However, of all hydatidiform moles less than 5% are followed by choriocarcinoma, and there has been no convincing morphological demonstration of choriocarcinomatous tissue arising directly from a hydatidiform mole. A number of workers have suggested that a marked degree of trophoblastic hyperplasia in a hydatidiform mole renders the subsequent development of choriocarcinoma more likely,[18,22,119,120] the presumption being that the hyperplastic trophoblast undergoes malignant change. This is an attractive concept, but the findings have not been substantiated[27,121-3] and there appears to be no significant relationship between molar trophoblastic hyperplasia and subsequent malignant transformation.

In about a quarter of cases choriocarcinoma is preceded by a spontaneous abortion. This is usually a presumptive association based on clinical history, and in very few patients has the abortus been examined histologically. It is, therefore, difficult to establish a direct tissue connection between the two events. I have personally studied a small series of choriocarcinomas preceded by spontaneous abortion, where histological material was available but no evidence of abnormal trophoblastic proliferation was seen in the abortion material in any of the cases. As Park[20] has pointed out, the great rarity of choriocarcinoma may account for the fact that no correlation has yet been found. He has suggested that the matter could best be resolved by a prospective study of the morphology of abortuses in an area such as the Philippines where the frequency of choriocarcinoma is sufficiently high to produce the data in a reasonable period of time. The best evidence for a link between choriocarcinoma and the preceding gestation is seen in relation to normal pregnancy, which precedes the onset in about a quarter of cases; rarely, the tumour has even presented clinically during the pregnancy itself. Two studies reported no abnormality in the placenta,[6,124] but a conclusive association was described by Brewer and Gerbie[125] who found foci of choriocarcinoma in the otherwise completely normal placentas of two patients, one at 26 weeks and the other at term, who died of disseminated choriocarcinoma. (They have also quoted a third, almost identical case in a personal communication.) Driscoll[126] reported finding an area of histologically typical choriocarcinoma in a term placenta, but there were no metastatic sequelae. In a review of the literature, Park[20] found reference to ten further cases of choriocarcinoma during pregnancy in which the uterus or placenta contained foci of tumour. Such reports, although small in number, offer the only direct evidence that choriocarcinoma may arise from apparently normal placental tissue. Recently, Bagshawe et al[127] have reported indirect evidence that choriocarcinoma may arise from a preceding normal pregnancy, by showing that primiparous women who subsequently developed choriocarcinoma had been immunised by paternal HLA antigens inherited by the child they had carried.

HETEROTRANSPLANTATION AND TISSUE CULTURE STUDIES

Because of its rarity, and the decrease in major surgery for the condition, material from choriocarcinoma has become less widely available for study. But heterotransplantation and <u>in vitro</u> tissue culture offer obvious advantages for studying the biology of human tumours, and also for testing the effects of therapeutic agents. The successful heterologous transplantation of malignant human cells was initially reported by Greene.[128] In 1959 Hertz[129] established lines of trophoblast cells derived from three human choriocarcinomas by serial transplantation in the hamster cheek pouch. The transplanted tumours were shown to retain the typical histological features of choriocarcinoma, and to exhibit gonadotrophic activity. These tumours have been extensively studied for purposes of chemotherapy screening,[130] ultrastructural analysis[52,54] and hormonal and immunological characteristics.[131] As a direct extension of Hertz's work Pattillo and Gey[132] established a continuous <u>in vitro</u> culture of trophoblast cells derived from one of the original choriocarcinomatous hamster cheek pouch explants. This cell line has also been extensively studied, with reports of ultrastructural, hormonal, chromosomal and electrophysiological characteristics.[133-5]

The usefulness of heterotransplantation techniques is limited by the immunological rejection reactions to tumour antigens, and frequent serial passage is required. This is, of course, overcome by <u>in vitro</u> techniques, but is a disadvantage if <u>in vivo</u> experiments are required. The discovery of the immunological characteristics of nude (congenitally athymic) mice has provided an in vivo model in which long-term tumour growth can take place. This has recently been utilised by Kim et al[136] who have established three choriocarcinomas, two of them gestational and one ovarian. Such a model will clearly be of immense value in the further study of the many fascinating characteristics of human trophoblastic disease.

EXPERIMENTAL MODELS

Choriocarcinoma appears to be exceedingly rare in animals, the first convincing account of a spontaneous choriocarcinoma being a metastatic uterine lesion in a rhesus monkey.[137] Several claims have been made that choriocarcinoma can be induced experimentally. The uterine tumour induced in pregnant rats by dimethylbenzanthracene[138] is now thought to be sarcomatous, however, and not a true choriocarcinoma.[6] A metastatic choriocarcinoma was found in one animal from a batch of pregnant armadillos given oral thalidomide,[139] and the development of a tumour resembling choriocarcinoma has been described in two out of 15 pregnant rabbits after electrocoagulative destruction of the lateral thalamic nucleus.[140] However, four groups of Japanese workers who reverted to the use of dimethylbenzanthracene in pregnant rats have all been able to produce histologically-confirmed malignant trophoblast with evidence of hormonal activity in some of the tissue.[141-144] It would now be of interest to attempt rather more natural studies. For example, trophoblastic neoplasia has a greatly increased frequency in developing countries, and Acosta-Sison[145] has suggested that malnutrition may be an aetiological factor. In a recent review of this aspect of trophoblastic disease, Reynolds[146] has suggested that specific nutritional deficiencies, such as thymidine precursors, essential in DNA synthesis, may lead to the development of hydatidiform mole. This is surely an area where the experimental rat model could be used to advantage.

SUMMARY AND CONCLUSIONS

If it is to provide a useful model for the study of normal and abnormal cell replication, a malignant tumour should fulfil certain criteria. Its clinical behaviour needs to be consistent, with a clearly defined effect upon the patient - usually the development of metastatic disease leading to death. Its behaviour should also be broadly similar to that of other human tumours, to provide a basis for comparative studies. While it should be possible to relate the structure of the tumour to the tissue from which it arises, it needs to be sufficiently dissimilar to enable normal and neoplastic cells to be differentiated. If an intermediate premalignant stage between the normal and neoplastic can be defined this also facilitates study. As with structure, the tumour should resemble the normal tissue in its functional aspects, yet be distinguished by clear differences between neoplastic and physiological activity. The possession of an easily measurable 'marker substance' is of immense value, and it is a considerable advantage if tumours of the same type can be induced in experimental animals or established in vitro.

Choriocarcinoma fulfils a number of these criteria. There are well defined cytogenetic differences between normal and malignant trophoblast, although a consistent pattern of chromosomal abnormality has not yet emerged. Hydatidiform mole is a closely associated lesion, and may provide a 'pre-malignant' link between normal and malignant trophoblastic proliferation. Malignant trophoblast possesses the capacity for continued and excessive growth, a property not shared by normal trophoblast. The placenta functions as an endocrine organ, and since choriocarcinoma shares this endocrine activity it secretes HCG, which has proved invaluable as a 'tumour marker substance' in monitoring therapy. Successful in vitro cell culture and heterologous transplantation models have been established, and the tumour can now be induced in experimental animals.

However, in other respects choriocarcinoma is far from ideal as a tumour model. Its very uniqueness as a neoplastic allograft sets it apart from other human tumours, making direct comparisons inappropriate. This is well illustrated by its clinical behaviour; the response of choriocarcinoma to cytotoxic agents has produced an enormous improvement in prognosis, a success unmatched in any other solid human tumour. Detailed studies of the structure and function of choriocarcinoma by light and electron-microscopy, tissue culture and biochemical analysis have shown remarkable similarities to normal trophoblast, with few significant differences. In fact choriocarcinoma possesses almost none of the conventional markers of malignancy, particularly in its morphological aspects. A further complication is that normal trophoblast itself is quite unlike any other normal tissue in behaviour, since it exhibits qualities of tissue destruction and invasiveness, including physiological 'metastasis'. In such circumstances the borderline between normality and neoplasia becomes considerably blurred.

Choriocarcinoma remains an enigma. Its treatment has been an unrivalled success, and for this reason alone it must warrant further study to provide an explanation for the differences between its behaviour and that of other tumours. In addition, evidence from the continued study of choriocarcinoma is certain to increase our understanding of the materno-fetal relationship, and good in vivo and in vitro model systems are already available for this purpose. At the same time choriocarcinoma has been shown to differ from other human tumours in so many respects that it must be doubtful whether useful comparisons can be made. Despite its many fascinating aspects, it would therefore be unwise to adopt choriocarcinoma as a model to improve our general understanding of normal and abnormal cell replication.

CHARACTERISTICS OF THE MALIGNANT CELL AND THE CELL CYCLE IN TUMOURS

Philip P. Dendy (Speaker) and Rosalind A. Meldrum

This paper gives a general view of the known properties of the human cancer cell and its cell division cycle. Because the subject is so broad, we have had to be selective - concentrating on solid tumours, to the exclusion of those originating in the reticulo-endothelial system, and restricting discussion of the immunological properties of tumour cells, which are considered in detail in the next section. Nevertheless, we hope this review will serve its prupose - to provide an informed basis for subsequent discussion of ways in which the placenta might be used for studying malignant processes.

There are various experimental sources of information on human tumour cells. First, and most important, are the methods of classical histology and cytology applied to human tumour biopsy specimens. Considerable weight can be attached to such observations, because the tumour cells have had no opportunity to respond to artificial laboratory stimuli, so they correspond closely with the in vivo state. However, the information obtained is essentially static in nature, and additional methods are required to study the dynamic behaviour of tumour cells, for example cell-cycle kinetics or cell-to-cell interactions. For human tumours, dynamic studies carried out entirely in vivo are difficult to perform, difficult to interpret, and - since they often require the administration of radioactive materials - frequently questioned on ethical grounds. Alternative methods have therefore been developed to study cancer cells, including short-term culture of human tumours; long-term culture of human tumour cell lines; transplantation of tumours into immune deprived animals (a method first developed for animal tumours but now successfully extended to human ones); spontaneous and induced tumours in animals studied both in vivo and in vitro; and virally transformed cells. By such methods, it has been possible to identify a number of features which may be used to compare and contrast normal and tumour cells. These features and some of the techniques used to study them can be summarised as follows:

> Morphological appearance, which may be studied - for example - by comparative histology, electron-microscopy, scanning electron-microscopy or short-term organ culture

Chromosome karyotype, which may be studied by banding techniques, and tumour-cell DNA values measured by microdensitometry or impulse cytophotometry

Biochemical properties, including glycolysis and respiration, patterns of enzyme activity, the presence or absence of normal or ectopic hormones, and biochemical changes associated with the cell surface

Growth behaviour, including studies in monolayer culture by time-lapse cinematography; growth of cells in semi-solid media, in suspension or as xenografts in immune deprived mice; density limitation of growth and/or contact inhibition; and invasion studies in organised tissues

Miscellaneous properties and tests, including: variations in the nuclear magnetic resonance or electron spin resonance signal; structuredness of the cytoplasmic matrix, antigenic tests, and perhaps a high level of reverse transcriptase and identification of the viral genome.

The properties listed above are based on *in vitro* studies, particularly on virus transformed cells, and a major purpose of this paper is to consider how accurately their results reflect the true behaviour of human tumour cells *in vivo*. Since cell division is absolutely fundamental to study of the cancer problem processes which are prerequisites of cell divisions - notably DNA synthesis - will first be considered under several headings before concluding with some details of tumour cell cycle kinetics. Although most readers will be familiar with the mammalian cell divisions cycle, the following summary may serve as a useful introduction. The main phases are shown schematically in Fig. 1. Following mitosis the cell enters the G_1 phase, which is very variable in duration for different cell types and may determine what happens in the rest of the cell cycle.[1] Alternatively, certain normal cell types (e.g. bone marrow stem cells and mature hepatocytes) can leave the cell cycle somewhere in the G_1 phase to enter a quiescent G_0 phase. This is a reversible change and under an appropriate stimulus, usually cellular depletion, these cells can return to the cycle. The S phase is the period of DNA synthesis, when the DNA content of the cell nucleus doubles (Fig. 1b), and this is followed by the G_2 phase in which the RNA and protein synthesis essential for cell division is completed. In normal cells, the S and G_2 phases commonly last for about eight and three hours respectively.

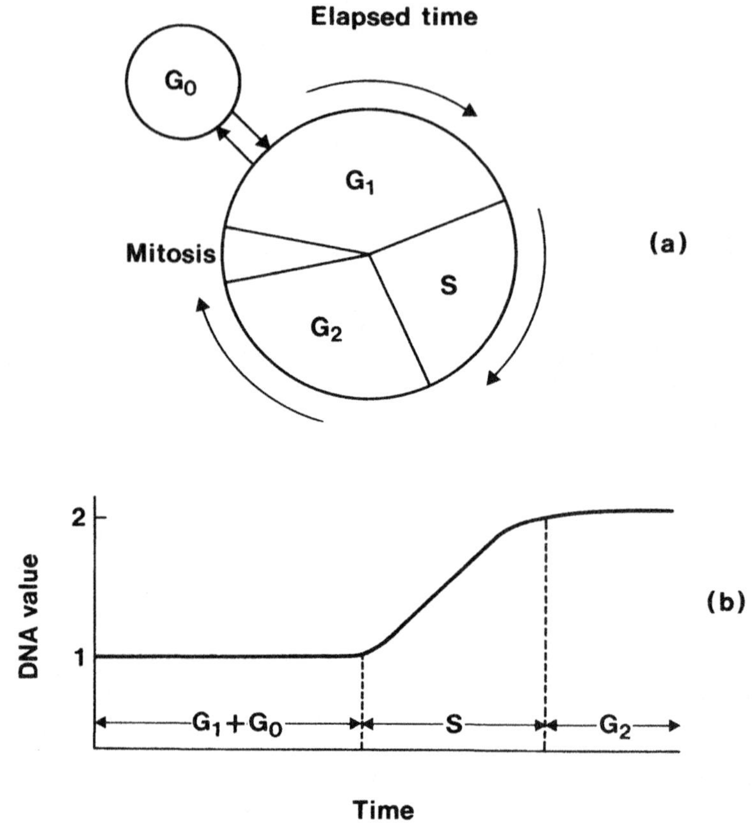

Fig. 1. Basic phases of the cell-division cycle in mammals (a), with graph showing how the nuclear DNA content changes during the cycle (b).

Cellular kinetics are often studied by methods employing tritiated (i.e. ^3H) thymidine, because thymidine is a specific precursor of DNA. Two procedures serve to illustate the value of this technique. First, if cells are exposed to tritiated thymidine for a period shorter than the duration of the S phase, say 15 minutes, the fraction of labelled cells shows the proportion actually synthesising DNA at that time. Second, if cells are exposed to tritiated thymidine for a period comparable to the duration of the whole cell cycle, the amount taken up shows what proportion of the whole cell population is actively dividing. In both cases the fraction of labelled cells is normally determined by autoradiography. The application of these and related methods to tumour cells are considered below.

THE HUMAN TUMOUR CELL

Morphological studies

There is an extensive literature[3] on the histological appearances of tumour cells, but a short technical note of particular interest has recently been published by Difruscio and Desa.[4] They have introduced the Papanicolaou stain as an alternative to haematoxylin-eosin stain for routine histological examination of the placenta. In addition to providing ready identification of certain categories of micro-organisms in infections of the placenta and its membranes, they suggest that the new technique provides excellent cytological differentiation - allowing ready recognition of many varieties of placental lesions. Among the more important cytological changes used to identify tumour cells is the relationship of the nucleus to the cytoplasm (e.g. altered nuclear cytoplasmic ratio, and altered position of the nucleus within the ctyoplasm). There are also a number of changes within the nucleus, including: variation in size between cells, increase in nuclear volume, alteration in shape, changes in the nuclear membrane such as furrowing and clumping, alterations in chromatin such as clumping and hyperchromasia, and abnormalities in the size, shape or number of nucleoli. When there are adequate histopathological findings to guide interpretation, it is generally possible to decide whether particular exfoliated cells are malignant or not.[5]

For many experimental systems, the application of these classical methods requires the growth or at least the maintenance of tumour material in vitro, either as a disaggregated cell suspension or monolayer, or as a more organised organ culture. Cultured cells may provide additional criteria of malignancy including degree of contact inhibition, piling up, colony formation, cohesiveness and focus formation. However, some traditional criteria, notably cell size and shape, become unreliable in culture. For example, the shape of single prostatic epithelial cells has been shown to vary from round to triangular,elongated or polygonal, depending on the conditions of attachment to the substrate.[6] In another study,[7] no correlation was found between malignancy and nucleolar size (expressed as a percentage of the nucleoplasmic area) for a range of cell types in monolayer culture; in vitro, nucleolar size appeared to be more closely correlated with nucleolar metabolism. Changes in metabolic activity when tumour cells are transferred from an in vivo to an in vitro environment probably invalidate a number of other cytological criteria of malignancy. Histologically, it is frequently possible to correlate the morphological appearance in short-term monolayer culture with the original tumour appearances,[8] and the degree of correlation can be improved if the monolayer of cells are trypsinised and fixed in suspension before staining.[9] Hajdu et al[10] used this technique to study cells from 52 human tumours, and the main cytological differences found between the two types of preparation are summarised in Table I. Recently, a similar comparison for melanoma cell lines has shown that the cytocentrifuge smear technique gave good cytological detail of the tumour cells which remained well preserved.[11] Furthermore these preparations had more features in common with melanoma cells studied in tissue preparations than did those from monolayer cultures, in which cellular appearances had changed as a result of artificial separation. It

TABLE I

Main cytological differences between tumour cells from monolayer culture and those trypsinised and fixed in suspension before staining

Features	Cells from monolayer preparation	Trypsinised, fixed smear of cell suspension
Shape of cytoplasm	Spindle	Round
Shape of nucleus	Oval	Round
Size of cell	Increased	Normal
Cellularity	High	Good
Organoid pattern	Absent	Present
Preservation	Good	Good
Cells in mitosis	Many	Few
Similar to *in vito*	No	Yes

It follows that classical cytological methods for tumour cell identification should only be applied to cells *in vitro* with great caution.

Much research effort has been devoted to electron-microscope study of tumour cells, the three principal methods[12] used in these studies being:

> *Thin sectioning* to obtain a two-dimensional image representing a single plane within the specimen
>
> *Negative staining*, which is useful for revealing selected aspects of membrane fine structure; isolated membranes are treated with a very soluble heavy metal salt (such as phosphotungstic acid) so that membrane components which are impermeable to the salt remain electron-lucent and stand out in negative contrast

Freeze fracturing, by rapid freezing and cleavage at low temperatures (-100 to -196°C); this process splits open membranes along planes of low mechanical resistance, and preparation of a heavy metal replica of the fractured surface enables the internal surfaces of the membrane to be examined.

Unfortunately, conventional electron-microscopy has so far provided no conclusive evidence that any cell membrane components are causally related to malignant behaviour. Typical of many reports are the conclusions of Weinstein et al,[13] who reviewed in detail the structure and function of intercellular junctions in cancer. There are two broad classes of junction: those with close contact between the surface membranes of neighbouring cells, and those in which the surface membranes are separated by an interspace, which frequently contains electron-dense proteinaceous material and typically measures some 15-35 nm across. There is much circumstantial evidence that cell junctions may be particularly important to the cancer problem. For example, they provide strong structural links bwtween cells, allow direct communication between cells (including the transfer of ions and small molecules without their entering the extracellular space) and, depending on the type of junction involved, may form an effective barrier to diffusion. Comparisons of normal tissues and tumours have shown that the junctions may differ in overall size, distribution at the cell surface, level of development and numerical density,[14] but the junctions themselves are generally indistinguishable at the ultrastructural level as viewed in the electron-microscope. A comprehensive review[13] of pathological reports indicates that junction deficiencies are common in tumours, but no consistent pattern emerged that might be correlated with either of the most important properties of tumour cells - invasiveness and ability to metastasise. Further studies of intercellular junctions should reveal more about their chemical nature and mode of interaction.

Introduction of the scanning electron-microscope, with its unique morphological applications[15] and capability for non-destructive X-ray microanalysis, provided important new histophysical techniques and a powerful impetus to tumour cell characterisation. A number of differences in surface morphology have now been reported between normal cells and cells transformed in vitro.[16] For example, the duct epithelium within dysplastic breasts or those containing benign neoplasms has been shown to differ quite clearly from the same tissue in carcinomatous breasts.[17] Duct cells from cancer patients varied more in size and shape and in the number, length and arrangement of the microvilli - with an increase in the number of rudimentary microvilli or 'knobs'. In particular, the surface microvilli showed a definite tendency to clustering, especially in the centre of the apical surface, and contained intracellular microvillous contacts. Moreover, ducts up to seven inches from the tumour showed similar changes. Extension of this technique to a micro-explant organ culture system, again using human breast carcinoma tissues, has revealed that fibroblasts can readily be distinguished from epithelial cells by: (1) almost complete absence of microvilli, (2) well-orientated subsurface microfilaments, (3) a ridged surface after critical-point drying, and (4) small tongue-like projections among cell-to-cell contacts.[18] A more important observation, for our purposes, was that - although ridge-like contacts were found in all non-malignant epithelium - an entirely different type of cell-to-cell contact between surface projections of widely variable diameter (0.5 - 1 000 nm) was observed both in cells from all breast carcinoma patients studied and from cultured carcinoma cell lines. Further more, the irregular distribution of microvilli noted above was confirmed.

Springer et al[19] used the scanning electron-microscope to monitor the changes in cell surface properties which occur when HeLa cells adapt from suspension culture to monolayer culture. They reported that the cells showed a step-wise response to the substrate which appeared to be cell-cycle independent. Their observations that cells in suspension, including tumour cells, have a highly villous surface and undergo an early change in surface topology to produce large globular processes with large areas for membrane attachment led them to suggest that these changes might represent an early stage in the metastatic process. Studies of the cell-surface properties of human tumours of various histopathological types (including carcinoma, malignant melanoma, rhabdomyosarcoma and glioblastoma) established in tissue culture have shown a high level of surface activity, but some detailed observations, e.g. a high surface density of microvilli, were also noted on exponentially growing normal human fibroblasts.[20]

In sum, we can say that scanning electron-microscopy has so far failed to provide a definite distinction between normal and tumour cells, though some significant and potentially characteristic differences have been identified. There is no evidence that any of these features is more prominent in any particular phase of the cell cycle, but there may be a relationship between the density of surface microvilli and overall proliferative activity. If tumour cells do have characteristic properties identifiable in the scanning electron-microscope, they may not be retained in monolayer culture, so the results of studies on such material must be interpreted with caution.

Karyotype and DNA value

Tumour cells frequently show chromosomal deficits, as shown by many workers - among them Miles,[21,22] who made detailed chromosomal analyses of both non-epithelial and epithelial solid tumours, and Miles and Wolinska[23] who analysed malignant effusions in a similar manner (Table II).

TABLE II

Comparison of cytological diagnosis with chromosomal analyses on specimens of malignant effusion

Cytological diagnosis	Cases	Chromosome status
Positive	20	Gross abnormalities
Positive	4	Ambiguous
Positive	11	Normal (or indistinguishable from treatment effect)*
Isolated malignant cells	2	Gross abnormalities
Isolated malignant cells	1	Ambiguous
Suspicious	3	Ambiguous
Suspicious	2	Normal (or indistinguishable from treatment effect)*
Negative	2	Gross abnormalities
Negative	5	Normal (or indistinguishable from treatment effect)*

* Studies complicated by previous radiotherapy and/or chemotherapy to many patients

In any extensive survey there are nearly always a small number of confirmed malignant cases in which the karyotype cannot be distinguished from diploid. For many years it was thought that this might simply reflect failure of the existing technology to detect small chromosomal rearrangements. However, even the introduction of chromosome banding techniques[24] has failed to resolve this problem completely. Sonta and Sandberg[25] have recently pointed out that few studies have yet been done on solid tumours because: (1) primary tumours have a low mitotic index, (2) banding is difficult due to the chromosomes being rather contracted, (3) cancerous chromosomes are often resistant to banding, and (4) long-term culture to overcome these problems may give spurious results. Three of the 15 primary intestinal tumours they studied gave diploid results, but the authors suggested that this might be due to the presence of normal cells, e.g. leucocytes, or to samples taken from a previously benign part of the tumour. However, most workers still feel that there are a few confirmed malignant tumours in which the cellular chromosomes are still indistinguishable from diploid.

There are obvious advantages to be gained from the increased resolution obtained with banding, and Mark[26] recently re-examined the whole question of the specificity of chromosomal abnormalities in human neoplasms in the light of additional evidence from banding studies. Studying three different categories of neoplasia (meningiomas, myeloproliferative disorders, and lymphoproliferative disorders), he found evidence of specific anomalies in meningioma, in the Philadelphia-chromosome positive type of chronic myeloid leukaemia, and in Burkitt's lymphoma. From this work and a review of a large number of other publications on the subject, he suggested that chromosomes 1, 8, 14 and 22 are more often involved in deviations associated with neoplasia than are the other chromosomes. He concluded that further intensive studies might reveal specific changes or patterns in some other tumour types. The following general conclusions appear to be justified by the evidence now available:

1. The majority of tumours contain cells with gross chromosomal abnormalities
2. Some tumours show the same karyotype in every cell, and distinctive marker chromosomes may be present throughout the tumour - both features strongly suggesting clonal development of tumour cell growth.
3. Other tumours show a broad spectrum of karyotype from one cell to another
4. There is no chromosomal change characteristic of malignancy
5. Correlation between prognosis and chromosome pattern is questionable
6. Diagnosis of malignant disease on the basis of karyotype examinations is not as accurate as traditional cytological methods, although it may be helpful in some circumstances.

Most studies of neoplastic transformation at the chromosomal level have been based either on <u>in vitro</u> studies of virus-induced changes or on cell hybridisation experiments, and Jones[27] has summarised some of the evidence that malignant cell transformation <u>in vitro</u> may be associated with the appearance of abnormal chromosome patterns. The degree to which malignant potential is expressed by transformed cells seems to depend on the balance between specific chromosomes responsible for the expression or supression of malignancy. It has been shown in studies of cells from chemically-induced mouse fibrocarcinoma, for instance, that when two copies of a specific marker chromosome are present, malignancy and antigenicity are suppressed - but both properties return if one copy of the chromosome is absent.[28] Karyotype analysis provides further information about established lines of human cells,[29] enabling two important questions to be answered: Does the tumour cell karyotype *in vitro* correlate well with findings *in vivo*? And does the tumour cell karyotype remain stable *in vitro*? With only a few exceptions both these questions can now be answered in the affirmative - supporting the idea that chromosomal abnormalities identified *in vitro* reveal the *in vivo* origins of dividing cells. It follows that when tumour cells show an abnormal karyotype, particularly if there is a marker chromosome, this provides a reliable, though technically time-consuming, method for studying the behaviour of human tumour cells in experimental systems (despite Sonta and Sandberg's view, quoted earlier,[25] that long-term culture may give spurious results).

Closely related to the question of abnormal karyotype is the evidence that tumour cells frequently contain an abnormal amount of DNA. If single cells can be stained with a chromophore which is both specific and stoichometric for a particular macromolecule, its quantity in each cell can be measured in various ways. A well-established method is to measure the DNA in the cell nucleus by microdensitometry after staining by the Feulgen reaction. Because errors may arise if the chromophore is not uniformly distributed, high-precision microdensitometers are generally used to scan the cell nucleus, as shown schematically in Fig. 2.

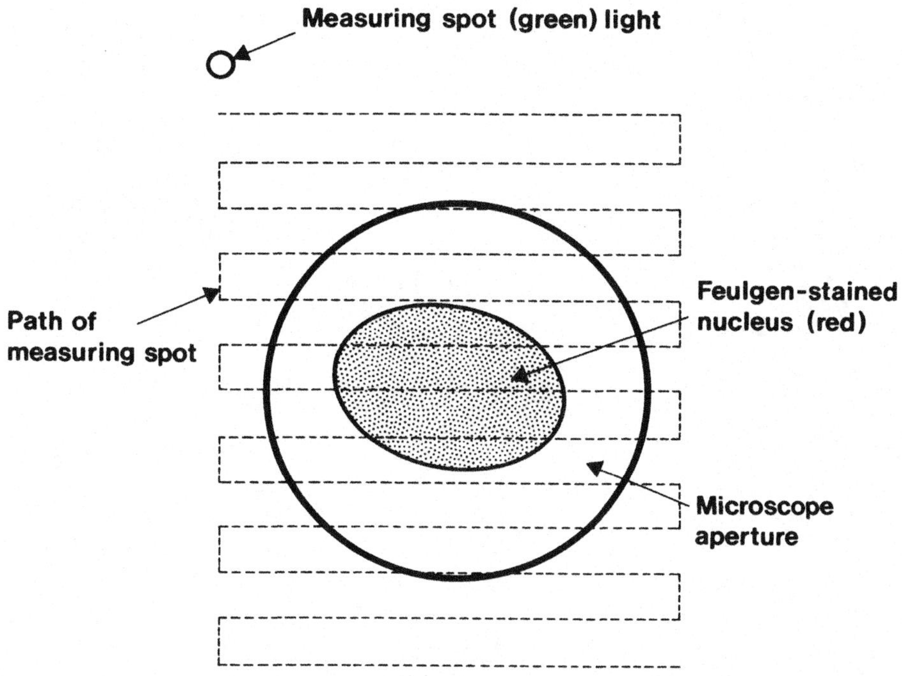

Fig. 2. Working principle of a scanning microdensitometer.

A relatively recent technique for rapid measurement of DNA values is impulse cytophotometry.[30] This requires a suspension of single undamaged cells; when stained with a fluorescent dye, such as ethidium bromide, each cell flowing through a measuring chamber is illuminated with an intense beam of laser light. The strength of the fluorescent signal is proportional to the amount of DNA in the cell nucleus, and the recorded values are stored automatically (Fig. 3). This technique has also been used extensively to study tumour-cell cycle kinetics and is referred to again later. An important advantage of making DNA measurements derives from the fact that - despite some doubts on the DNA value of small lymphocytes[31] - normal

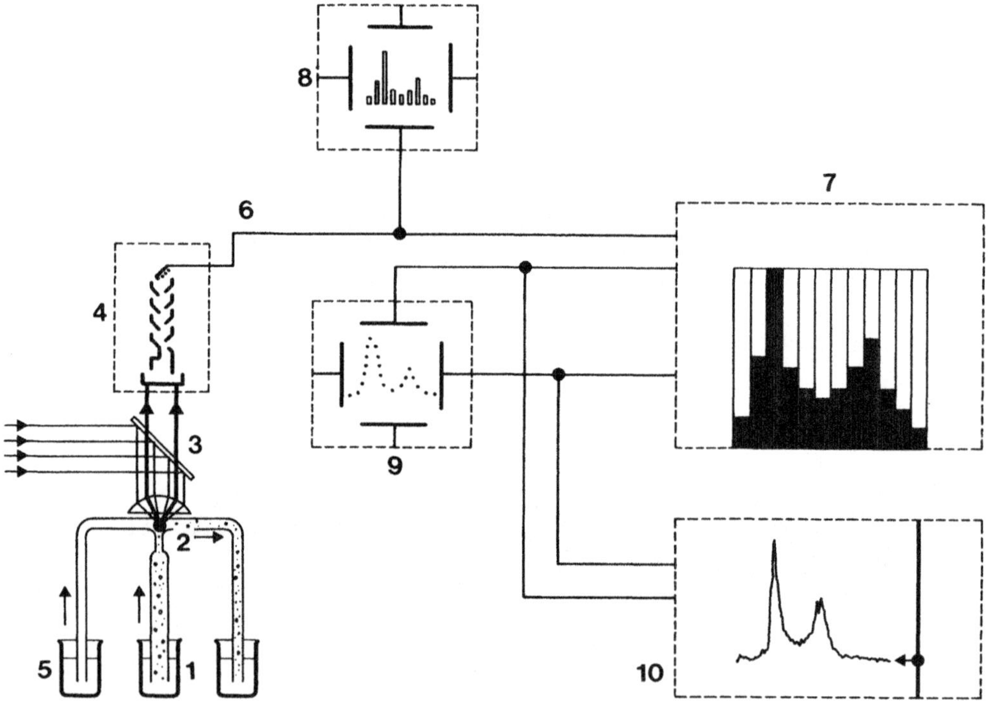

Fig. 3. Basic design of the ICP 11 (Phywe) Pulse Cytophotometer. A beam of laser light enters the system from the left to illuminate cells in the measuring chamber, 1 sample contained, 2 measuring region, 3 dichroic reflector, 4 photomultiplier, 5 particle free cleansing liquid, 6 amplified signal, 7 multichannel analyser, 8 and 9 cathode-ray oscilloscopes, and 10 final display.

cells in the same phase of the cell cycle are now widely believed to have the same DNA value in different parts of the body. An easily identifiable exception is the occasional appearance of cells with simple multiples of that value, examples being adult liver cells and, occasionally, normal adult ovary cells. This consistency has important advantages when comparing and contrasting the nuclear DNA values of normal and tumour cells:

1. A biological standard is readily available to provide the normal diploid DNA value
2. The presence of nuclei with tetraploid and occasional octaploid DNA values in adult liver provides a ready check on the linearity of the relationship between staining and DNA content
3. Normal tissue, for comparison, does not have to come from the same organ as the tumour cells
4. If normal human tissue is difficult to obtain, animal tissue can be used by applying a constant to convert the diploid DNA value for, say, a mouse liver cell to the corresponding human value.

Following earlier work on DNA values in different species[32] and in selected human tumours,[33-35] Bohm and Sandritter[36] reviewed the whole subject of cytophotometric measurement of DNA values in human tumour cells and included their own experience with 250 tissue smears prepared from unfixed human tumours of various types. Their main conclusions were that benign human tumours have identical diploid stem lines, indistinguishable from normal cells in DNA content, whereas cells from the vast majority of malignant tumours exhibit nuclear DNA values which are more or less beyond the diploid DNA content. Although it is well established that the cells in some malignant tumours have normal DNA values, the exact percentage of such tumours is uncertain. Bohm and Sandritter[36] reported that only 4% of all the malignant tumours they investigated had a diploid stem line, while others[37-39] have found higher and lower rates for particular tumour types. It remains to be seen whether these are true differences or determined, at least in part, by normal cells being examined in some supposedly neoplastic specimens. Many of the discrepancies are almost certainly a result of sampling problems, since there is a definite inverse correlation between abnormal DNA values and histological degree of differentiation. This has been noted on several occasions and is well summarised in the results obtained with an impulse cytophotometer by Tribukait and Esposti.[40] They correlated DNA values and morphology for neoplastic and non-neoplastic urothelium and showed that while 7 out of 17 malignant but highly differentiated tumours (41%) showed no abnormal DNA peak, only 5 out of 28 (18%) moderately differentiated, and 1 out of 38 (3%) poorly differentiated tumours failed to show such a peak. Similar results have been reported in bladder tumours by Fossa et al,[41] who also found that patients with diploid tumours had a higher survival rate than those with non-diploid tumours.

A good correlation has generally been reported between chromosome number and modal DNA value. Atkin[42] studied both parameters for 23 ovarian neoplasms and found that all high DNA values corresponded to high chromosome numbers, all low DNA values except one corresponded to a low chromosome number, and only one normal DNA value corresponded to a low chromosome number. Moreover, there was very good correlation between the actual chromosome number and the estimated chromosome number based on DNA measurement. The ratio between estimated and actual chromosome numbers was generally slightly higher than one (indicating that the amount of DNA per chromosome was slightly above normal) but in only one case was the ratio outside the range 0.95 to 1.15. A simultaneous chromosomal and nuclear DNA study of uterine adeno-carcinoma and its metastases also showed good agreement.[43] Several workers have considered the significance of chromosomal changes and changes in nuclear DNA values to the development and prognosis of malignant disease. Bohm and Sandritter[36] found that well-differentiated tumours generally showed a well-defined DNA stem line - which was absent from undifferentiated anaplastic tumours. They also suggested that since undifferentiated tumour histology and widely-scattered DNA values were more frequently found at autopsy than at surgery, their presence indicated a late stage in the progression of malignant disease. These results, taken in conjunction with the evidence that some malignant tumours contain cells with normal DNA values and karyotypes, leads to the tentative conclusion that changes in DNA value and karyotype may be a secondary consequence of malignant transition, not a primary cause.[44,45] While gene changes must frequently, if not always, be involved in the induction of cancer, gross morphologically-recognisable chromosome changes may be a prerequisite for only a small number of human cancers. Bohm and Sandritter[36] suggest that direct determination of the DNA content should give more important information about tumours, biologically and functionally, than can be obtained from chromosome counts. However, although we shall shortly suggest practical reasons why DNA measurement may be preferable at present, there is no <u>a priori</u> reason for choosing one rather than the other.

Interpretation of DNA measurements is complicated if cells are undergoing division at the time. A normal cell in mid S-phase will <u>appear</u> to have an abnormal DNA value because it is in process of doubling its DNA content (see Fig. 1) This may represent a particularly serious problem if the proliferating fraction is higher than normal. For example, Sprenger et al[46] found that routine photometric prescreening for the detection of cervical carcinoma produced an unacceptably high proportion of false positives, due to inflammatory activation of cell proliferation. Using the same technique, Johannisson et al[47] found a significant decrease in the mean DNA content per cell nucleus following six to seven months of exposure to progesterone (from a releasing device) and suggested that the proliferative activity of the endometrium was being suppressed. In human solid tumours, the tritiated-thymidine labelling index is generally low, with quite marked variations depending on the site and histological grade of the tumour. Hainau and Dombernowski[48] cultured human

TABLE III

Tritiated thymidine uptake (expressed as mean indices) by cells from human bladder tumours of different histological types and malignant grades. (Adapted from Hainau and Dombernowski[48]).

Tumour type	Thymidine uptake, according to grade of malignancy				
	0	I	II	III	IV
Controls	0.12				
Transitional epithelium tumour (papillary)	4.2	3.6	6.9	21.6	
Transitional epithelium tumour (solid)				17.4	24.2
Squamous cell carcinoma			20.5		

bladder tumour material with tritiated thymidine for four hours followed by fixation and autoradiography to show that the labelling index was correlated with the histological grade of malignancy (Table III), indices in excess of 20% being recorded for some tumours. Another approach to interpretation of DNA values has been by statistical analysis - a method adopted by Lederer et al[49] in an attempt to derive diagnostic information from the spread of DNA values in malignant testicular teratoma. But it is hard to see how this could provide consistent results in the absence of information about the proportion of cells in the S phase. This problem may be accentuated by culture in vitro, where there will generally be increased proliferative activity.

In our own work with short-term cultures of normal malignant human tissues, we have adopted a technique for identifying S phase cells autoradiographically after labelling the culture with tritiated thymidine immediately before fixation. The value of this additional information is illustrated in Figs. 4a and b, which show histograms of DNA values for the nuclei of actively-growing normal human embryonic skin and muscle cells. When the cells in S phase are identified, two well-defined peaks corresponding to the G_1 and G_2 phase cells can be clearly distinguished (their spread being due to instrumental and other errors in the measuring procedure). An

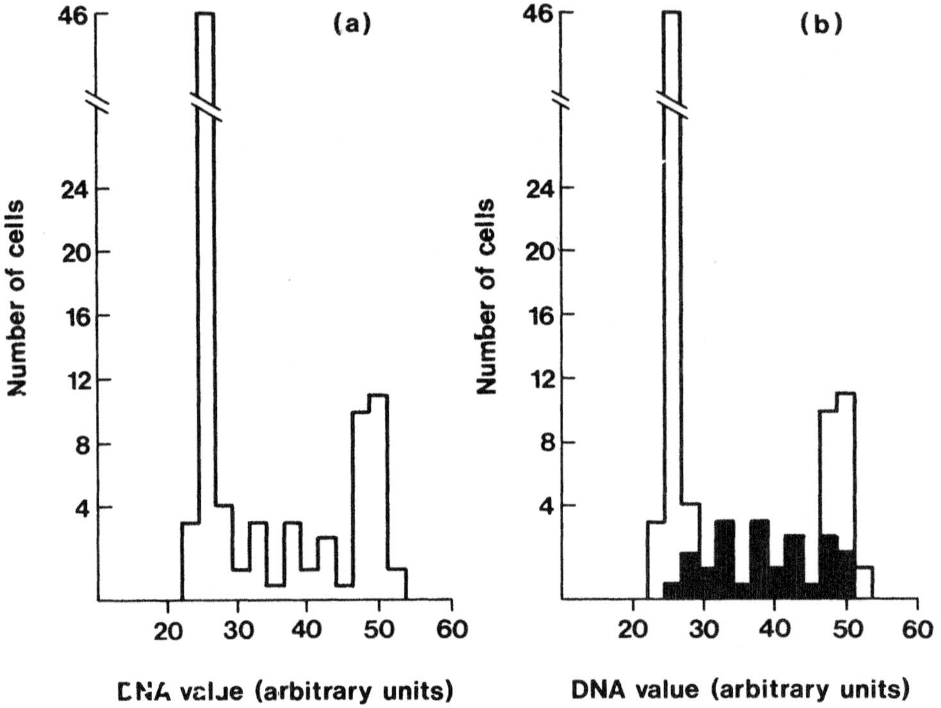

Fig. 4. Distribution of DNA values for actively-growing human embryonic skin and muscle cells, without identification of S phase cells (left) and after identification of S phase cells by tritiated thymidine plus autoradiography (right), shown black.

important advantage of combining microdensitometry and autoradiography in this way is that they can be used to monitor the progress of tumour cells in culture - as shown in Fig. 5. for cells derived from a highly anaplastic abdominal tumour. Before culture, there was a cell population with normal DNA values and probably two populations with abnormal values. After 10 days in culture, the normal population had disappeared and an appreciable proportion (about 21%) for the tumour cells were in the DNA-synthetic S phase. After 22 days in culture, the percentage of cells in S phase had fallen again, and a higher proportion appeared to have G_2 phase DNA values.

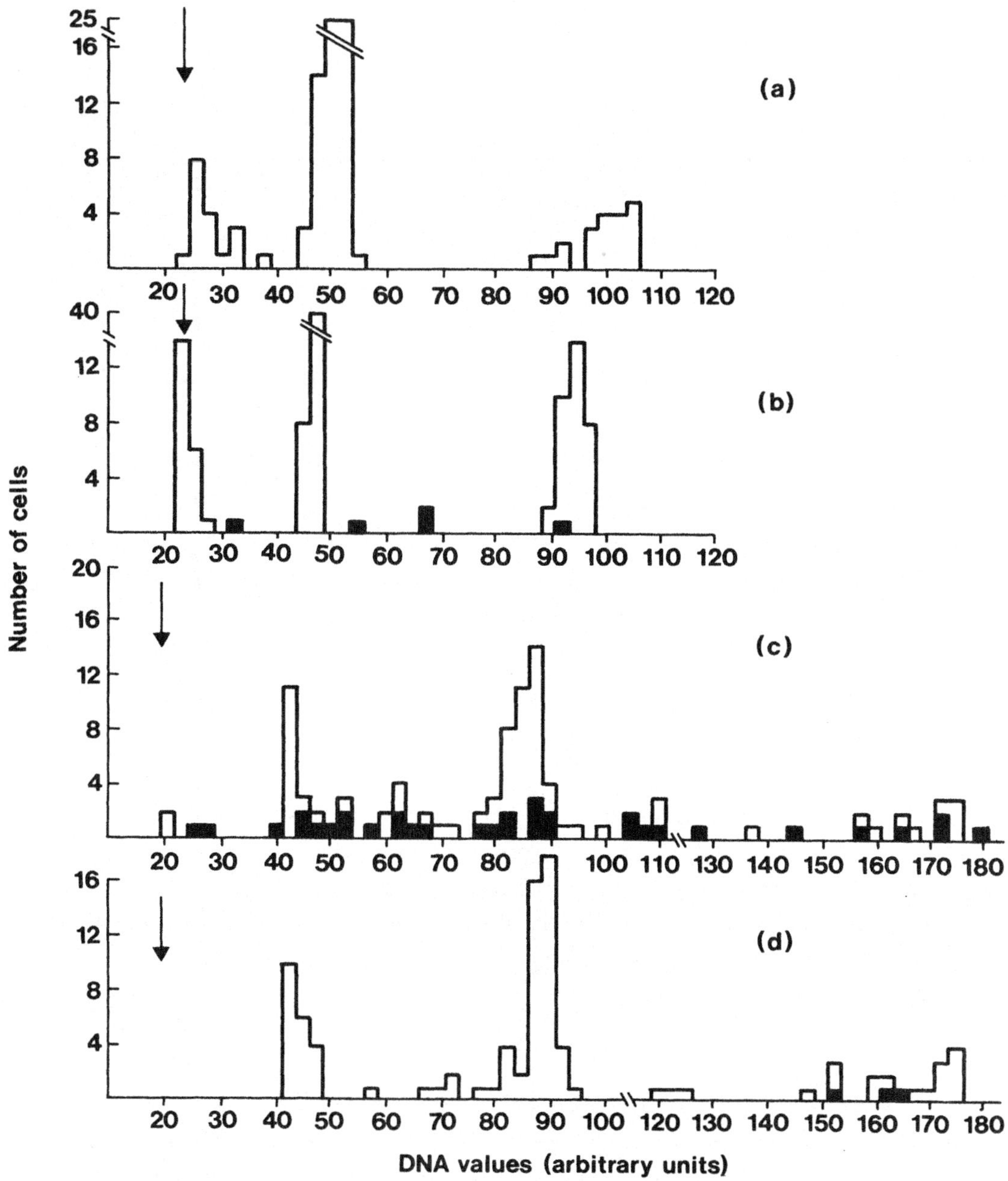

Fig. 5. DNA values (with identification of S phase cells as black areas) for cells derived from a human abdominal tumour, after tissue disaggregation (a), and after 3 (b), 10 (c), and 22 days in culture (d). The normal diploid DNA value to be expected from measurements on adult liver cells at the same time is arrowed on each diagram.

On the basis of these measurements, the cells in culture at that time could be identified as the tumour-cell component of the mixed-cell biopsy originally taken into culture.

To summarise this section, we can say that in many situations an abnormal karyotype or DNA value provides a specific and reproducible criterion of malignancy at the cellular level. The method of tumour-cell identification by combined microdensitometry and autoradiography has a number of important advantages for experimental work:

1. It is based on a cellular property that is a known indicator of malignancy for many tumours
2. It can be readily quantitated and has a fairly high level of accuracy
3. Unlike chromosomal studies which can be used only on dividing cells, it can be used to measure all isolated cell nuclei
4. Since it is applied to single cells, it gives an indication of the proportions of tumour and normal cells in a mixed population
5. If biopsy specimens are maintained or grown *in vitro*, it may be used to monitor the behaviour of the tumour cells and their relative proportions in a mixed-cell population.

Two future developments would be of value. The first is the need for a more automated method; this might be based on the impulse cytophotometer if a suitable technique could be developed to remove cells in the S phase by means of a cell-cycle phase specific drug. The second need is for an analagous method for identifying malignant cells in the rather smaller number of tumours which show no abnormality in DNA value.

Biochemical properties

Quantitative techniques have been developed to study a wide range of cytochemical and biochemical properties - in addition to the nuclear DNA content - including RNA, proteins, polysaccharides, lipids and sulphydryl groups.[50] The application of many of these techniques in different biological situations has been reviewed,[51] but none of them has yet found much application in cancer research because of failure to identify characteristic features of malignant cells. However, one purpose of this meeting is to take a new look at the cancer problem, and it is important to keep these methods in mind since many of them are excellent in appropriate situations.

Since the application of established techniques to recognition of tumour cells has not been very successful, it may be preferable to identify properties which seem to be characteristic of such cells and then develop suitable techniques for measuring them. One aspect of deviant biochemical behaviour which has produced promising results is the study of isoenzyme patterns. (Isoenzymes can be defined as a biochemically distinct class of catalytically active proteins with the same specificity of bond cleavage or alteration, but occupying several zones following electrophoresis. Isoenzymes generally show variations in other properties too, and a good survey of the techniques used in their study, together with a review of the properties of human alkaline phosphatases, has been published by Fishman and Ghosh[52].) Since the early report, in a patient with bronchogenic carcinoma, of an isoenzyme of alkaline phosphatase which appeared to be of tumour origin, a number of other workers have shown that this is quite a general phenomenon. For example, Miki et al[53] were able to separate the alkaline phosphatase in gastric carcinoma tissue from 23 patients into three separate bands by polyacrylamide-gel disc electrophoresis. At least one of these species appeared to originate in the tumour cells.

The relevance of this work to the placenta is that some of the isoenzymes of alkaline phosphatase, which are thought to be of tumour origin, have properties very similar (if not identical) to those of alkaline phosphatases in human serum during certain stages of pregnancy. Two related reports have discussed the relevance of developmental genes to neoplastic transformation. In the first, Fishman et al [54] showed by biochemical, immunological and electrophoretic techniques that the alkaline phosphatase isoenzyme pattern during phase 1 (weeks 6 to 10) of human trophoblastic development is quite different from that after 14 weeks, being heat sensitive and inhibited more by L-homoarginine but much less by L-phenylalanine during the earlier period. Between about 11 and 13 weeks there is a mixture of the two patterns. In the second paper, Fishman[55] suggested that there is a close relationship between this 'early' alkaline phosphatase, which has been named chorionic alkaline phosphatase, and human chorionic gonadotrophin. For some years now a similar close relationship has been recognised between term placental isoenzyme and the Regan isoenzyme found in some tumours. Fishman accordingly re-examined earlier work on ascites fluids from 22 ovarian malignancies with the results shown in Table IV. These data suggested that when human chorionic gonadotropin alone was detected, the active genes in the tumour were those normally functional before ten weeks of gestation; and when only the Regan isoenzyme was detected, the genes normally active after 15 weeks were functioning. Presence of both compounds indicated activity in both sets of genes, a condition also observed in normal placental development. Numerous reports on the use of various tissue serum enzyme assays in primary cancer diagnosis, or to follow the course of the disease, have recently been reviewed by

TABLE IV

Presence of various isoenzymes in 22 different ovarian malignancies, (adapted from Fishman[55])

Regan isoenzyme	Human gonadotropin Present	Human gonadotropin Absent
Present	9	4
Absent	6	3

Schwartz.[56] Another biochemical property of malignant and transformed cells is a raised level of plasminogen activator, which catalyses the conversion of plasminogen to plasmin. The local presence of plasmin can then be identified by degradation of an opaque fibrin monolayer in the same region. The technique can be roughly quantitated by comparing plaque diameters with those produced by known amounts of urokinase, and quantification by measuring the release of radioactivity from ^{125}I labelled fibrin has also been considered. Two practical problems in this approach are that wide variations in plasminogen activator concentration have been reported between one part of a tumour and another and that several normal cells and tissues, notably macrophages, are also capable of producing plasminogen activator.

These reports and many others lead to the conclusion that no biochemical properties specific and exclusive to tumour cells have yet been identified. It is therefore useful to think of the problem in terms of molecular inbalance, and Weber[57] has tried to correlate this with a degree of neoplasia. By examining in detail several different chemically-induced hepatomas which exhibited a broad spectrum of malignancies, he was able to identify three types of alteration in metabolic behaviour:

1. Malignancy-linked changes which correlated positively or negatively with tumour growth rate
2. Ubiquitous changes occurring in the majority of tumours but in a discontinuous fashion, and
3. Coincidental changes which varied continuously but showed no correlation with malignant behaviour.

Weber[57] listed over 60 biochemical discriminants that correlated with growth rate in hepatomas - many of them associated with the known increase in the level of DNA metabolism in tumour cells, so they may not be truly tumour specific. He also emphasised the need to try and correlate the changes in biochemical parameters with metabolic advantage to tumour cells. For instance, he suggested that the observed decrease in important enzymes for glyconeogenesis and the elevated levels of enzymes involved in glucose catabolism lead to increased glycolysis and a greater availability of precursors, notably ribose and NADPH, required for nucleic acid metabolism. There are several difficulties in extending this approach to human tumours, both because the system is much more restrictive and because their natural history is more variable. Some parameters will not be measurable, for example, if the methods used are not very sensitive and tissue supply is limited; inconsistencies in the results can then be expected. If correlation with malignancy is attempted, then the results will be open to widely differing interpretations - since histology, growth rate, net growth rate after cell loss (see below, under 'Cell cycle in tumours'), capacity to metastasise, and survival can all be used as criteria of malignancy. However, they are not always (indeed, one could almost say they are infrequently) correlated one with another. Most biochemical studies of human tumour-cell properties have been disappointing.

Studies on tumour-cell properties which may be related to specific hormonal behaviour have focused on mammary carcinoma, with most work being done on organ culture and tumour fragments. An early report which showed great promise was that of Salih et al,[58] who cultured breast tumours in media containing different concentrations of 17beta-oestradiol. On the basis of histological appearance and total dehydrogenase activity they were able to divide cases into quite distinct oestrogen-dependent and oestrogen-independent categories. They also reported that there then seemed to be a good correlation between <u>in vitro</u> steroid dependence and clinical progress on anti-oestrogenic therapy. In a later paper, the same group[59] suggested that the dependence of mammary tumour growth on prolactin could be evaluated in a similar manner. However, two more recent papers[60,61] have reported failure to confirm these findings. No significant hormone effects could be demonstrated in organ cultures of human breast carcinoma.

A slightly different approach to a similar problem has been proposed by Woods et al,[62] who have been looking for the milk protein lactalbumin and for oestrogen receptors in human breast carcinomas. On the basis of their own and other findings, they have suggested that the presence of oestrogen receptors alone does not guarantee response to endocrine therapy. However, detection of lactalbumin in the same tumour is taken as evidence that the oestrogen has not only bound to the cell receptor but has also modified DNA transcription. The frequency of detection of both oestrogen receptors and lactalbumin was quite close to the known response rate for mammary tumours to endocrine therapy. A closely-related study is that of Horne et al,[63] who used an enzyme-bridge immunoperoxidase technique to look for the presence of pregnancy-specific beta-glycoprotein and human placental lactogen in human tumours. A retrospective study of patients treated surgically between 1962 and 1966 suggested a good correlation between mean survival time and the presence of one or other of these protein hormones, especially pregnancy-specific beta-glycoprotein (Fig. 6). Both these approaches are now being subjected to prospective clinical trials.

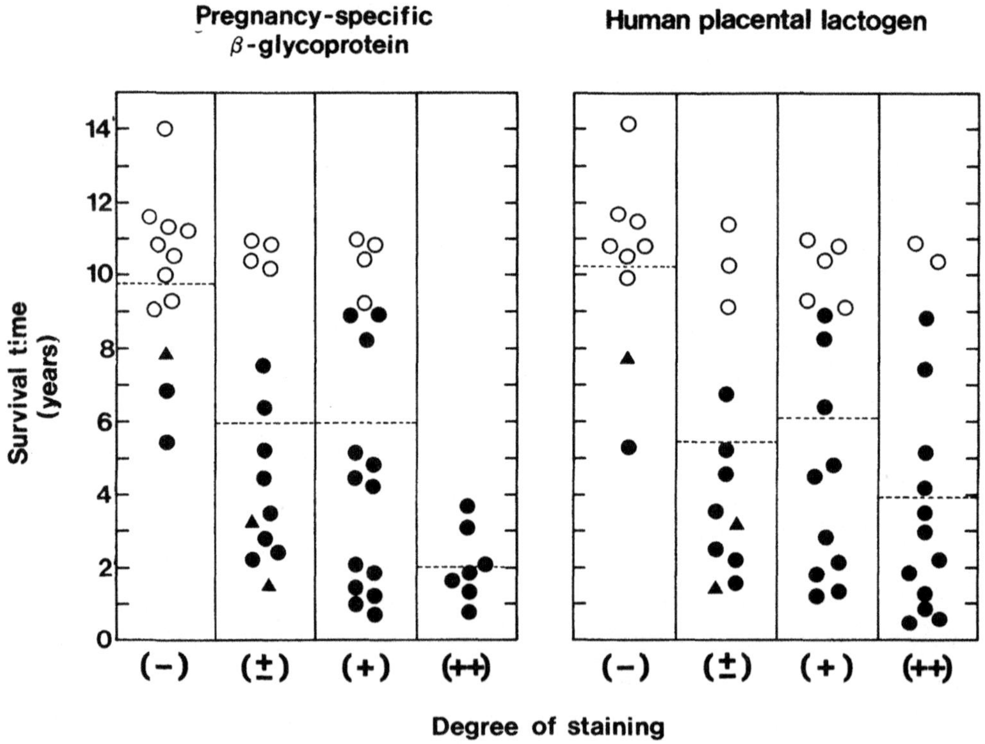

Fig. 6. The relationship between survival time and the degree of staining of pregnancy proteins, in patients with breast cancer (from Horne et al[63]) O alive and well ● dead ▲ death not due to breast cancer.

We generally favour the use of median rather than mean survival time, because it is less affected by one or two long-term survivors. However, the difference would be slight in this case, and neither method is very satisfactory when less than 50% of the patients have died, as in each of the left-hand columns.

Clearly there is much to be learned from this type of study on biopsy or surgical material about the variability of human tumours and maintenance of such cells in culture would be an advantage. However, technical problems have frustrated almost all attempts to establish monolayer cultures from human mammary carcinoma. Trempe[64] successfully established two cell lines from malignant pleural effusions secondary to breast cancer, but attempts with solid tumours - particularly scirrhous infiltrating duct carcinoma - have not been a success. Within a short time in culture, the fibroblastic component literally strangles the epithelial outgrowth, and attempts to avoid this problem by growing the cells on feeder layers have also proved disappointing.[65] Culture of this type of material would be invaluable in learning to combat breast cancer, and further intensive efforts are justified to improve cell separation techniques and enhance the viability of human mammary tumour cells in vitro.

By way of introduction to the next section - on tumour growth - two biochemical properties of the cell surface need to be considered. In each instance the possibility of a difference between tumour and normal cells was first suggested by work with virally-transformed cells. First came the observation[66] of increased agglutinability of tumour cells with plant lectins, e.g. concanavalin-A. Second, changes in surface glycoproteins (subsequently shown to be due to the presence of higher molecular weight glycopeptides in fucose-containing trypsin-labile glycoproteins) were reported in virally-transformed cells by Buck et al.[67] Both reports led to an intensive search for similar properties in human tumours. Van Beek et al[68] reported changes in molecular weight in the L-fucose-containing surface glycopeptides for tumour cells obtained from the peripheral blood of patients with active leukaemia or leukaemic transformation of lymphosarcoma. They emphasised that the observation related to only a minor part of the sialoglycoprotein cell surface and not to its total sialic acid content. Subsequent studies have shown that the presence of this high molecular weight component in tumour cells is, like its absence from the most similar control cells, a very widespread phenomenon and possibly universal. No more precise biochemical difference has been identified and this may be a general non-specific change in a whole group of molecules. On the other hand, the precise relevance of concanavalin-A agglutination tests to studies on human tumours remains controversial. Indeed, Smets et al[69] have shown that, in vitro, high concanavalin-A agglutinability can be dissociated from changes in surface glycoprotein of the type under discussion, which makes it unlikely that both properties can be closely correlated with malignancy.

Tumour cell growth behaviour

The cell surface plays a dominant role in cell growth and movement, and several studies have been made using time-lapse photography on cultured cells.[70] Ambrose[71] reported that normal BHK fibroblasts displayed a single fan-like pseudopodium, whereas transformed BHK-21 fibroblasts showed several independent pseudopodia. Fine microvilli formed in much the same way so that both normal and tumour cells showed similar movement in culture. The tumour cells, because they had several pseudopodia, tended to change direction of movement more frequently than the normal cells. Ambrose suggested that the larger size of tumour cells was due to the increased negative charges on their cell surfaces - which repel each other and cause the membrane to expand. The surface-change density of tumour cells has been extensively studied by electrophoresis. Among reports of other changes, Abercrobmie[72] found that sarcoma cells showed more tendency to pile up than to form normal fibroblastic monolayers, while Bell[73] made observations on normal and transformed T3T3 cells - noting that the tumour cells criss-crossed each other but normal cells did not. Tumour cells were not able to move over the exposed surfaces of other cells but infiltrated underneath them, remaining in contact with the substrate. Projan and Tanneberger[74] tried to confirm some of these observations for freshly-cultured human tumour cells and found that although malignant cells showed some contact inhibition of movement, it was less effective than in normal cells. Residual contact inhibition was very variable from one tumour-cell culture to another indicating considerable individuality of each histological type or, more probably, of each individual tumour. Decreased contact inhibition of movement may therefore not be a reliable index of malignancy; Turbitt and Curtis[75] found that contact inhibition differed with the age of the culture and with the density of cultured cells. Density-dependent inhibition of growth of normal cells in culture has been demonstrated, and many studies have shown that virally-transformed cells generally have a higher terminal density than their normal counterparts.

Studies on human tumour cells have been much more fragmentary. Westermark[76] found that a proportion of neoplastic human glial cells in culture were still sensitive to growth restraint induced by cell density, though the effect was never as complete as among normal cells. All neoplastic lines reached higher terminal cell densities than corresponding normal cells. (When investigating this phenomenon it is important that strict feeding regimes are followed, so that decrease in cell growth cannot be attributed to depletion of nutrients). To the pathologist, invasiveness provides an important distinction between benign and malignant tumours. Most in vitro studies of invasiveness have been on confrontations between embryonic and adult cells in monolayer, 90% of such studies being evaluated by light microscopy.[77] Adhesion of malignant cells to their substrate is believed to be the key initial event in invasion. The importance of the nature of the substrate has been demonstrated by studying adhesion of HeLa cells, hepatomas and transformed BHK-21 fibroblasts to substrates of connective tissue, mesenchyme and the basal and apical sides of epithelium.[78] The adhesion of non-malignant BHK cells to the same substrates was also studied, and all cells were found to adhere to substrates of connective tissue, mesenchyme and the basal side of epithelium. The apical side of intact epithelium proved to be non-adhesive, while perforated epithelium allowed adhesion only at the site of perforation; but HeLa cells adhered to the apical side of epithelium in the presence of dilysine. From this Ridder et al[78] concluded that long-range electrostatic repulsion might be responsible for the non-adhesive character of epithelia. Measurements of the forces required to separate pairs of comparable normal and malignant cells have been made by Coman,[79] who suggested that malignant cells showed less mutual adhesiveness than normal cells - and these observations have since been confirmed under standard conditions of agitation or aspiration.[80,81] Considerable evidence of a morphological and structural basis for the reduced mutual adhesiveness of tumour cells has been provided by electron-microscopy,[82] but adhesion studies do not yet permit a clear distinction between normal and tumour cells. Penetration also plays a very important role in invasiveness, as shown by comparing penetration of the chorioallantoic membrane of hen eggs by several cell lines with malignancy - assessed by the ability of the cells to form tumours in animals of the same strain from which the cells had been derived.[83] From Table V it can be seen that the degree of penetration corresponds closely with the degree of malignancy.

TABLE V

Depth of penetration into the chorioallantoic membrane by various cell types. The first three are considered non-malignant, the others being listed in increasing order of malignancy. (Adapted from Easty and Easty[83]).

Cell type	Percentages of cells penetrating to depths shown			
	0-30 μm	40-70 μm	80-120 μm	130-160 μm
BHK 21	99.5	0.5		
L	99.5	0.5		
Peritoneal Macrophages	96	4		
P4	97.3	2.7		
GP hepatoma	99	1		
SP	93	6.5		
Walker	55	37	8	
P4 T	52	4	2.4	
PyY	69	23	9	
SV109	88	8	3	1
H-P melanoma	72	15	11	2

However, as long ago as 1935 Santesson[84] noted that while the more anaplastic carcinomas actively infiltrated normal fibroblasts, highly-differentiated mammary tumours did not do so, but simply pushed them back. It should not be assumed that tumour cells are always invasive.

The interaction of normal squamous epithelium, normal connective tissue, and intra-apithelial neoplasia from human uterine cervix in monolayer culture has been studied by Willbanks et al,[85] who found that normal epithelium caused retraction and detachment of normal fibroblasts and of intra-epithelial neoplastic cells. But invasion of normal epithelial sheets by the neoplastic cells was never observed. They concluded that the different cell types in this system compete for the substrate and that the dominant cells appear to be those of normal cervical epithelium. The interactions of several malignant and normal cell types with human decidua graviditatis are summarised in Table VI, from which it can be seen that the malignant cells caused considerable destruction of the decidual cells. Several authors have reported the destruction of normal cells in the region of tumour cell invasion. In

TABLE VI

Interactions of malignant and normal cell types with human decidua graviditatis (after Schleich et al[86])

Cell type (Normal cells below)	Effect on decidua graviditatis Adhesion to surface	Migration over surface	Invasion	Injury
HeLa	+++	+++	+++	++
AFi sarcoma	+	-	+++	+++
Lymphoblastoid cells	+	-	+++	+++
HeLa clone S3	++	++	-	++
FL (amnion)	+	++	-	+
Girardi heart	+	+	-	-
Fetal lung	+	-	-	-
Endometrium	+	-	-	-
Normal lymphocytes	+	+	(+)	-

- none + detecable ++ moderate +++ intense (+) questionable

studies of normal human kidney cells and virus transformed KB cells in culture, Kruse and Patterson[87] found that there was marked inhibition of RNA and DNA synthesis in normal cells that were in direct contact with malignant ones. Mareel et al[88] studied the interactions of malignant and non-malignant cells with chick blastoderm cells, and found that repair of the lower layer of the chick blastoderm was inhibited at the site of transplanted malignant cells, but not at the site of transplanted normal cells. They proposed this transplantation method as a means of distinguishing malignant from normal cells. The properties of migration and invasion are of course not confined to tumour cells. Their behaviour should be compared and contrasted with that of primitive normal cells, e.g. primitive germ cells[89,90] during embryological development. Another tumour-like property is the ability of malignant cells to grow in semi-solid media, but normal cells do sometimes form colonies in agar, so this may not provide a reliable criterion for distribution between cell types. However, colony formation in agar has been shown to be a suitable method for monitoring cell survival after chemotherapy.[91]

To summarise this section so far, we can say that the characteristics of growth behaviour discussed - namely, abnormal cell movement, decreased contact inhibition, growth to a high terminal cell density, invasiveness and destruction of normal tissues, and growth in soft agar - are all frequently associated with malignant cells. However none provides a universal marker for malignancy because there are exceptions to each.

'Tumorigenicity' (i.e. the ability of transplanted cells to form tumours in animals of the same strain, 'the sygeneic host') is generally considered to be the best test for epithelial transformation in animal systems, and growth may now be obtained from human tumour cells implanted in immunosuppressed or genetically athymic nude mice. However, there are a number of problems associated with this technique. For example, growth of human tumour cells in nude mice may be taken as evidence of malignancy but not as proof.[92] Also, different tumour cell types show considerable variability in growth rate - which is often very slow. The xenograft method does not therefore provide a system for quick assessment of drug effects, for instance, although it may provide a method for validating predictive tests for drug sensitivity based on short-term culture. Before the xenograft system can be employed extensively for investigations in human tumours, data are required on whether prolonged serial passage alters the characteristics of the human primary from which they were derived. Houghton and Taylor[93] found that histological integrity was maintained for up to ten serial passages of human colo-rectal tumour xenografts. The passaged tumours also retained human lactate dehydrogenase and glucose-6-phosphate dehydrogenase isoenzyme patterns and a human chromosome constitution. However, the cell kinetics of these xenografts differed from those of the primary tumour from which they were derived.[94] Thus the xenograft technique offers a powerful new method for the study of human tumour cells but further work is required to determine how faithfully the cells retain their in vivo properties.

Miscellaneous tests for tumour cells

Three physical techniques now being used to study cancer cells and tissues need to be considered. The first is nuclear magnetic resonance (NMR), which enables the degree of structure of tissue water to be assessed by measuring the spin-lattice relaxation time (T_1) of the magnetic moments of hydrogen nuclei in applied magnetic fields, as first suggested by Damadian.[95] Reduced structuring of tissue water associated with abnormalities such as tumours would be expected to produce an increase in the T_1 value. NMR studies have now been performed in normal and malignant tissues by many groups[96,97] and an increase in the T_1 of the tumour over the corresponding normal tissue from the same patient has generally been observed. Although there are notable exceptions, and there is sometimes considerable overlap of results from normal and malignant samples of the same tissue from different patients, Koutcher et al[98] reported successful discrimination between normal and malignant tissues in 84 out of 89 colon, breast and lung samples. They also reported that histologically normal tissue adjacent to malignant colonic tissue showed comparable elevation of the NMR malignancy index. By combining the NMR technique, which gives an average for intra- and extra-cellular water, with immersion refractometry for determination of intracellular water alone, Gordon and Ross (personal communication) have demonstrated a definite increase in intracellular water in experimentally-induced rat liver tumour cells, compared with normal cells from non tumour-bearing animals. In addition, a smaller increase in intracellular water was shown in non-neoplastic liver cells from tumour-bearing rats. Intracellular water content and NMR values correlated well, and it was concluded that an appreciable portion of the increase in water content of malignant liver must be intracellular. In general, though, it is unlikely that changes in NMR signal will ever provide an absolute marker of malignancy, if the effect is due solely to changes in water content - which are almost certainly secondary. Other pathological states, such as inflammatory reactions, can also give rise to increases in tissue water which are probably indistinguishable from malignancy when tested by NMR alone. Nevertheless, the technique may give useful information in certain circumstances.

Closely related to NMR is the technique of electron spin resonance spectroscopy in which energy is absorbed from a magnetic field applied across a sample by unpaired electrons. Two mechanisms by which carcinogenesis could cause changes in electron pairing are changes in free radical concentrations and variations in paramagnetic ion concentration in the tissue. Some experimental evidence for both these mechanisms has been reported. Slater[99] investigated normal and malignant human tissues, and found greatly reduced free-radical signals in two samples of cervical cancer, compared with the corresponding normal tissues. More recently Dodd and Silcock[100] investigated the electron spin resonance signal due to paramagnetic ions in rat Yoshida sarcoma (an implanted muscle tumour) and found changes in the tumour, thought to be associated with inflammatory or immune reactions, within one day of implantation. Further signal changes were found during development of the tumour, and the presence of metastases in the regional lymph nodes was readily demonstrated. However, these features have not been found to reflect properties of tumours in general, and the future role - if any - of electron spin resonance in the diagnosis of malignancy remains uncertain.

The third technique, developed by Cercek and Cercek,[101] is the use of fluorescence polarisation to study the structure of the cytoplasmic matrix. Cells in suspension are treated with fluorescent dye and exposed to polarised light at a frequency which will excite fluorescence, the degree of fluorescence polarisation produced being directly related to the level of structure in the cytoplasmic matrix. Using the equipment shown schematically in Fig. 7, measurements of the light transmitted are made alternately when the polariser is vertical and horizontal. When untreated lymphocytes from different patients were studied, no significant differences were found in the polarisation value, P. If the cells were first treated with phytohaemagluttinin, however, the normal cells showed a 20 to 50% decrease in P, but those

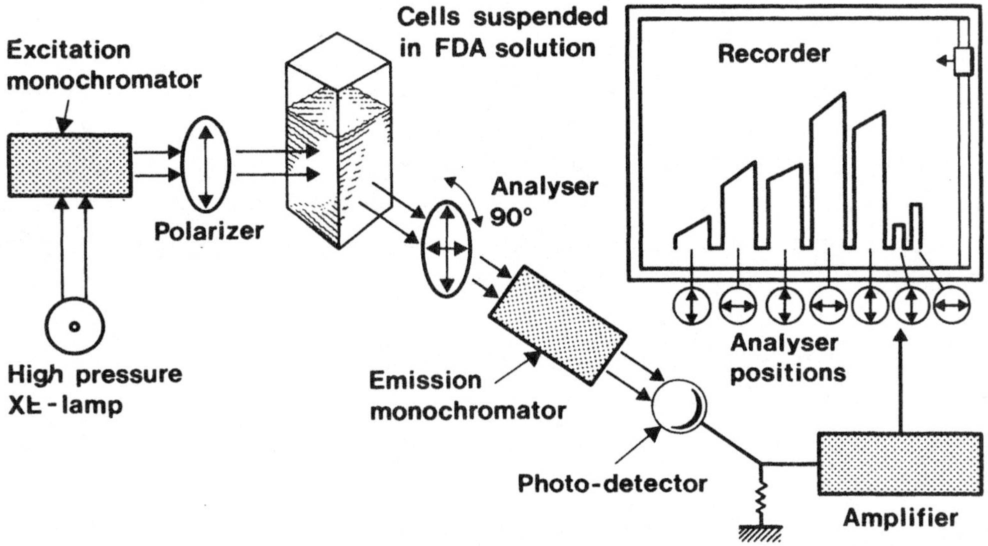

Fig. 7. Stages in fluorescence polarisation for the study of biological structures (from Cercek and Cercek[101]).

from cancer patients were little affected. By contrast, if the cells were first treated with cancer basic protein those from cancer patients showed a decrease in P, but the normal cells were unaffected. By calculating the response ratio between these P values, malignant conditions could be almost completely separated out. Since the lymphocytes were chosen from a very broad spectrum of malignancies, this may be a useful technique for detecting human cancers and leukaemias.

Other possibilities for recognising tumour cells include identification of the viral genome, the possibility of a high level of reverse transcriptase, and antigenetic tests. All these subjects are extremely complex, not infrequently controversial (e.g. arguments for and against the viral origins of cancer) and have little practical application to human tumour cells at present. The fact that none of them has anything in common with the three methods outlined above highlights the broad spectrum of disciplines now attacking the problem of the cancer cell.

THE CELL CYCLE IN TUMOURS

Since tumour growth is the macroscopic consequence of uncontrolled cell division, a study of the cell division cycle of tumour cells may be fundamental to our understanding of the problem. Furthermore, the effects of both ionising radiation and chemotherapeutic drugs on a cell population will depend on the distribution of the proliferating cells in the cell cycle and on the proportion of non-cycling cells. More knowledge of this and a better understanding of tumour cell kinetics ought to lead to improved treatment schedules. The various stages of the cycle of human tumour cells follow the same sequence as those of the normal cell (Fig. 1), and the S phase can be identified autoradiographically in tumour cells, as in normal ones, by means of a radioactive DNA precursor (usually tritiated thymidine). The percentage of labelled cells in the whole population, the labelling index (LI), gives the proportion of cells that were in S phase during contact with the tracer. Like normal cells, tumour cells are recognisable in mitosis, the percentage of the entire population in this phase constituting the mitotic index (MI). The features of tumour-cell population kinetics which have been most frequently studied <u>in vivo</u> are:

1. The mitotic cycle of the proliferating cell
2. The size of the non-proliferating cell pool (if any) and the capacity of these cells to return to the cycle and
3. The extent of cell loss.

As intimated in the introduction, measurements of the cell cycle and the duration of its phases are restricted in human tumours for ethical reasons. A major concern has been that because tritiated thymidine is incorporated specifically into DNA, and the mean range of the emitted beta-particles in tissue is only about 1 μm, the DNA strands themselves would receive excessive radiation. It has been confirmed that tritiated thymidine is more harmful to cells both in vitro and in vivo than, say, tritiated water of equal radioactivity. However, a number of workers, including one of the authors (Dendy, unpublished), have looked into this question, and the enhancement factor is probably only about ten - somewhat less than feared. Straus et al[102] have recently reported that, after giving tritiated thymidine intravenously to nine patients with advanced malignant disease, most of the dose was found to have been rapidly excreted; only about 20% of tritiated thymidine was incorporated into the DNA. They also stated that since most of the energy resides in rapidly proliferating tissue, the energy deposition per cell will be limited by cell division. These considerations led them to conclude that the importance of studying cell kinetics in patients with cancers justified the doses of tritiated thymidine required. However, their own calculations show that the dose rate to the nucleus could be as high as 0.041 Gy (4.1 rads) per day, which means that the effective biological dose is not inconsiderable. The question of giving tritiated thymidine intravenously to patients for cell-cycle kinetic studies therefore remains extremely controversial.

Because of these problems, a new method recently described by Chang et al[103] is of particular importance. This enables the percentage of cells in S phase in human tumour biopsies to be estimated by means of an antinucleoside antibody technique. The method can be applied to frozen sections (which have had no chance to adapt to in vitro conditions) and is based on the fact that antinucleoside antibodies - rabbit anti-guanosine immunoglubulin conjugated to horseradish peroxidase, in this instance - will react specifically with single-stranded DNA which is exposed for binding only during S phase. The authors showed excellent correlation between the labelling index obtained by this method and that produced by tritiated thymidine exposure in fine-needle aspirates of human tumours. The method is applicable to biopsies from mammary and head and neck tumours, but has not yet been applied to other types of tumour.

Some determinations have been made of human tumour cell kinetics in vivo, the most commonly used method for assessing the duration of the cell cycle and its phases being the percentage labelled mitoses (PLM) curve. This is obtained by scoring the percentage of labelled mitotic cells at regular time intervals after injection of tritiated thymidine. Theoretically, after a time interval corresponding to the G_2 phase, all cells entering mitosis should be labelled (since they would have been in S phase at the time of injection). After a further period equivalent in duration to the S phase the percentage of labelled mitoses suddenly drops

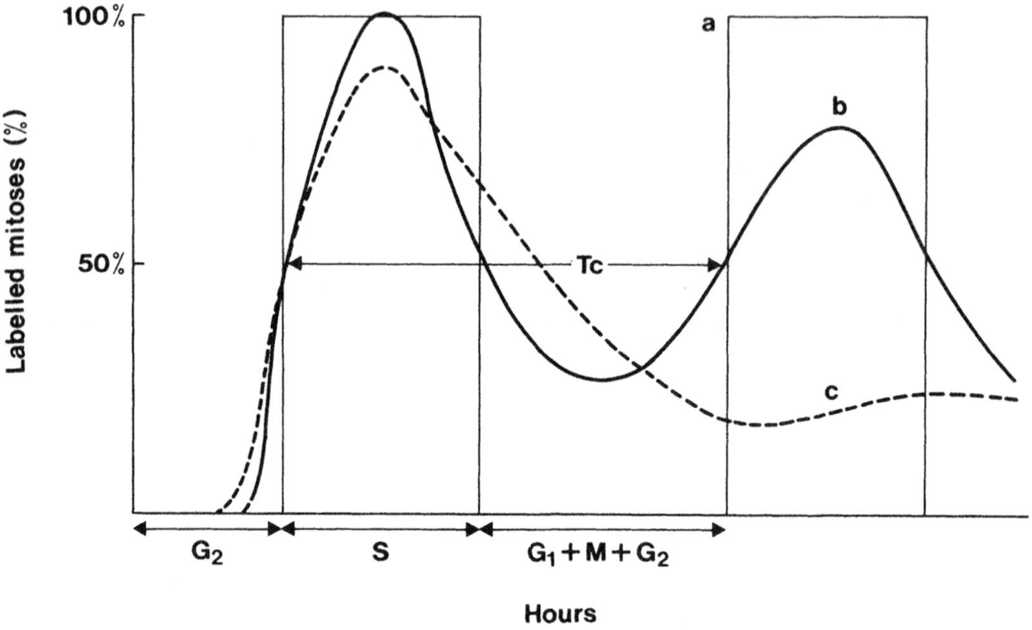

Fig. 8. The percentage of dividing cells which are labelled changes with time after a short exposure to tritiated thymidine. Theoretical percentage neglecting time spent in mitosis (a), compared with findings for an established cell line in vitro - e.g. HeLa (b), and for an actively-growing tumour in vivo (c).

to zero. The curve will however return to 100% when the labelled cells pass round the cycle once more (Fig. 8). When measurements are made on a cell line which has been maintained in culture for some time, the results approximate quite well to the theoretical behaviour. An estimate of the cell-cycle duration may then be made by determining the time interval between the 50% point on the ascending limb of the first curve and the same point on the second curve. However, for human tumours labelled in vivo, the second peak of the PLM curve is often ill-defined.[94,104] This makes it impossible to estimate the duration of the cell cycle or its phases with any accuracy. Another limitation is that such investigations can be performed only on large, easily accessible tumours with a high mitotic index - which are probably not representative of all human solid tumours. Tubiana and Malaise[1] have reviewed data for 31 such tumours. The median cell-cycle time was about two days, but the main feature was variation in all relevant measurements. Some of these are shown in Table VII, and similar variations were recorded for the lengths of the cell-cycle phases. The cell-cycle time and S-phase duration did not appear to vary with

TABLE VII

Doubling times (DT) and labelling indices (LI) for various human tumours. From this data and other information, the growth fraction (GF) and cell loss factor can be estimated (from Tubiana and Malaise[1]).

Histological type	DT (days)	LI (%)	GF (%)	Cell loss factor (%)
Embryonal tumours	27	30	90	93
Malignant lymphoma	29	29	90	94
Mesenchymal sarcoma	41	15	15	76
Squamous cell carcinoma	58	8	25	89
Adenocarcinoma	83	2	6	56

histological type - which did, however, correlate with the labelling index and doubling time. The spread of cell-cycle times is generally wider in human solid tumours than in experimental tumours.[105,106] For instance, ascitic tumours in animals have a lengthening of the cell cycle during growth; and this, together with other differences in cell kinetics, makes them questionable models for human solid tumours.

Since in vivo studies are restricted in man, tissue culture might be a way to provide more detailed studies of tumour cell kinetics. This has proved to be the case with measurements of the cell cycle by time-lapse cinematography, particularly when combined with autoradiography,[107] and there are various methods by which cells growing in culture can be synchronised into the same phase of the cell cycle.[108] However, several of the techniques used on cells established in culture cannot yet be applied to tumour cells recently explanted from a patient.

The work of Hoshino et al[109] is of considerable interest because it permits comparison of in vivo and in vitro data. These workers took biopsies from several human gliomas which had been labelled in vivo with tritiated thymidine, before culturing pieces of tumour tissue and measuring the labelling index after different periods in culture (Table VIII). In general, the labelling index in primary cultures agreed with that found in the original tumours but gradually decreased during the culture period. This suggests that a greater proportion of the cell population became capable of cycling after the cells were transferred to in vitro conditions, since division of cells which had not been labelled in vivo then reduced the proportion of labelled cells. A 'double labelling' technique using tritiated (^{3}H) and ^{14}C

TABLE VIII

The change in labelling index for various brain tumour cells maintained in culture. The figures given are generally averages of more than one independent measurement made during the periods shown (adapted from Hoshino et al[109]).

Tumour type	Average labelling index of biopsy specimen	Percentage of labelled cells after: 1-4 days	5-9 days	10-20 days
Glioblastoma	8.1	8.0	6.0	3.2
Glioblastoma	4.5	4.5	4.7	1.3
Astrocytoma	5.4	5.0	3.6	1.3
Astrocytoma	2.2	2.9	0.8	-
Secondaries in brain	6.3	(0.1)	5.0	2.2

thymidine was also used to study cells transferred from primary explant into secondary cultures, and the labelling indices of transferred cultures again contrasted sharply with those of the primary cultures. The pulse labelling index was very high during the first few days after passage, indicating that the transferred cells proliferated at a higher rate - which dropped one week after passage. A similar pattern was also observed with long-term established human glioma cultures. Hoshino[110] has earlier shown that the duration of the S phase in human glioma cells was fairly constant through passage in culture and close to its duration in vivo. This finding has been largely confirmed by Lepont[111] who obtained nearly pure populations of G_1 cells (identified by DNA content) from mouse Ehrlich ascites, which he subsequently cultured without observing any difference in the duration of the cell cycle in these cells from those of the original population. There are very few other reports of this type of correlation being attempted. Clearly more research is necessary to establish how the kinetic behaviour of cells in culture compares with their behaviour in vivo.

At any one time, a significant fraction of the cells in a tissue are not engaged in active proliferation. This may have a considerable effect on the response of the tumour to radiotherapy or chemotherapy. The growth fraction (GF) was defined by Mendelsohn[112] as the ratio between the number of cycling cells and the total number of cells in a tissue. A number of methods and models have been constructed to estimate the GF in tumours,[112-14] and a few direct measurements have been made on experimental solid tumours. When the growth rate slows down as the tumour gets bigger, the GF appears to diminish slightly,[115] and it is also smaller in slowly growing tumours.[114] Using continuous thymidine infusion, Clarkson et al[116] found the GF to lie between 15 and 90% in ascitic tumours. And Bennington,[117] using a single pulse of tritiated thymidine, reported a GF of about 50% in the most actively proliferating areas of squamous carcinoma of the human cervix. Closely related to the idea of a growth fraction are the concepts of G_0 phase and tumour stem cells. The existence and kinetic behaviour of stem cells have been well documented in normal tissues, especially in the haemopoietic system; some of these cells, while retaining the potential for replication, are not in cycle and have been assigned to the G_0 phase. The possibility that some tumour cells are in a G_0 phase has frequently been discussed, but the durations of cell-cycle phases, especially the G_1 phase, are so heterogeneous in solid tumours and sometimes so prolonged that a cell-cycle time cannot be properly defined (see Fig. 8). Therefore the fact that the labelling index with continuous administration of tritiated thymidine may fail to reach 100% within the course of an experiment does not enable a cell which might be in the G_0 phase to be distinguished from one which is in cycle, but has an extremely long G_1 phase. Even if it is conceded that a G_0 phase exists in solid tumours, there is no evidence either way on whether or not cells that entered it could return to the cell cycle.

Numerous attempts have been made to relate cell-cycle time to tumour-volume doubling time. For an exponentially growing population there is a direct relation between the two, but the volume-doubling time is longer, often considerably longer, than the cell-cycle time *in vivo*, because not all the tumour cells are in cycle at once and because there is cell loss from tumours. The term 'cell loss' includes not only cell death within the bounds of the tumour but also cell migration to other parts of the body via lymph or blood or exfoliation into body cavities and fluids. An estimate of cell loss is obtained by comparing the potential doubling time of the population of tumour cells (i.e. the time required to bring about 100% increase in the number of cells if losses did not occur) with the actual doubling time. The potential doubling time may be assessed by measurement of the thymidine labelling index coupled with estimates of the length of the DNA synthetic period,[118] or by measurement of the mitotic index,[119] the rate of cell loss usually being expressed as a fraction of the cell birth rate. Estimates range from 50 to 90% of new cell production in human tumours.[118-19] Cell losses from human solid tumours can clearly be considerable - which helps to explain why the doubling times average as much as 30 to 90 times longer than the duration of the cell cycle.[1]

Turning briefly to clinical aspects, it must be admitted that the precise relevance of tumour cell-cycle kinetic parameters to prognosis remains uncertain. Tubiana and Malaise[1] concluded that there is a significant correlation between tumour growth rate and survival, but in a recent study of head and neck cancer

Nervi et al[120] could find no correlation between response to treatment and any of the kinetic parameters studied (growth rate, intermitotic time, growth fraction, cell loss and DNA content), even when the cancers were grouped according to their clinical growth characteristics. Similarly, attempts to synchronise pulses of drug or radiation therapy to solid tumours, so that they are given when a high proportion of cells are in a sensitive phase of the cell cycle, have been largely unsuccessful. Limited success has been reported by Price et al[121] and Stathopoulos et al[122] for head and neck cancers, but it can be argued that this improvement was due to better protection of the normal cells rather than a more effective attack on the tumour cells. The method cannot be expected to be generally effective for solid tumours in which only a small percentage of cells are in cycle at any one time.

One clinical applicaion of cell-cycle kinetic studies which is yielding more promising results is an attempt to monitor tumour response to therapy. For reasons already discussed, this is extremely difficult, but introduction of the impulse cytophotometer has renewed interest. Several groups are working on either myeloblastic or lymphocytic leukaemia, and one of the earliest reports came from Hillen et al[123] who used pulse cytophotometry to look at DNA distributions in cells from freshly aspirated bone marrow. They found that the presence of a high percentage of cells in S phase was associated with a good prognosis for chemotherapy with cytosine arabinoside - either alone or in combination with thioguanine or daunomycin. This percentage remained high at the time of complete remission, but a later drop in the percentage S phase cells was early evidence of a relapse. More recently, Smets et al[124] have shown a positive correlation between cytophotometric changes and clinical effects following chemotherapy for 17 out of 19 patients with leukaemia and lymphosarcoma. Pulse cytophotometry gave a correct indication of drug insensitivity for five patients - which suggests that this might provide the basis for a drug sensitivity test. However, while pulse cytophotometry is being applied to study of cell-cycle kinetics in various increasingly sophisticated in vitro systems, a number of technical problems, notably tumour sampling, tissue disaggregation and separation of normal from tumour cells has limited its use from human tumours to a few rather specialised, though important, cases.

CONCLUSIONS

The foregoing survey of current knowledge of tumour cells and of their cell-cycle kinetics was written with a view to stimulating further research in the areas where it is most needed. Although the many features that have so far been considered are for the most part fairly typical of tumour cells, none of them constitute unequivocal markers. Moreover, many are based on experimental systems that have not been fully validated for human tumour cells. When Billiau et al[125] cultured 47 sepparate human tumours, most of them sarcomatous, although some of the cultures showed evidence of tumour origin, including aberrant karyotypes, none complied with the currently accepted in vitro criteria of malignancy such as lack of topo-inhibition and high-density growth. A similar picture was revealed by Smith et al[126] when they tried to characterise human tumour cells in tissue cultures derived from osteogenic sarcomas. The parameters measured were saturation density, cell morphology, growth pattern, growth on contact inhibited monolayers of normal fibroblastic epithelial cells, and tumorigenecity in immunosuppressed mice. While each tumour cell line showed some, none showed all of the abnormal growth properties usually associated with malignant transformation. Over the course of many years, Pontén has made a careful study of more than 100 biopsies from human brain tumours, 25 of which gave glioma cell lines. Reviewing this work recently[127] he reported equivocal findings from nearly all his tests for tumour cells - including plating in agarose, agglutination with concanavalin-A, production of plasminogen activator and the presence or absence of actin cables. The only consistent feature was that tumour cells always grew to a higher terminal saturation density. Pontén has suggested that there may be limitless variation in the phenotypes expressed in different glioma cells and that the essence of malignancy is the ability to retain such altered phenotypic aberrations for several generations. If this is correct, then study of individual phenotypes should reveal the particular methods of counteracting growth employed by different tumours. On the same reasoning, several attempts have been made to develop individualised chemotherapy from the results of predictive tests on the patient's own tumour cells.[128]

If in vitro work with human tumour material is planned, features of malignancy will be required at the single cell level that satisfy certain criteria. The tests concerned should be:

1. Applicable to tissue cultures
2. Easy to perform soon after exploration
3. Quantitative both for degree of malignancy and for the proportion of malignant cells in the cell population, and
4. Specific, with few false positives or false negatives.

At the same time

5. The findings should correlate well with tumorigenesis.

The results of our own work, and those of others, show that when human tumour cells have an abnormal karyotype or DNA value this provides a reasonably stable criterion of malignancy, even when the cells are taken into culture. Of the two,

DNA measurements can be obtained more quickly and easily than karyotype studies so this may be the best single specific marker currently available, but - as indicated above - multiple criteria will frequently be necessary. It is clear that future work on tumour-cell properties must concentrate more on the diverse nature of human tumour cells recently removed from patients and less on animal model systems.

The problem of defining cancer cells is greatly complicated by changes in other cells and tissues - either away from the site of the tumour (as noted with scanning electron-microscope and nuclear magnetic resonance studies) or in cells not thought to be malignant (as with the structuredness of cytoplasmic matrix). Furthermore, Smith et al[126] have reported that although skin fibroblasts from osteosarcoma patients appeared normal in vitro, they showed a greater ability than normal fibroblasts to grow in immunusuppressed mice. Closely related is the work of Azzarone[129] and his colleagues[130] who also studied skin fibroblasts from patients with tumours. Compared with fibroblasts from healthy subjects, these cells showed better growth in low serum concentrations, better growth in soft agar, and growth to a higher saturation density - all properties usually associated with tumour cells. Although the possibility of tumour cell contamination in the fibroblast cultures cannot be entirely excluded, the balance of evidence suggests that fibroblasts from patients with neoplastic disease have an above-normal tendency to malignant transformation. The implication of these reports is that changes at the cellular level associated with malignant disease may extend far beyond those regions histologically identifiable as tumour.

Studies of cell-cycle kinetics for human tumours have so far been rather disappointing. The work is immensely difficult because of the extremely heterogeneous behaviour of the cells and the ethical problems associated with in vivo studies; the method developed by Chang et al[99] which may permit in vitro assay of human tumour-cell kinetics could therefore be very important.

No differences in cell-cycle behaviour such as might be exploited for either diagnosis or therapy have yet been identified between normal and tumour cells. The reciprocal relationship between loss of control of cell division in tumours and the orderly enhanced control of cell division during embryological development probably deserves further study, while attempts to monitor responses of solid tumours to therapy by investigating cell-cycle kinetics are beginning to produce some promising results. The length of this article - which only touches some aspects of the problem of characterising malignant cells - is indicative of the immense amount of work already done on human tumour cells and their cell-cycle behaviour. Much more remains to be done and fresh approaches using new techniques would be welcome.

We acknowledge with thanks permission from the undernoted authors to reproduce or adapt their data:-

S.I. Hajdu (Table 1), C.P. Miles (Table II), B. Hainau (Table III), G.C. Easty (Table V), A. Schleich (Table VI), M. Tubiana (Table VI), T. Hoshino (Table VIII), Phywe Ltd., Gottingen, W. Germany (Fig. 3), C.H.W. Horne (Fig. 6), and L. Cercek (Fig. 7).

We would like to thank the Head of Department, Professor J.R. Mallard, for his encouragement of our own contribution to this work. Financial support from the Cancer Research Campaign is also gratefully acknowledged.

QUESTIONS FOR THE FUTURE

Following this detailed review of the characteristics of malignant cells - and by way of a link with the subsequent contribution on future prospects for cancer research - it may be helpful to consider ten forward-looking questions that Philip Dendy put to the meeting as a basis for discussion, together with some of his own comments:

1. Which of the approaches noted above - human or animal, in vivo or in vitro - deserve further intensive study?

2. What alternative systems for studying the cancer problem are available? How, for example, might the placenta be used?

3. Is a more intensive study of cell-to-cell interactions and intercellular junctions required? What are the prospects for elucidating the chemical nature of intracellular junctions?

4. Is short-term monolayer culture a worthwhile technique for studying the properties of human tumour cells? And, if so, how can it be improved?

5. Are any of the properties, so far attributed to tumour cells, sufficiently characteristic to be exploitable for cancer management, or do we need an entirely fresh approach?

6. Can we expect any useful information from a study of tumour cell-cycle kinetics in the foreseeable future?

7. Do G_0 phase cells exist in solid tumours, or is this a misleading concept?

8. Are there significant differences in drug sensitivity between the cells from different tumours? And does a primary tumour and its metastases show the same chemosensitivity response spectrum?

9. What new physical techniques can be used to study the cancer problem?

10. What are the prospects for prevention, earlier detection, cure?

Without seeking to answer his own questions, Philip Dendy concluded by stressing the value of bringing research workers and clinicians together from a very wide range of disciplines to consider such fundamental problems. In writing the foregoing review, Rosalind Meldrum and he had both been impressed - like many other workers - by numerous similarities between tumour and embryonic cells. Yet there is a crucial difference. Embryonic cells know when to switch off the cell cycle; tumour cells have forgotten. Should research be directed towards a 'tumour cell re-education programme' - so that the processes of dedifferentiation that the tumour cell has undergone might be halted and reversed? If that could be accomplished, and applied clinically, a tumour at any site - and even the patient who presents with advanced malignant disease and multiple secondaries - should be amenable to cure.

DISCUSSION

Prospects for cancer research

'Some 15 years ago', said Peter Beaconsfield 'Bob Harris was brave enough to commit to paper his idea on the prospects for cancer research over the next decade (Cancer, Pelican Books, 1962). In brief, he considered it then under four main headings:

1. Hormone dependence
2. Techniques for virus studies
3. Chemotherapy, and
4. Immunological aspects.

Time has shown that his informed guesswork was remarkably good - which may have something to do with his accepting my invitation to repeat the exercise and outline his prospects for the next ten years.'

R. J. C. Harris took the structural differences between normal and cancer cells (outlined by Philip Dendy) as his starting point, and commented that most past attempts to distinguish them had become bogged down because the karyotype looked the same. However, in the case of virus transformation, it became possible to detect a number of spots in the resulting cancer cells which showed physical evidence of integrated virus DNA. Everyone then looked forward to finding one chromosome, and even a single spot on it, which gave rise to neoplastic change. That is no longer a reasonable expectation. 'Too many things have been shown to happen in too many spots. I believe,' Dr. Harris went on, 'that the way is opening now, for the first time - through the technique known as genetic manipulation - for us to find out exactly what these altered spots in virus transformed cells imply. The only assumption required is that the virus DNA sits at a particular spot because local conditions there are favourable to the production of specific effects - and those can now be investigated.

'In the so-called shotgun experiment, used for genetic manipulation, enzymes are employed to split the total genome of a tissue into small portions. Each small portion can be incorporated into a vector of some kind, a phage or a plasmid, and thus used to transform bacteria. It is then possible to clone the particular piece of DNA - producing not merely litres but even hundreds or thousands of litres . Biologically there is no limit, but in the United Kingdom the Health and Safety Executive have laid down the limits of what they regard as safe experimentation. In other countries - which may be broader-minded or less conscious of the possible consequences of making large quantities - libraries of human DNA have been set up. Some of these consist of thousands of small pots containing bit 1, bit 2, bit 3, bit 4, and so on - each representing human genes, in effect, but referred to as 'bits' because they have not yet been identified. Various means of identification are already available, though it will take time to work through all the material, and research in this field should help to clarify the structural differences between malignant and normal cells. By studying the bits of oncogenic DNA that become integrated into the genome, it ought to be possible to find out why certain sites are preferred, what is adjacent to the oncogenic bit, whether a normal bit has been dropped from the cell's own DNA to make room for it and, if so, what has been dropped. The sites concerned are likely to be specific, not on one chromosome but in certain parts of the total genome. This would need to be done on normal tissue of some kind, and perhaps those interested in the placenta could say whether it is suitable for the purpose. It could probably be handled in the same way for different species, to provide reference material for man, mouse, guinea pig, rat and so on. Before long, a picture should begin to emerge of the functions performed by particular bits of DNA at particular sites - both in normal cells and in the course of malignant transformation by oncogenic viruses.

'But what about all the human cancers that have nothing to do with viruses, or do not appear to have. If you want a real prediction, my personal impression is that, when this genetic manipulation starts on human cells, we shall find remnants of any number of oncogenic viruses that have cropped up during man's evolutionary history, but which are no longer readily recognisable as such now. They might just be identified by their 'fingerprints' that still persist. I am always very perturbed to read about so-called 'nonsense' DNA. Is this simply a means of concealing ignorance on the part of those who use the term, or does it really mean DNA that has no function. It offends me, evolutionarily, to think that something which does nothing is still retained. That would be remarkably uneconomic and unevolutionary, but one can only speculate on the origins, present physiological functions and possible pathological role of such DNA fragments - pending the outcome of future research.' Dr. Harris also speculated that it might become possible to study teratogenesis directly in feto-placental preparations, rather than whole pregnant animals, and went on to propose vaccine studies towards the end of pregnancy. In monkeys, for instance, which attain immunological competence in the last third of gestation, active immunisation against oncogenic and other agents might be accomplished by modifying the immune balance between placenta and fetus.

Areas of cancer research

Satisfactory discussion of cancer research is made difficult both by the vast size of the subject and by the natural tendency of experts to pull in different directions dictated by their own personal interests. As chairman, Peter Beaconsfield therefore sought to impose some order on the discussion by dividing research into three areas: pre-DNA synthesis, i.e. the availability, supply, and formation of precursors, together with the numerous factors that influence those processes, the stage of DNA synthesis, i.e. replication and repair, and the post-DNA phase. Taking the field as a whole, more money, more time, more scientific resources and more thought have been devoted to cancer research than to almost any other biological topic, yet no specific morphological, chemical or physical differences have been shown between carcinomatous and normal tissues. A major reason for this failure may be the fact that by far the greatest volume of work has been done on the post-DNA phase: immunological aspects of cell behaviour, biochemical and other characteristics of tumour cells, studies of oncodevelopmental proteins - the so-called markers - and even epidemiological research. All these are, in Peter Beaconsfield's view, peripheral to the main issue, a classic example of locking the stable after the horse has gone. But they can be studied by familiar techniques, and that is probably why such vast resources - in brains, money and time - have gone into the investigation and measurement of processes that are in reality end results. What we need to know is what initiates neoplasia in the cell about to undergo malignant change.

Therapeutic and prophylactic advance also lag far behind research expenditure. Overall, the death rate from cancer has changed little in the past few decades, and the prognosis is improved in only a few very specialised instances, such as the reticuloses, prostatic carcinoma, and choriocarcinoma. There is clearly a wide disparity between input and output in cancer research, but is it really more difficult to find out why some cells continue replicating indefinitely when others stop than it was to get a man to the moon and back? The truism that getting the right answers depends on asking the right questions applies to cancer research no less than to other scientific projects.

DNA and neoplasia

Taking up the question of DNA's role in neoplasia, Jan Pontén proposed a simplified approach to human malignant tumours. In terms of function, the DNA of a tumour (or normal) cell can be divided into at least three portions. The first contains the 'obligate' genes, i.e. those necessary for cell survival. Secondly, there must be a portion of the genome where functions that are not essential for survival can be 'modulated' by switching genes on or off - a process that necessarily plays a part in differentiation. And thirdly, a large portion of the genome must be 'inactivated' in one way or another. Division of genetic material into these three classes appears to be widely applicable, and their studies in 25 different glioma lines have led Jan Pontén and his colleagues to several important conclusions:

1. There is no evidence that the 'inactive' portion of the genome ever becomes activated; if it is inactive in the normal astrocyte, it remains inactive in the malignant astrocyte. However, the obligate and modulated portions of the genome present a picture of disorder in malignant astrocytes. Different genes, as manifested in the phenotype, are active in all 25 lines studied, - producing an individual fingerprint of disorder in each tumour. This confirms that no single defect leads to cancer, or more specifically to gliomas. The network of controls concerned in the obligate and modulated portions of the genome, is disrupted at different spots - and that disruption of control may itself be an important feature of malignant change.

2. Each malignant tumour's properties appear to be largely determined by the portion of the genome responsible for the normal features of the tissue of origin. Thus, choriocarcinoma resembles chorionic tissue, gliomas resemble astrocytes and so on. It is therefore impossible to generalise about the structure of tumours - or about their behaviour. The pattern of invasion of choriocarcinoma, for example, corresponds to the invasive behaviour of normal chorionic cells, and differs from that of other tumours.

3. In one respect, however, it is possible to generalise about malignant cells, since they all share a capacity for infinite proliferation. But where, asked Jan Pontén, does the relevant genetic control (and/or lack of it) reside in the genome? At one spot? Or is infinite proliferation due to a combination of changes? And what underlies the unique ability of such cells to escape programmed death or ageing?

In reply to this last question, Peter Beaconsfield pointed out that most carcinoma cells die without replicating. Those that are very disturbed in structure cannot replicate, only those of more 'normal' appearance continuing to do so. In any cancer, a proportion of the cells is always dying, and the host is able to deal with some of the remainder. Also, tumour cells usually replicate more slowly than normal ones. If all tumour cells were capable of replicating like normal ones and none died, every ten cycles of cell division would increase the tumour mass by a factor of 2^{10}. Another feature of malignant tissues mitigating their proliferative capacity is the fragility of some of their constituent cells, making them less resistant to changes in the extracellular environment. Drawing attention to this as a cause of the high death rate among malignant cells, Jan Pontén suggested that it could be influenced by drugs and other factors. At the same time, a proportion of the malignant cells would retain a capacity for infinite replication - and transmit it genetically to enough daughter cells to at least maintain their numbers.

With regard to the differences in different glioma cell lines, especially in respect to their 'modulated' or differentiated functions, Richard Gardner likened tumour growth to very vigorous clonal selection. Studies of X-chromosome inactivation mosaics have generally shown that tumours appear to originate from only one cell, or possess only one of two phenotypes. How then, he asked, is it possible to be sure that the 25 different types of glioma studied do not simply represent malignant change undergone by 25 different types of normal astrocyte? Agreeing with the implication of the question, Jan Pontén said that the hundreds or thousands of different astrocytes in the brain could well possess the potential to produce as many different gliomas. Hamish Munro then pushed the argument further by suggesting that malignant cells might be repeating what happened in the first animal cell -

which 'threw away a lot of DNA, and became dependent, like social security, on its neighbours.' This can be duplicated in cultures of E.coli. This wild type grows more slowly, because it has to make all its own tryptophan and histidine pathways by comparison with mutants that lack tryptophan or histidine - and therefore do not have to make the relevant DNA, RNA, or protein. Cell division in the latter therefore goes on faster. Could the malignant cell - possibly by living on necrotic portions of local cells, getting nucleotides transferred across gap junctions, and the like - have become less demanding for energy? By reducing the number or complexity of reactions required, malignant cells might have the advantage of needing less labour for each cell division. While agreeing that this was quite possible, Jan Pontén reiterated his view that the disorder of neoplasia always works against the malignant cell. It is usually a fragile cell, and liable to develop lethal variants, so it will always be subject to high death rates.

Referring to the prospects for genetic engineering as a means of cancer research, Jan Pontén foresaw complications arising from the vast amount of work that would be required to study countless bits of DNA - most of which must be completely irrelevant to neoplastic change. The task is indeed a formidable one, but R.J.C. Harris stressed its potential value - not least as a way of finding out what the 'nonsense' DNA was actually doing in cells, even if that action has ceased by the time they are studied. Similar considerations may apply to virus-induced tumours, when virus DNA becomes intergrated into the cell genome. Moreover, that alone will not necessarily produce true tumour cells, as Eva Klein showed by reference to Burkitt's lymphoma. It is well established that experimental intergration of its causative EB virus into the lymphocyte genome drives lymphocytes so chronically that cell lines can be established from them. But these cell lines are not, as they were first thought to be, identical with those derived from actual lymphoma cells. The picture is further complicated by the observation that integration of EB virus into lymphoblastic cell lines appears not to happen at a definite site on the genome. This has been shown mainly for nasopharyngal carcinomas, which are also caused by the EB virus. But perhaps the most crucial finding reported by Eva Klein is that production of tumour cells by this virus requires a highly-specific secondary chromosomal change - translocation of chromosome 14. This appears to be crucial, since some lymphomas are negative for EB virus yet marked by chromosome-14 translocation. In other words, for the EB virus to act carcinogenically, it has not only to infect the cell but also to induce a specific secondary chromosomal change. And once that has happened the continued presence of the virus may not be essential. It is of interest that a similar marker, translocation on chromosome 15, has been found in thymal tymour cells from leukaemic mice.

Genetic primary lesion

All the evidence quoted above points to the primary lesion of cancer being in the DNA, a view with which Peter Beaconsfield agreed in general, while stressing the need to seek more detailed information. The crucial questions - only partially elucidated for virus-induced tumours like Burkitt's lymphoma, and hardly at all for others - that he would like to see answered are: What changes take place in the genetic material? And how can they best be studied? These are not new questions, he went on. When Boveri wrote, in 1914, that the primordial cell of a malignant growth is a somatic cell that contains, as a result of an abnormal process, a definite and wrongly combined chromosome complex', he was referring to what we should now call a change in DNA. This suggestion was further elaborated by Rous in 1940 who was the first to propose that carcinogenesis might be a two-stage process. Research is greatly influenced by current beliefs, and if those now engaged in thinking about cancer and working on it would agree, at least tentatively, that neoplasia results from a permanent change in the genetic code - whatever the reasons for this might be - then the direction of research as well as the concentration of effort would be chanelled along these lines. Noting that he had drawn attention to this need in 1964, Peter Beaconsfield maintained that brains to carry out the necessary research are more difficult to find than money. But since there will never be sufficient of either to study all the possibilities, priorities in probabilities need to be established - instead of dissipating both brains and money in the study of late effects peripheral to the main issue, i.e. features of cancer and cancer cells in the post-DNA phase. Related to this, there has long been unnecessary caution about using the word 'mutation' to describe the underlying DNA change. Spontaneous somatic mutation simply means that a non-germ cell has undergone a permanent transmissable change. 'Spontaneous' reveals to the initiated that we do not know what caused it - as with 'idiopathic' in general medicine. In essence, a mutation is properly defined as a change in the sequence of base pairs in the DNA molecule. If the primary lesion is found to be on the DNA, and if it passes from mother to daughter cell, and if that change is permanent, then cancer is a mutation according to the dictionary definition.

Peter Beaconsfield continued: 'Any abnormality that is transmissable and permanent must be so as the result of a signal coming from the DNA. Whether the genetic signal which results in neoplastic transformation invokes uncontrolled replication or interferes with mechanisms repressing replication, or both, the abnormality is indeed permanently transmissable and can therefore only come from one or more mutations in the genetic material. There are many examples of just one gene change resulting in a mutation and of neoplastic transformation induced by direct penetration of DNA. Changing a single gene in a fruit fly makes a leg grow where an antenna should be. Some chemical pollutants have a similar effect on buterfly genetics, changing wing colour permanently. More to the point, there is experimental evidence that specific chromosomes are responsible for supressing malignancy in human cells. A tentative effort has already been made to effect some kind of molecular analysis of so-called 'oncogenes', but this will have to be followed by both atomic and energy analyses of cancer DNA before we can begin to understand the genetic mechanisms that underlie malignant change.

'There are many theories which try to explain what makes a cell replicate without restraint. All of them are unsatisfactory because in formulating them their authors have not gone far enough back in cell function. Much evidence from biological experimentation and mathematical computation supports the contention that changes in DNA arrangements are responsible for uncontrolled growth. The initiation of such neoplastic transformation appears to result from single or multiple insults to the genetic material when conditions are conducive to change. The DNA molecule must be 'unzipped' to make it susceptible to physical, chemical, or biological injury. Whether the resulting transformation of the cell's genetic material produces an immediate neoplastic change, or whether a second stimulus is also required will depend on the current functioning of the repressor and repair DNA systems. When studying the effects of certain antimetabolites on animals with experimentally-induced ascites cell tumours we gave daily injections of the compound in question, subcutaneously between the scapulae or into the lactating mammary gland. Of the 100 or so animals so treated, three developed lumps at the injection site - one in the scapula group and two in the mammary group. Unless the DNA had been unzipped to effect repair after the injection injury the metastatic cancer DNA could not have inserted itself locally and produced a new tumour. No lumps appeared in the control groups.

'If we are prepared to accept - both on logical grounds and from direct evidence - that DNA is the site of the primary neoplastic lesion, then we should re-examine the different theories of cancer in that light. In essence, these fall into two broad groups: those concerned with abnormal regulation of cell reproduction, and those concerned with abnormal cell reproduction itself. I consider this division artificial,' said Peter Beaconsfield. 'To produce a permanent transmissible change of either sort, there has to be an underlying genetic modification'. He therefore put forward a unified theory of uncontrolled cell replication as a natural event which can arise in three circumstances:

1. By chance. All body cells, except in the central nervous system, are replaced over a period of about two years. The liver cells are replaced the most slowly, and the red blood cells and mucosal linings most rapidly. Our bodies are

composed of some 10^{20} cells, about 2% of which are replicating every day - so the active process affects trillions of cells. On sheer probability, something must go wrong somewhere sometime in the course of so much mitotic activity. Again, probability dictates that some of the mitotic errors will result in the transformation of normal cells into tumour cells. Moreover, most cells go through more than a million biochemical reactions per second, making our supposedly sophisticated methods of recording chemical reactions by photolysis look coarse and clumsy by comparison. Yet it is a mathematical fact that the larger the number of components and the more numerous the different functions being carried out the less are the chances of an error passing right through the system or, if it does, of its having any functional importance - confirming the old saying about safety in numbers. Back in 1963, the mathematician Professor Aldo Andreotti expressed no surprise that experimental research on cancer had not yet produced a major breakthrough. The enormous number of cellular reactions just referred to and the atomic complexity of cell structure means that such a collosal number of experiments would be required to investigate the primary lesion or lesions as to make a comprehensive study technically extremely difficult, if not impossible, to set up. Furthermore, the fundamental differences between normal and cancer cells are very probably of such a kind and so miniscule in degree as to appear insignificant to anyone but a physicist familiar with massive differences of scale between cause and effect. The number of atoms involved in the construction of a cell is practically incalculable, and the functional reactions so numerous that mutation would almost never occur - without sufficient time coupled with the interaction of internal and external factors. This leads us to the second circumstance in which uncontrolled cell replication may arise.

2. With ageing. As age increases, so does the incidence of abnormality in cell replication and repair systems. Progressive changes in metabolic function and protein synthesis take place, together with a tendency for the frequency of errors to rise. So far as carcinogenesis is concerned, the production of mutations is greatly influenced by a variety of other cellular events whose effects are cumulative - and may also influence the way in which genetic mutations are expressed. Maturing and ageing of cells as well as heredity play a vital part in mutation and thus in evolutionary processes - including the evolution of normal cells into cancer cells characterised by uncontrolled replication.

3. Through environmental influences. Probably the most important of the three circumstances leading to uncontrolled cell replication are physical and chemical factors in the interval and external environment. Either might accelerate or promote normal cell replication thereby increasing the probability of chance

errors. Also some of these factors can be injurious to the cell as a whole, increasing the need for repair processes, and even disturbing the different repair systems. Any fault here can produce an error in the DNA which is then incorporated into the molecule as a mutation, the strand having been opened up or 'unzipped' by reason of its activity in replication or repair, and thus predisposed to change or 'trauma'. Clearly such an injury has to be located where activity is (or is about to be) taking place, for activation to occur. For an order to be transmitted from DNA, a gene has first to be 'unzipped' and turned on; it is at this time that mutation takes place. After the mutation has occurred, uncontrolled cell replication may start at once or the potential for it may lie dormant depending on the length and strength of the stimulus and the general state of the cell. Alternatively, the injury to the DNA, and thus the abnormality it causes, may be repaired (or perhaps compensated for), while - at the opposite extreme - the cell bearing a mutation may be unable to survive the damage and dies without replicating. If a mutation lies dormant, as may apparently happen for an indefinite period, it comes into effect only when conditions are conducive or when other influences remove or diminish the repressor and feedback mechanisms restraining its expression - the cell's defences against error have broken down. Unrestrained replication is of course only one possible outcome.

'Biological observations,' said Peter Beaconsfield in conclusion, 'give credence to this unified concept that the errors underlying malignant transformation should be viewed as natural events occurring through chance, abetted by ageing and/ or environmental influences. They also point strongly to the primary lesion being a disturbance of DNA base pairs. Mathematical computation not only shows that the pattern of errors is in line with this view, but may also eventually help to reveal why particular types of error take place. The physical structure of matter and the statistical physics of energy, together with quantum theory and quantum jumps, form part of the study of nucleic acid function we have to make if we are going to try to break the alterations in the genetic code that transforms normal cell replication into malignancy. Studying the many reasons why some people do and others do not develop cancer under apparently identical circumstances may establish the importance of external factors and even of some internal ones. But it will be most unlikely to resolve the essential point - the location and the type of the fundamental genetic lesion which forms the initial abnormality. Statistical physics could well provide the key to that. From a structural viewpoint there is plainly a molecular basis for cancer, but from an energy viewpoint there has to be an atomic basis for tumour occurrence. For cancer cells to continue replicating without stopping, not only must their genetic code be different from normal DNA; they must also have a distinct energy pattern.'

Somatic mutation?

While Jan Pontén agreed that genetic mutation underlies neoplastic change, Richard Gardner suggested that somatic mutation in a cell need not necessarily imply a change in its DNA. At their face value, experiments involving mouse teratocarcinoma cells that have been perpetuated by transplantation to syngeneic adults for 12 years or so appear to have undergone permanent neoplastic transformation: in an adult host they will grow progressively until the animal is killed. Yet if those cells are transplanted back into a very early embryo at the blastocyst stage, they will form 50% or more of the somatic tissue of the mouse, and even give rise to functional spermatozoa. Similar observations have also been made in plants. Instead of assuming a unitary mechanism for all somatic mutation, several possibilities could be considered: that viruses can alter DNA in such a way as to cause a genetic mutation, that changes in a cell's DNA might occur for endogenous reasons, and that gene expression might be modified to produce somatic mutation without any alteration in the genetic code itself. Putting teratocarcinoma cells into syngeneic mice may be like transplanting an eskimo into the Sahara desert; the cell cannot thrive in that environment. But if the malignant cells are put into an environment to which they can respond, that could well be what enables them to differentiate into a normal range of somatic and germ cells. This distinction failed to convince Peter Beaconsfield, however. In reality, he said, the question depends on our understanding of terminology. Is there a real difference between abnormal cell replication and abnormal regulation of cell replication? Both depend on getting a signal from somewhere. If abnormal replication can arise from environmental stimuli, it can only be maintained through successive generations by a consistent signal from somewhere - and that somewhere has to be the DNA, whether we speak of abnormal cell replication or abnormal regulation of cell replication, In either event, if the change is permanent, it has to involve a DNA locus.

Pointing out that genetic mutations in the DNA itself are relatively rare events, Richard Gardner sought to clarify the distinction from somatic mutations due to changes in gene expression, by reference to a botanical example. Cells taken from tobacco and certain other plants can be grown in monolayer culture at low density. In order to get proliferation of these cells, certain growth factors have to be present. Yet if all the growth factors are withdrawn following establishment of the culture, some single cells will carry on proliferating to form quite large clones. They are then growing independently of external controls, something like neoplastic cells, but the frequency with which they revert to the non-proliferating state is several orders of magnitude more frequent than the mutation rate. When they are proliferating, these cells actually synthesise the very growth factors they need. To produce such rapid changes in their behaviour, the cells must be switching the genes that control endogenous production of the relevant growth factors on and off with equal rapidity. As Richard Gardner pointed out, reversible changes on this time scale would be hard to explain in terms of genetic mutation, unless one postulates very highly permutable regions of DNA that can mutate to and fro at high frequency. In his view, it is much more likely that the reversible change producing these somatic mutations takes place in the pathways of gene expression. But Rebecca Beaconsfield queried whether such change should be described as a mutation at all - in the dictionary sense of alteration in a base pair. Agreeing that there is no evidence of such an alteration in the botanical example, cited above, Richard Gardner drew a parallel with the many heritable, stable changes in the genotypes of cells from many animal systems that are normally described as mutations - without there being any evidence of a change in the gene content or the genetic information within the cells in question. There is in fact no evidence either way - which Peter Beaconsfield did not find surprising. Although mutations are usually regarded in crude terms, such as gross injury from ionising radiation, the DNA strand is so long and the nucleotides are so small that a change in base pair sequence could be very hard to find - as if, in a crocodile of children in school uniform stretching from London to Brighton, just two changed partners. The course of future investigative work and the therapeutic possibilities will depend greatly on whether or not true mutations are found to underlie particular somatic changes in cell structure and/or function.

Criteria of malignancy

Discussion then returned to the properties of malignant cells, with Gerald Easty concluding that no single feature has yet been described that would characterise a cell as potentially or actually malignant - apart, perhaps, from the ability of cultured cells to go on proliferating indefinitely in vitro. This is probably the best single criterion available at present, but it involves delays, not all malignant cells can be made to grow in culture, and the conditions are artificial. Whether malignant transformation is due to a single change or - as Dr. Easty believes more probable - by a cascade of disturbances in control, we are still faced with the problem of how they are perpetuated. Suppose, for example, that a cancer patient could be kept alive, instead of dying from the tumour, would it go on proliferating indefinitely? Although much work has concentrated upon the proliferative aspects of malignancy, some benign tumours grow very much faster. Perhaps more characteristic of a malignant tumour is its ability to spread. Placental studies may be particularly relevant here, since the trophoblast not only invades but also 'knows' when to stop invading other tissues. If we could stop malignant cells invading and spreading, the tumour would in effect be rendered benign and comparatively easy to remove.

So how is the invasiveness of trophoblastic tissue controlled? The picture is not yet clear, but David Billington concluded from the fact that the syncytium is derived from the cytotrophoblast that the latter is a terminal cell with a pre-determined lifespan. While this suggests that the very small quantity of cytotrophoblast left towards the end of pregnancy might limit the invasiveness of the syncytium, Harold Fox objected that a substantial amount of cytotrophoblast still remains at a later stage - compared with the relatively early stage when it ceases to be invasive. There appears to be little invasion beyond six to ten weeks of human pregnancy and - significantly - there is evidence of its being brought to an end on the trophoblastic tissue's own initiative, with only slight variations at different 'host' sites. This may well prove to be a fruitful field for future research, and Gerald Easty drew particular attention to another (already touched upon earlier) - the behaviour of normal epithelium and how it differs from that of the corresponding carcinoma cells. In principle, such studies should be more relevent to human cancer, which is about 85% epithelial in origin, than the more familiar work on fibroblasts in culture. In practice, though, Dr. Easty said he had found it extraordinarily difficult to make morphological distinctions _in vitro_ between normal epithelial cells and neoplastic cells derived from them. Moreover, normal epithelial cells in a growth phase do not show the clear-cut phenomenon of contact inhibition of growth described in normal fibroblasts. _In vitro_ work, the only practical method at present, on epithelial cells from the kidney, skin, and ductal epithelium of the breast has shown that mitosis can take place even in very densely populated regions, so that multilayers of cells are formed without any fancy media or special perfusion techniques. In other words, the criteria which have been developed to distinguish neoplasia in fibroblasts do not, in Dr. Easty's view, apply generally to epithelial cells. More needs to be known about what regulates and controls epithelial growth _in vitro_ - subject to his proviso that it may tell us little of nothing about what happens _in vivo_...

Interdisciplinary discussion and collaboration often enables _in vitro_ findings to be viewed from a range of _in vivo_ standpoints, and Sir William Henderson particularly noted this as an important feature of the symposium. It also means that different disciplines have different lines of research to offer, a notable example being the associated fields of virus-induced malignancies and genetic manipulation, referred to earlier by R.J.C. Harris. Sir William took the view that while this certainly presented new opportunities for research, there might be a danger of over-reacting to the so-called hazards of genetic manipulation. That could be prejudicial to its potential benefits - many of which lie in the agricultural field, especially on the plant side. Although it is too early to judge whether we have overdone precautionary controls, Sir William thought it paradoxical that Britain had originally taken a much more relaxed view of the possible risks than, for instance, the United States - yet we have now become the only country with legislation controlling genetic research. It is plainly important that such controls should not unduly impede research, especially in a field like malignancy where a variety of genetic mechanisms may be involved. But Sir William did sound a note of additional caution that like should be compared with like in interpreting experimental findings. Studies of cell proliferation in plants may, for instance, be of questionable relevance to neoplasia in man or other animals.

'Cancer DNA'

The theme of genetic research was taken up again by Peter Beaconsfield, with reference to so-called 'cancer DNA', coded for neoplastic cell proliferation. 'Breaking the code, especially in higher animals, is fraught with tremendous technical difficulties', he said. 'The problems as I see them fall mainly into three categories: to extract pure DNA in its naturally occuring form, to loosen up the coiled strand so as to examine at least part of its length, and to locate and decipher the locus (or loci) responsible for the cancer process. The methods we use at present are unsatisfactory, as well as insufficient, for this kind of work. The technical problems of extracting undisturbed DNA, identifying the locus where changes have taken place and deciphering and identifying the transcriptional changes in the DNA have yet to be solved. The physico-chemical changes are likely to prove so miniscule that present methods of measurement could not detect them.

'Back in 1962, John Kovach pointed out to me that DNA should be extracted by less traumatising methods than ultracentrifugation and complex chemical interactions if we were to avoid altering intermolecular forces and structures. He suggested the use of ion exchange methods, similar to the techniques used for viral extractions, and I realised that such methods could be adapted for purification and concentration as well as extraction of DNA. Also, by varying the concentration of the eluate in the ion exchange column it should be possible to separate the cancer DNA from the normal as it is likely to have a less stable atomic state. No matter how small the physical and chemical differences between normal and cancer DNA, they should each demonstrate their own characteristic absorption band, energy equation, and potential difference. But localising and then reading the cancer code is almost a new discipline and certainly one for which an ordinary biomedical researcher will need a lot of expert help. The special techniques employed in genetic engineering could bring us much closer, and probably solve some of the problems, but we would also need the collaboration of a high energy physicist and a theoretical mathematician, plus an advanced computer expert. Here at last is one biomedical problem that really does need a computer!

'Turning to two clinical aspects, cancer DNA is likely to differ from normal DNA in a number of ways. One of these will be its antigenic properties, which, however slight, are always present. This weak antigenecity could be enhanced - for example, with haptones - and thus open up new prospects for therapy. The difference between normal and cancer DNA has been worked out from mathematical computations, which point to a distinct difference between the two, both in changed base sequence and in energy variant. These two distinct differences together produce a new and different order of life - unrestricted and confused. The second clinical aspect concerns metastases. These are often found long before the primary tumour is demonstrable and when there is no direct evidence of the latter's invasiveness. Personally, I have never been impressed by the widespread but largely unsubstantiated view that metastases are caused by dissemination of malignant cells as such. I would like to suggest that part of the cancer DNA from certain malignant cells gets out of the nucleus and is carried around the body until it arrives in an area where the DNA is unzipped for some reason. Here, if the circumstances are right, it becomes incorporated into normal DNA, producing a change in base sequence. Moreover, probability calculations suggest that dissemination of cancer DNA may be considerable, in affected individuals, but that it can set up secondary neoplasia only when local conditions are such that it can gain entry and become incorporated into the normal DNA. This is how I interpret the interscapular tumours in my laboratory animals, referred to earlier in this discussion.

'All the foregoing is an oversimplified look at a complex problem', Peter Beaconsfield went on. 'But I submit that the problem is capable of solution if treated as a multidisciplinary project, and I would like to suggest it be tackled in the following way. So that the main goal does not become obscured by side issues, the director should be a clinician. The urgency that is inseparable from a clinician's attitude to his daily work - because he deals with people's problems at first hand - is exactly the atmosphere in which this kind of consumer-oriented research needs to be carried out. Furthermore, the director must be able to convince the super-specialists whose help he needs that the project matters sufficiently for them to abandon their own work temporarily so as to collaborate on this project. I am sufficiently convinced of the validity of my belief that cancer arises from recognisable changes in the genetic code to be willing to translate it into practical terms. To confirm this concept in practice, I would first need a physical chemist to perfect and streamline procedures for obtaining DNA in its pure natural form. This done, I would require a high-energy physicist, as such people are used to recording minutiae. Together with a theoretical mathematician of ingenuity and imagination, he should be able to reduce the areas of localisation of the abnormal DNA to some extent, or at least sufficiently for a computer expert to be able to make a programme. Such super-specialists would need very specific information, direction, and guidance to make the best use of their expertise, since the goal would be outside their own fields and not of their own choosing. However, without their special knowledge and equipment it would be impossible to find out what we need to know.

'Up to the present my difficulty in setting up a project of this kind has been in assembling specialists of the calibre required. Many are immersed in their own work or wasting their talents in government 'defence' establishments. A biological mini-Manhattan project to crack the cancer DNA code would have a beneficial spin-off in rehabilitating the public repute of science and scientists (badly needed ever since Hiroshima). It should also put limited research resources to better use than endlessly investigating the destructive power of the atom - which monopolises about 50% of the top scientific capacity of the West and an even larger share of total research expenditure.'

The need to bring physical and biological studies together was also stressed by Marcellino Dianzani, who stressed that even the slightest impurities would be likely to affect the detailed observations required when investigating a substance as complex as DNA. He also reported on one possible means of carrying out such studies, discussed at a CIBA Symposium a few days earlier. This concerned the relationship between protein structure and the passage of an electron flux along two-dimensional protein molecules. Whether this particular technique can be applied to three-dimensional DNA remains to be seen, but that possibility at least serves to emphasise the importance of sophisticated physical methods in DNA research. And Peter Beaconsfield expressed the hope that work on the lines indicated by R. J. C. Harris and himself would lead to some of the answers sought.

However, Richard Gardner felt that such work need not necessarily focus on the DNA itself. There is a continuity of organisation between DNA and other cell constituents which means that each studied in isolation may reveal little or nothing of its normal function in the intact cell or tissue. This may be a problem in all sorts of regulation. An example very difficult to explain in terms of conventional DNA theory comes from the single-celled paramecium, which has longitudinal rows of cilia that beat in one direction along its body surface. If, by careful microsurgery, the orientation of one of those ciliary rows is reversed, all the progeny produced by fission of that paramecium, for literally hundreds of generations. also have one row of cilia reversed. There is certainly no nucleic acid that can be detected in the base of the cilia, so, in this particular case, there may be some template organisation that is perpetuated quite reproducibly, in a polarised way, outside the nuclear genome. On conventional views, all the proteins that go to make the cilia must be transcribed correctly from parts of the genome - yet at some stage the instructions must be reversed. This highlights the need to study not only DNA itself but also its actual effects in situ under different circumstances. As regards the possibility that some sort of cellular template change might modify genome instructions, Peter Beaconsfield said he hoped something of the sort might prove to be a causative mechanism in neoplasia - since it could well be easier to investigate, and perhaps treat, than the genetic mutations he believes to underlie malignant change.

Referring to an earlier comment that it was unfortunate that research in the field had been seduced by the relative ease of making genetic studies on E.coli, Peter Beaconsfield went on to say that if the placenta had been used the initial difficulties would undoubtedly have been greater but the model would have resembled human tissues far more closely. He then summarised the merits of the placenta as an experimental animal. It can be obtained at all stages of development, including embryonic, and all the mechanisms and the stimuli that affect cell replication can be studied in vivo, in vitro, and in tissue culture. Like all somatic cells, those of the placenta are replaced by replication, and they can be used to search for the initial signal of abnormal replication, whether this is in the DNA itself or due to some other error. The placenta could also be used for studying the regulation of genetic expression and the way gene repressors operate. Having all the regulatory mechanisms and enzymes it is a suitable tissue to study DNA excision repair systems. Moreover, the placenta represents a large biopsy specimen from all mothers and offspring affected by those hereditary diseases which are characterised by defective repair enzyme systems. Of particular research interest would be the hereditary conditions whose victims are known to be 'cancer prone'.

Invasiveness - of trophoblast and neoplasms

Another aspect of placental studies, raised by Olga Genbačev, concerns the differences between malignant cells and invasive placental trophoblast reported by previous speakers. But one feature was not mentioned earlier: the fact that in the syncytoptrophoblast there is no cell membrane separating the invasing placental cells. That might, she suggested, be connected with the cessation of further proliferation when the cytotrophoblast becomes syncytial. Do choriocarcinoma cells show comparable behaviour with loss of cell membranes in the syncytial type? The answer, provided by Robert Aitken, appears to be 'yes'. But it is not true that trophoblast invasion depends upon its syncytial form as David Billington pointed out. Some of the most aggressively invasive trophoblast is cellular in nature, there being quite substantial species differences. The crucial question though, and the one Olga Genbačev proposed as a subject for research in human placental tissue, is whether the mechanisms bringing trophoblastic proliferation to an end can be identified. The factors responsible are probably distinct from those that regulate invasiveness, since the two processes do not appear to be directly linked. Both look promising fields for further investigation, alongside more fundamental genetic studies - with the placenta providing material for all three.

Collaboration between malignant cells?

Taking up the reference in Richard Gardner's paper to inactivation of the X-chromosome in the early embryo, Hamish Munro queried whether the affected cells lose their capacity to synthesise certain molecules. If so, do unaffected neighbouring cells have the capacity to transfer the deficient compounds to them via gap junctions. Some such mechanism might allow a cancerous growth to thrive by cooperation with other cell populations - despite deficiencies in its own metabolism. Whether metabolic cooperation of this sort, which has been observed in vitro, actually takes place in vivo remains uncertain, according to Richard Gardner, nor is there any direct information on whether cancer cells with defects in major pathways would die sooner if there were no cooperation from neighbouring normal cells. If such a mechanism does operate, however, it would obviously work best in a very small clone of malignant cells with a relatively large proportion of normal cells in the immediate vicinity. With tumour growth, contacts with normal cells would become less and the efficiency of any exchange mechanism would be reduced - though it is worth bearing in mind that intercellular transmission via gap junctions could pass through several intermediate cells on a journey from, say, a normal cell to a defective neoplastic one. The whole field of relationships between neoplastic and normal cells, and among the latter, also calls for more research - in much of which placental tissues could be employed.

The way ahead?

Before asking the speaker and other participants for their conclusions on the most worthwhile future direction of cancer research, with special reference to placental studies, Peter Beaconsfield said he had been warned that cross-fertilisation between disciplines would not be easy. So it had proved. 'We have not moved into each other's special fields. We are all making suggestions within our own disciplines - which may not be inevitable but certainly limits collaboration at the practical level and, perhaps more important, fails to fire the imagination. When

I tried to be more adventurous, about research into cancer DNA, no-one either actively supported or seriously challenged my deliberately provocative proposals. Do please tell us now, with rather less reserve, how you would like to see future work develop.' Richard Gardner responded by stressing the need for a system that would enable cells to be studied at the earliest possible stage in the neoplastic process. The widely-used in vitro model using viruses to transform cells suffers from the relationship between in vitro transformation of cells and its in vivo counterpart - manifest malignancy - not being entirely clear and straightforward. Moreover, material from manifest in vivo tumours already appears to be many steps removed from the initial neoplastic event. Best of all, of course, would be a system to study the earliest neoplastic change, under conditions as natural as possible, in human tissue.

An opportunity that comes close to satisfying some features of this ideal may be afforded by the few human neoplastic conditions with which virus infection and/or chromosome changes are known to be associated. With EB virus infection of lymphocytes, for example, the course of malignant transformation can be studied, bearing in mind that a secondary chromosomal change also appears to be required. Emphasising these aspects of her earlier remarks on the subject, Eva Klein expressed the view that work in this field should at least come close to the fundamental causes of the admittedly unusual types of human neoplasia in question. With both a chromosome change and (presumably) viral DNA involved, there might well be opportunities for Peter Beaconsfield's proposed genetic studies.

Continuing the genetic theme, Eric Newsholme raised the question of control of DNA synthesis - which is presumably suppressed at all stages of the cell cycle other than the S phase. In other words, the enzymes responsible must somehow be totally inactivated for the rest of the time. There may be a parallel here in the suppression of phosphorylase activity in muscles at rest - and its immediate response to exercise in order to mobilise glycogen. These changes are known to be controlled by an interconversion system and possibly also by the existence of a substrate cycle, but we know little of the regulatory mechanisms that control the process of replication. Studies of how DNA synthesis is switched on and off, how messenger RNA works at particular sites on the DNA and how repression operates should all provide valuable information on control of the cell cycle. And understanding of normal control mechanisms should help to shed light on what goes wrong with them in neoplasia. Here, it is often hard to distinguish cause and effect. For instance, the observation that dividing cells - in tumour or placental tissue - demand more energy could be viewed the other way round. Suppose, said Eric Newsholme, that a tumour cell had lost some of its ability to control both energy formation and energy wasting. The feedback mechanisms for limiting energy formation might have been lost, or equally the cell could have lost the ability to dispose of surplus energy (perhaps by the still hypothetical process of 'futile cycling'). What would the cell then do with its surplus energy? Might it not instruct itself to divide? The alternative would, after all, be cell death. This proposal, that neoplastic cell division could be secondary to failure of energy regulation, has wider implications. It suggests that the replicative capacity of neoplastic cells could conceivably be normal - but responding to other abnormalities in the cell. Though pure hypothesis, this does serve to emphasise the importance of studying control mechanisms. It is also in line with Peter Beaconsfield's plea for more research effort to go into the earliest phases of neoplasia.

Moving on to features of neoplastic tissue, Dorothy Villee drew a parallel with those of embryonic tissues, with particular reference to similarities between the transient zone in the adrenal gland of the human fetus and human adrenal carcinomas. The former grows very rapidly and the latter are highly anaplastic. But more specifically, her detailed work on the steroid biosynthetic pathways has revealed patterns which are identical in the anaplastic adrenal carcinomas of children and in the fetal transient zone. Could it be that certain embryonic cells remain in a state of limbo until some unknown trigger turns them into very rapidly replicating cells once again? Maybe, but Richard Gardner expressed reservations about many of the parallels drawn between tumours and embryonic cells. And Peter Beaconsfield pointed out that fetal cells could not really stay in limbo; they would have to replicate if they were to survive over a period of years - a point that Dorothy Villee confirmed.

However, Alan Browne pointed out that latency between cause and apparent effect cannot be wholly ruled out. Venereal infection with the herpes virus of type A in young women appears to be related to carcinoma of the cervix many years later. Presumably the virus gets into the cervical cells, lies dormant, and is eventually activated by some unknown factor(s) to produce a florid carcinoma. The mechanism here seems to be that the infected cell continues to replicate normally over the intervening period, until repressor signals or feedback mechanisms are removed and virus replication can take place - perhaps 20 or 30 years later. In other words, the potentially carcinogenic virus appears to stay in limbo in host cells that have to continue replicating. There are of course other examples, as Hamish Munto reminded participants, including X-ray skin burns causing epitheliomas at precisely the same sites many years later - after thousands of normal cell divisions. The trigger mechanism here may be related to ageing, with 'deprogramming' of the affected cells. With the adenocarcinoma of the vagina in adolescent girls induced by stilboestrol treatment in utero, which takes about 15 or 20 years to develop, the trigger appears to be hormonal. But then gradual accumulation of DNA errors, perhaps caused in various ways, and accruing over a long period, could play a part in latency between cause and effect in all such cases. The seemingly specific trigger in a particular type of tumour may be more in the nature of a last straw - or even coincidental... Referring to the concept of the 'immortal strand', Richard Gardner suggested that anything which caused sustained tissue disorientation or increased stem cell activity might increase the rate at which errors accumulate. Perhaps, said Hamish Munro in a light-hearted but nonetheless pointed reference to Burns Night, all these ideas form part of an 'immortal memory'. But in parts of Scotland, and particularly in Glasgow the accent is such that the toast becomes 'the immoral memory' - serving to remind us that accumulated errors may be due to past sins of commission.

One thing at least is clear from this concluding part of the discussion - that latency should be added to the other positive opportunities for research into the initial phases of neoplastic change, noted earlier. Studies of human tissues known to have been exposed to a potentially carcinogenic influence - whether chemical, radiation or virus - should sooner or later yield valuable information about the nature of the changes their cells are harbouring. Quite probably these changes will prove to be in the DNA itself, which lends further emphasis to Peter Beaconsfield's plea for research to focus on the search for so-called 'cancer DNA'. But that search should not be confined to mutations that might be expected to induce neoplasia and/or remove controls on cell proliferation. Bearing in mind Eric Newsholme's notion that a cell's energy-control problems might induce mitosis, the possible secondary (or tertiary) effects of any mutations, alone or in combination, would have to be considered. The technical difficulties of identifying mutations in 'cancer DNA' might prove to be no more than the first step in unravelling the tangled skein of carcinogenesis. However that may eventually prove to be, more thought of this kind plainly needs to go into asking the right questions for cancer research to answer, if we are to get a better return on research investment. In that research the placenta may well have an increasing part to play.

REFERENCES TO PAPERS IN SECTION II

ORIGIN AND FORMATION OF THE PLACENTA

R. J. Aitken, Rebecca Beaconsfield and Jean Ginsburg

1 Graham, C.F. (1970) Experimental early parthenogenesis in Mammals, in Schering Sympsium on Intrinsic and Extrinsic factors in Early Mammalian Development Vol 6 (Ed G. Raspe) New York: Pergamon.

2 Tarkowski, A.K., Witowska, A. and Mouricha, J. (1970) Experimental parthenogenesis in the mouse. Nature 226, 162.

3 Gibbons, A.F. and Chang, M.C. (1973) Indirect effects of X irradiation on embryonic development; irradiation of the exteriorized rat uterus. Biol. Reprod. 9, 133.

4 Gamow, E.I. and Prescott, D.M. (1978) The cell life cycle during early embryogenesis of the mouse. Exp. Cell Res. 59, 117.

5 Enders, A.C. (1971) The fine structure of the blastocysts. Biology of the Blastocyst Ed. Blandan R.J. Chicago: University of Chicago Press, 71.

6 Gardner, R.L., Papaioannou, V.E. and Barton, S.C. (1973) Origin of the ectoplacental cone and secondary giant cells in mouse blastocysts reconstituted from isolated trophoblast and inner cell mass. J. Embryol. Exp. Morph. 30, 561.

7 Hartig, A.T. and Rick, J. (1954) Pre-implantation stages of the human ovary, a description of four normal and four abnormal specimens ranging from the second to the fifth day of development. Contrib. Embryol. Carneg. Inst. 35, 199.

8 Gardner, R.L. and Papaioannou, V.E. (1975) Differentiation in the trophectoderm and inner cell mass. The Early Development of Mammals, Ed. Balls, N. and Wild, A.E.,p.197, Cambridge University Press,

9 Barlow, P., Owen, D.A.J. and Graham, C. (1972) DNA Synthesis in the preimplantation mouse embryo. J. Embryol. Exp. Morph. 27, 431.

10 Luthardt, F.W. and Donahue, R.P. (1973) Pronuclear DNA synthesis in mouse eggs. Exp. Cell Res. 82, 143.

11 Woodland, H.R. and Graham, C.F. (1969) RNA Synthesis during early development of the mouse. Nature 221, 327.

12 Epstein, C.J. (1969) Gene expression and macromolecular synthesis during preimplantation embryonic development. Biol. Reprod. 12, 82.

13 Petzold, U., Daines, W., Gottschewski, G.H.M. and Neuhoff, V. (1972) Das Protein muster in friihen Entwick Lungsstadien des Kaninchens. Cytobiologie 5, 272,

14 van Bkerkon, J. and Manes, C. (1974) Development of pre-implantation rabbit embryos in vivo and in vitro. 11. A comparison of qualitative aspects of protein synthesis. Develop. Biol. 40, 40.

15 Wales, R.G. (1975) Maturation of the mammalian embryo. Biochemical aspects. Biol. Reprod. 12, 66.

16 Barbehenn, A.K., Wales, R.G. and Lowry, O.H. (1974) The explanation for the blockage of glycolysis in early mouse emrbyos. Proc. Nat. Acad. Sci. 71, 1056.

17 Brinster, R.L. (1971) Protein synthesis and enzyme constitution of the pre-implantation mammalian embryo in Regulation of Mammalian Reproduction Ed. Segal, S.J., Crozier, R. and Corfman, P.A., Charles C. Thomas, Ill.

18 Fridhandler, L. (1961) Pathways of glucose metabolism in fertilised rabbit ova at various pre-implantation stages. Exp. Cell Res. 22, 303.

19 Dickmann, Z. and Dey, S.K. (1974) Steroidogenesis in the pre-implantation rat embryo and its possible influence on morula-blastocyst transformation and implantation. J. Reprod. Fert. 37, 91.

20 Edwards, R.G. (1977) Early human development from the occyte to implantation, p.175 in Scientific Foundations of Obstetrics and Gynecology Ed. Philipp, E.E., Barnes, J. and Newton, M. W. Heinemann, London.

21 Dorland, R.M., Biggers, J.D. and Lechene, C.P. (1976) Kinetic aspects of rabbit blastocoele fluid accumulation: an application of electron probe micro-analysis. Dev. Biol. 50, 201.

22 Tuft, P.H. and Boving, B.G. (1970) The forces involved in water uptake by the rabbit blastocyst. J. Exp. Zool. 174, 165.

23 Dalcq, A.M. (1957) Introduction to General Embryology. Oxford University Press. London.

24 Tarkowaski, A.K. and Wroblewska, J. (1967) Development of blastomeres of mouse eggs isolated at the 4 and 8 cell stage. J. Embryol. exp. Morph. 18, 155.

25 McLaren, A. (1976) Mammalian Chimaeras, Cambridge University Press, London.

26 Mintz, B. (1965) Experimental genetic mosaicism in the mouse. In, Preimplantation Stages of Pregnancy, G.E.W. Wolstenholme and M. O'Connor p.194, Churchill London.

27 Hillman, N., Sherman, M.I. and Graham, C. (1972) The effect of spatial arrangements on cell determination during mouse development. J. Embryol. exp. Morph. 28, 263.

28 Gardner, R.L. and Johnson, M.H. (1972) An investigation of inner cell mass and trophoectoderm tissues following their isolation from the mouse blastocyst. J. Embryol. exp. Morph. 18, 179.

29 Gardner, R.L. and Johnson, M.H. (1973) Investigation of early mammalian developments using interspecific chimaeras between rat and mouse. Nature. New Biol. 246, 86.

30 Gardner, R.L. and Johnson, M.H. (1975) Investigation of cellular interaction and deployment in the early mammalian embryo using interspecific chimaeras between the rat and mouse. In, Cell Patterning. CIBA Foundation Symp. 19, pp. 183. Associated Scientific Publishers, Amsterdam.

31 Gardner, R.L. and Rossant, J. (1976) Determination during embryo-genesis. In, Embryogenesis in Mammals. CIBA Foundation Symp. 40, pp. 5. Elsevier Press, Amsterdam.

32 Rossant, J. (1975) Investigation of the determinative state of the mouse inner cell mass. 1. Aggregation of isolated inner cell masses with morulae. J. Embryol. exp. Morph. 17, 467.

33 Solter, D. and Knowles, B.B. (1975) Immunosurgery of mouse blastocyst. Proc. Nat. Acad. Sci. 72, 5099.

34 Handyside, A.H. and Barton, S.C. (1977) Evaluation of the technique of immunosurgery for the isolation of inner cell masses from mouse blastocysts. J. Embryol. exp. Morph. 37, 217.

35 Handyside, A.H. (1978) Time of commitment of inside cells isolated from preimplantation mouse embryos. J. Embryol. exp. Morph. 45, 37.

36 Hastings, R.A. and Enders, A.C. (1975) Junctional complexes in the preimplantation rabbit embryo. Anat. Rec. 181, 17.

37 Ducibella, T., Albertini, D.F. Anderson, E. and Biggers, J.D. (1975) The preimplantation mammalian embryo: characterization of intercellular junctions and their appearance during development. Dev. Biol. 45, 231.

38 Cross, M.H. (1973) Active sodium and choloride transport across the rabbit blastocoele wall. Biol. Reprod. 8, 566.

39 Cross, M.H. (1974) Rabbit blastocoele bicarbonate: accumulation rate. Biol. Reprod. 11, 654.

40 Biggers, J.D. and Borland, R.M. (1976) Physiological aspects of growth and development of the preimplantation mammalian embryo. Ann. Rev. Physiol. 38, 95.

41 Boyd, J.D. and Hamilton, W.J. (1952) Cleavage, early development and implantation of the egg In, Marshalls Physiology of Reproduction Vol. 2, Ed. Parkes, A.S. Longmans, London.

42 Steptoe, P., Edwards, R.G. and Paurdy, J.M. (1972) Human blastocysts grown in culture. Nature 227, 132.

43 Perry, J.S. and Rowlands, I.W. (1962) Early pregnancy in the pig. J. Reprod. Fert. 4, 175.

44 Aitken, R.J. (1977) Embryonic diapause. In, Development in Mammals Vol. 1, Ed. Johnson, M.H., North Holland, Amsterdam.

45 Viaxhodd, T.L.W. (1854) Entwickelungsgeschichte des Rehes. J. Richer'shce Buchhandlung, Giessen, Germany.

46 Short, R.V. and Hay, M.F. (1966) Delayed implantation in the roe deer (Capreolus capreolus). In, Comparative Biology of Reproduction in Mammals, Ed. Rowlands, I.W., Academic Press, London.

47 Sadlier, R.M.F.S. (1969) The ecology of reproduction in wild and domestic animals, Methuen, London.

48 Lataste, M.F. (1891) Des variations de durée de la gestation chez les mammifères et des circonstances qui determinent ces variations: théorie de la gestation retardée. C.R. Soc. Biol. (Paris) 9, 21.

49 Norris, M.L. and Adams, C.E. (1971) Delayed implantation in the Mongolian gerbil, Meriones unguiculatus. J. Reprod. Fert. 27, 486.

50 Sharman, G.B. (1954) Reproduction in marsupials. Nature 173, 202.

51 Sharman, G.B. (1970) Reproductive physiology of marsupials. Science 167, 1221

52 Tyndale-Biscoe, C.H., Hearn, J.P. and Renfree, M.B. (1974) Control of reproduction in macropodid marsupials. J. Endocr. 63, 589.

53 Canirenc,R., Bonnin-Laffarque, M. and Lafus-Boue, M. (1971) Realisation expérimentale précoce de l'ovo implantation chez le Blaireau européen (Meles meles) pendant la periode de latence blastocystaire. C.R. Acad. Sci. (Paris) 273, 1855.

54 Pearson, O.P. and Enders, R.F. (1944) Duration of pregnancy in some mustelids. J. Exp. Zool. 95, 21.

55 Holcomb, L.C., Schaible, P.J. and Ringer, R.K. (1962) The effects of varied lighting regimes on reproduction in the mink. Mich. Agr. Exp. Sta. Quart. Bull. 44, 666.

56 Wright, P.L. (1963) Variations in reproductive cycles in North American mustelids.In, Delayed Implantation, Ed. Enders, A.C., pp. 77, University of Chicago Press, Chicago.

57 Belyaer, D.K., Pereldik, N.S. and Portnova, N.T. (1951) Experimental reduction of the period of embryonal development in sables. (Martes zibellina). J. Gen. Biol. 12, 260.

58 Mead, R.A. (1971) Effects of lighting and blinding upon delayed implantation in the spotted skunk. Biol. Reprod. 5, 214.

59 Canirenc, R. (1960) L'ovo-implantation differée des animaux sauvages in, Les fonctions de nidation uterine et leur troubles, Masson, G. Paris.

60 McLaren, A. (1973) Blastocyst Activation In The Regulation of Mammalian Reproduction. p.321 Ed. Segal, S.J., Crozier, R., Corfman, P.A. and Condliffe, P.G. Springfield, Illinois.

61 Weitlauf, H.M. (1974) Metabolic changes in the blastocysts of mice and rats during delayed implantation. J. Reprod. Fertil. 39, 213.

62 Aitken, R.J. (1974) Delayed implantation in the roe deer (Capreolus capreolus) Ph.D. Thesis, University of Cambridge.

63 Aitken, R.J. (1974b) Delayed implantation ir roe deer (Capreolus capreolus). J. Reprod. Fert. 39, 225.

64 Aitken, R.J. (1974c) Calcium and zinc in the endometrium and uterine flushings of the roe deer (Capreolus capreolus) during delayed implantation. J. Reprod. Fert. 40, 333.

65 Aitken, R.J. (1975) Ultrastructure of the blastocyst and endometrium of the roe deer (Capreolus capreolus) during delayed implantation. J. Anat. 119, 369.

66 Aitken, R.J. (1976) Uterine secretion of fructose in the roe deer. J. Reprod. Fert. 46, 439.

67 Canirenc, R. and Bonnin-Laffargue, M. (1963) Inventory of problems raised by the delayed ova implantation In the European badger (Meles meles L.) in, Delayed Implantation,Ed. Enders, A.C., pp. 115. University of Chicago Press, Chicago.

68 Surani, M.A.H. (1975) Hormonal regulation of proteins in the uterine secretion of ovariectomized rats and the implications for implantation and embryonic diapause . J. Reprod. Fert. 43, 411.

69 Adams, C.E., Hay, M.F. and Mann Lutwak, C. (1961) The action of various agents upon the rabbit embryo. J. Embryol. exp. Morph. 9, 468.

70 Murray Jr., F.A., Bazer, F.W., Wallace, H.D. and Warnick, A.C. (1972) Quantitative and qualitative variation in the secretion of protein by the procine uterus during the estrous cycle. Biol. Reprod. 7, 314.

71 Daniel Jr., J.C. (1972) Local production of protein during implantation in the rabbit. J. Reprod. Fert. 31, 303.

72 Renfree, M.B. (1972) Influence of the embryo on the marsupial uterus. Nature 240, 475.

73 Wyatt, C., Heap, R.B. and Perry, J.S. (1976) Protein synthesis in co-culture of blastocyst and endometrium explants during blastocyst steroidogenesis in the pit. J. Int. Cong. Endocr. Hamburg. Abstr. 226, 109.

74 Squire, G.D., Bazer, F.W. and Murray Jr., F.A. (1972) Electrophoretic patterns of porcine uterine protein secretions during the estrous cycle. Biol. Reprod. 7, 321.

75 Roberts, G.P. and Parker, J.M. (1974) Macromolecular compnents of the luminal fluid from the bovine uterus. J. Reprod. Fert. 40, 291.

76 Roberts, G.P. and Parker, J.M. (1976) Fractionation and comparison of proteins from bovine uterine fluid and bovine allontoic fluid. Biochim. Biophys. Acta. 446, 69.

77 Gibbons, R.A., Bixon, N. and Roberts, G.P. (1977) Uterine secretions in the cow and sheep. Biochem, Soc. Trans. 5, 452.

78 Beier, H.M. (1968) 'Uteroglobin': a hormone-sensitive endometrial protein involved in blastocyst development. Biochim. Biophys. Acta 160, 289.

79 McGaughey, R.W. and Murray, F.A. (1972) Properties of blastokinin: amino acid composition, evidence for subunits and estimation of isoelectric point. Fert. Steril. 23, 399.

80 Beats, M. (1977) Physio-chemical characterization of uteroglobin and its interaction with progesterone.In, Development in Mammals Vol. 2, Ed. Johnson, M.H.,North Holland, Amsterdam.

81 Beats, M. and Baier, R. (1975) Binding of progesterone to the proteins of the uterine luminal fluid. Identification of uteroglobin as the binding protein. Biochim. Biophys. Acta 392, 346.

82 Beats, M. and Rungger, D. (1975) Translation of the messenger RNA for rabbit uteroglobin in Zenopus oocytes. FEBS Letters 59, 305.

83 Bullock, D.W., Woo, S.L.C. and O'Malley, B.W. (1976) Uteroglobin messenger RNA. Translation in vitro. Biol. Reprod. 15, 435.

84 Kirshnan, R.S. and Daniel, J.C. (1967) 'Blastokinin': inducer and regulator of blastocyst development in the rabbit uterus. Science 158, 490.

85 Arthur, A.T., Cowan, B.D. and Daniel Jr., J.C. (1972) Steroid binding to blastokinin. Fert.Steril. 23, 85.

86 Rahman, S.S.U., Velayo, N., Domres, P. and Billiar, R.B. (1975) Evaluation of progesterone binding to uteroglobin. Fert. Steril. 26, 991.

87 Beier, H.M. (1970) Hormonal stimulation of protease inhibitor activity in endometrial secretion during early pregnancy. Acta endocr. Copenh. 63, 141.

88 Johnson, M.H. (1974) Studies using antibodies to the macro-molecular secretions of the early pregnant uterus in, Immunology in Obstetrics and Gynecology. Ed. Centaro A., pp. 123, Excerpta Medica, Amsterdam.

89 Beier, H.M. (1976) Uteroglobin and related biochemical changes in the reproductive tract during early pregnancy in the rabbit. J. Reprod. Fert. Suppl. 25, 53.

90 Noske, I.G. and Feigelson, M. (1976) Immunological evidence of uteroglobin (blastokinin) in the male reproductive tract and in non-reproductive ductal tissues and their secretions Biol. Reprod. 15, 704.

91 Beier, H.N., Kirchner, C. and Mootz, U. (1978) Uteroglobin-like antigen in the pulmonary epithelium and secretion of the lung. Cell. Tiss. Res. (in press).

92 Beier, H.M., Bohn, H. and Muller, W. (1975) Uteroglobin-like antigen in the male genital tract secretions. Cell. Tiss. Res. 165, 1.

93 Feigelson, M., Noske, I.G., Goswami, A.K. and Kay, E. (1977) Reproductive tract fluid proteins and their hormonal control. Ann. N.Y. Acad. Sci. 286, 273.

94 Denker, H.W. (1976) Mechanismen der Implantation des Saugetierembryos und ihre experimentelle Beeinflussung. Hahil. schrift Medizin. Fakult. RWTH Aachen.

95 Danile Jr., J.C., (1973) A blastokinin-like component from the human uterus. Fert. Steril. 24, 326.

96 Daniel Jr., J.C. (1972) Blastokinin in the northern fur seal. Fert. Steril. 23, 78.

97 Cowan, D.R. (1944) Decreased mutual adhesiveness, a property of cells from squamous cell carcinomas. Cancer Res. 4, 625.

98 McCutcheon, M., Cowan, D.R. and Fontaine, B.M. (1948) Studies on invasiveness of cancer. Cancer 1, 460.

99 Tjernberg, B. and Najicik, J. (1965) Cannulation of lymphatics leaving cancerous nodes in studies on tumour spread. Acta Cytol. 9, 197.

100 Easty, G.C. and Mercer, E.H. (1960) An electron microscopy study of the surfaces of normal and malignant cells in culture. Cancer Res. 20, 1608.

101 De Ridder, L., Mareel, M. and Vahaet, L. (1975) Adhesion of malignant and non-malignant cells to cultured embryonic substrates. Cancer Res. 35, 3164.

102 Parr, B.M. and Parr, E.L. (1974) Uterine luminal epithelium: protrusions mediate endocytosis, not apocrine secretion in the rat. Biol. Reprod. 11, 220.

103 Nilsson, B.O., Bergström, S., Hakansson, S., Lindquist, I., Ljungkvist, I., Lundkvist, O. and Naeslund, G. (1978) Ultrastructure of implantation. Upp. J. Med. Sci. Suppl. 22, 27.

104 Hertig, A.T. (1968) Human Trophoblast. Charles C. Thomas, Springfield, Ill.

105 Falck-Larsen, J. and Knoth, M. (1971) Ultrastructure of the anchoring villi and trophoblastic shell in the second week of placentation. Acta Obstet. Gynecol. Scand. 59, 117.

106 Falck-Larsen, J. (1978) Aspects ultrastructuraux de l'ovo-implantation humaine. In, L'Implantation de l'Oeuf Ed Du Mesnil du Buisson, F., Psychoyos, A. and Thomas, K., Masson, Paris

107 Martinez-Manantou, J., Cortez, J., Giuer, J., Aznar, R., Casazola, J. and Rudel, H. (1966) Low doses of progestogen as an approach to fertility control. Fertil. and Steril. 17, 49.

108 Kirby, D.R.S. (1969) The extra-uterine mouse egg as an experimental model. Advanc Biosci. 4, 256.

109 Sherman, M.I., Strickland, S. and Reich, E. (1976) Differentiation of early mouse embryonic and teratocarcinoma cells in vitro: plasminogen activator production. Cancer Res. 36, 4208.

110 Ossowski, L., Quigley, J.P., Kellerman, G.M. and Reich, E. (1973) Fibrinolysis associated with oncogenic transformation; requirement of plasminogen for correlated changes in cellular morphology, colony formation in agar and cell migration. J. Exp. Med. 138, 1056.

111 Smith, A.F. and Wilson, I.B. (1974) Cell interaction at the maternal-embryonic interface during implantation in the mouse. Cell. Tiss. Res. 152, 525.

112 El-Shershaby, A.M. and Hinchliffe, J.R. (1975) Epithelial autolysis during implantation of the mouse blastocyst: an ultra-structural study. J. Embryol. exp. Morph. 33, 1067.

113 Amoroso, E.C. (1952) Placentation. in, Marshall's Physiology of Reproduction. Vol. 2 Ed. Parkes, A. S. Longmans, London.

114 Samuel, C.A. (1971) The development of pig trophoblast in ectopic sites. J. Reprod. Fert. 27, 494.

115 Petropoulos, E.A. (1973) Maternal and fetal factors affecting the growth and function of the rat placenta. Acta Endocrinologia 73, Supplement 176.

116 Heuser, C.H. and Streeter, G.L. (1941) Development of the macaque embryo. Carnegie Contrib. Embryol. 29, 15.

117 Houston, M.L. (1969) The villous period of placentogenesis in the baboon (Papio sp) Amer. J. Anat. 126, 1.

118 Ginsburg, J. and Jeacock, M.K. (1964) The placental barrier p. 86.In, Absorption and distribution of drugs. Ed. Binns, T.B. E. & S. Livingstone, Edinburgh.

119 Ramsey, E.M., Houston, M.L. and Harris, J.W.S. (1976) Interactions of the trophoblast and maternal tissues in three closely related primate species. Amer. J. Obstet. Gynec. 124, 647.

120 Hertig, A.T. and Rock, J. (1946) Two human ova of the pre-villous stage having a developmental age of about seven and nine days respectively. Contrib. Embryol. Carneg. Inst. 31, 65.

121 Boyd, J.D. and Hamilton, W.J. (1970) The human placenta. W. Heffer & Sons Ltd. Cambridge.

122 Beer, A.E. and Billingham, R.E. (1974) Host response to intraunterine tissue, cellular and fetal allografts. J. Reprod. Fert. Suppl. 21, 59.

123 Hamilton, W.J. and Boyd, J.D. (1960) Development of the human placenta in the first three months of gestation. J. Anat. 94, 297.

124 Brosens, I., Robertson, W.B. and Dixon, H.G. (1967) The physiological response of the vessels of the placental bed to normal pregnancy. J. Path. Bact. 93, 569.

125 Fauve, R.M., Hevin, B., Jacob, H., Gaillard, J.A. and Jacob, B.F. (1974) Anti-inflammatory effects of murine malignant cells. Proc. Nat. Acad. Sci. 71, 4052.

126 Southern, A.L., Kobayashi, Y., Bremner, P. and Weingold, A.B. (1965) Diamine oxidase activity in human material and fetal plasma and tissues and parturition. J. Appl. Physiol. 20, 1048.

127 Buffoni, F. (1966) Histaminase and related amino oxidases. Pharmacol Rev., 118, 1163.

128 Benda, M.R. and Minaret, L.F. (1960) Histaminase sérique et cancer. Bull Mem. Soc. Med. Hôp. Paris, 76, 184.

129 Baylin, S.B. (1977) Histaminase (Diamine oxidase) activity in human tumors: an expression of a mature genome. Proc. Nat. Acad. Sci. 74, 883.

130 Lin, C.W. and Kirley, S.D. (1976) Histaminase as an onco-placental enzyme: biochemical and immunological evidence.p. 469 In Onco-Developmental Gene Expression. Ed. Fishman, W.H. and Sell, S. Academic Press, New York.

131 Brettner, A. (1964) Sum Verhalten der Sekundären Wand der Utero-placentargefasse bei der decidualen Reaktion. Acta Anat. 57, 367.

132 Pijnenborg, R., Robertson, W.B. and Brosens, I. (1974) The arterial migration of trophoblast in the uterus of the golden hamster. (Mesocricetus auratus). J. Reprod. Fert. 40, 269.

133 Pijnenborg, R., Robertson, W.B. and Brosens, I. (1975) The role of ovarian steroids in placental development and endovascular trophoblast migration in the golden hamster. J. Reprod. Fert. 44, 43.

134 Brosens, I. (1975) p.64 in Human Placentation Ed. Brosens, I., Dixon, G. and Robertson, W.B., Excerpta Medica, Amsterdam.

135 Brosens, I., Robertson, W.B. and Dixon, H.G. (1967) The physiological response of the vessels of the placental bed to normal pregnancy. J. Path. Bact. 93, 569.

136 Adcock, E.W., Teasdale, F., August, C.S., Cos, C., Meschia, G., Battaglia, F.C. and Naughton, M.A. (1973) Human chorionic gonadotrophin: its possible role in maternal lymphocyte suppression. Science, 181, 845.

137 McManus, L.M., Naughton, M.A. and Martinez-Hernandez, M. (1976) Human chorionic gonadotrophin in human neoplastic cells. Cancer Res. 36, 3476.

138 Murgita, R.A. and Tomasi, T.B. (1975) Suppression of the immune response by alpha-feto-protein. II The effect of mouse alpha-feto-protein on mixed lymphocyte reactivity and mitogen-induced lymphocyte transformation. J. Exp. Med. 141, 440.

139 Goeken, N.E. and Thompson, J.S. (1976) Immunosuppressive properties of human alpha-feto-protein, and human cord plasma albumin. p.307 in Onco-Developmental Gene Expression. Ed. Fishman, W.H. and Sell, S. Acad. Press.

140 Drydsdale, J.W. and Singer, R.M. (1974) Carcinofetal human isoferritins in placenta and He La cells. Cancer Res. 34, 3352.

141 Bohn, H. (1976) Isolation and characterization of placental specific proteins SP_1 and PP_5. p.117 in, Protides of the Biological Fluide Ed. Peeters, H. Brügge, Belgium.

142 Stimson, W.H. (1976) Studies on the immunosuppressive properties of a pregnancy associated alpha-macro-globulin. Clin. Exp. Immunol 25, 199.

143 Fishman, W.H., Nishiyama, T., Rule, A., Green, S., Inglis, N.R. and Fishman, L. (1976) Onco-developmental alkaline phosphatase isozymes. p.165 in, Onco-Developmental Gene Expression. Ed. Fishman, W.H. and Sell, S. Acad. Press.

144 Horne, C.H., Towler, C.M., Pugh-Humphreys, R.G., Thomson, A.W. and Bohn, H. (1976) Pregnancy specific beta-1-glycoprotein - a product of the syncytiotrophoblast. Experientia, 32, 1197.

CHORIOCARCINOMA AND RELATED GROWTH ANOMALIES

Christopher W. Elston

1 Novak, E. and Seah, C. S., (1954). Choriocarcinoma of the uterus. Study of 74 cases from the Mathieu Memorial Chorionepithelioma Registery. American Journal of Obstetrics and Gynecology, 67, 933.

2 Brewer, J.I., Rhinehart, J.J. and Dunbar, R.W. (1961) Choriocarcinoma. A report of the 5 or more years survival from the Albert Mathieu Chorionepithelioma Registry. American Journal of Obstetrics and Gynecology, 81, 574.

3 Li, M.C., Hertz, R. and Spencer, D.B. (1956) Effect of methotrexate therapy upon choriocarcinoma and choricadenoma. Proc. Soc. expl. Biol. & Med., 93,361

4 Hertz, R., Bergenstal, D.M., Lipsett, M.B., Price, E.B. and Hillbish, T.G. (1959) Chemotherapy of choriocarcinoma and related tumors in women. Ann. N.Y. Acad. Sci., 80, 262.

5 Hertz, R., Ross, G.T. and Lipsett, M.B. (1964) Chemotherapy in women with trophoblastic disease: choriocarcinoma, chorioadenoma destruens, and complicated hydatidiform mole. Ann. N.Y. Acad. Sci., 114, 881.

6 Bagshawe, K.D. (1969) Choriocarcinoma, The Clinical Biology of the Trophoblast and its Tumours. London: Arnold.

7 Bagshawe, K.D., (1976) Endocrinology and treatment of trophoblastic tumours. Journal of Clinical Pathology, 29, Supplement (Royal College of Pathologists) 10, 140.

8 Hertz, R. (1978) Choriocaroinoma and Related Gestational Trophoblastic Tumors in Women. Raven Press, New York.

9 De Vita, V.T., Jr., Young, R.C. and Canellos, G.P. (1975) Combination versus single agent chemotherapy: a review of the basis for selection of drug treatment of cancer. Cancer, 35, 98.

10 Richart, R. (1961) Studies of placental morphogenesis. I. Radioautographic studies of human placenta utilizing tritiated thymidine. Proceedings of the Society for Experimental Biology and Medicine (New York), 106, 829.

11 Galton, M. DNA content of placental nuclei. Journal of Cell Biology, 13,183

12 Carter, J.E. (1964) Morphologic evidence of syncytial formation from the cytotrophoblastic cells. Obstetrics and Gynecology, 23, 647.

13 Enders, A.C. (1965) Formation of syncytium from cytotrophoblast in the human placenta. Obstetrics and Gynecology, 25, 378.

14 Tighe, J.R., Garrod, P.R. and Curran, R.C. (1968) The trophoblast of the human chorionic villus. Journal of Pathology and Bacteriology, 93, 559.

15 Boyd, J.D. and Hamilton, W.J. (1970) The Human Placenta. W. Heffer & Sons, Cambridge.

16 Teacher, J.H. (1903) On chorionepithelioma and the occurrence of chorionepitheliomatous and hydatidiform mole-like structures in teratomata. Journal of Obstetrics and Gynaecology of the British Empire, 4, 1-64, 145-199.

17 Ewing, J. (1910) Chorioma: a clinical and pathological study. Surgery, Gynecology and Obstetrics, 10, 366.

18 Hertig, A.T. and Mansell, H. (1956) Tumors of the female sex organs. Part 1. Hydatidiform mole and choriocarcinoma. In Atlas of Tumor Pathology, Section 9, Fascicle 33. Washington, D.C.: Armed Forces Institute of Pathology.

19 Ober, W.B., Edgcomb, J.H. and Price, E.B., Jr. (1971) The pathology of choriocarcinoma. Annals of the New York Academy of Sciences, 172, 299.

20 Park, W.W. (1971) Choriocarcinoma: A study of its Pathology. London: Heinemann. Philadelphia: Davis.

21 Elston, C.W. (1978) In The Pathology of the Placenta by H. Fox. Holt-Saunders, Philadelphia, London, pp 368-425.

22 Hertig, A.T. and Sheldon, W.H. (1947) Hydatidiform mole: a pathologico-clinical correlation of 200 cases. American Journal of Obstetrics and Gynecology, 53, 1.

23 Elston, C.W. (1970) A Histopathological Study of Trophoblastic Tumours: with special reference to the Cellular Reaction to Choriocarcinoma. MD Thesis, University of London.

24 Gore, H. and Hertig, A.T. (1967) Problems in the histologic interpretation of the trophoblast. Clinical Obstetrics and Gynecology, 10, 269.

25 Sutherland, A.M. (1951) An unusual case of chorionepithelioma of the uterus. J. Obstet. Gynaec. Brit. Emp., 58, 29.

26 Meyer, R. (1930) Mola hydatiformis (Blasenmole) und Chorionepithelioma malignum uteri. In Handbuck der speziellen pathologischen Anatomie und Histologie, ed. by O. Lubarsch and F. Henke. Springer-Verlag, Berlin, Vol. 7, pt. 1, p. 625.

27 Smalbraak, J. (1957) Trophoblastic growths. A clinical, hormonal and histopathologic study of hydatidiform mole and choriocarcinoma. Amsterdam: Elsevier.

28 Bloom, H.J.G. and Richardson, W.W. (1957) Histological grading and prognosis in breast cancer. British Journal of Cancer, II, 359.

29 Black, M.M., Opler, S.M. and Speer, F.D. (1955) Survival in breast cancer cases in relation to the structure of the primary tumour and regional lymph nodes. Surgery, Gynecology and Obstetrics, 100, 543.

30 Delfs, Eleanor (1957) Quantitative chorionic gonadotrophin. Prognostic value in hydatidiform mole and chorionepithelioma. Obstetrics and Gynecology, 9,1.

31 Ring, A.M. (1972) The concept of benign metastasizing hydatidiform moles. American Journal of Clinical Pathology, 58, 111.

32 Tow, W.S.H. (1966) The classification of malignant growths of the chorion. Journal of Obstetrics and Gynaecology of the British Commonwealth, 73,1000.

33 Brewer, J.I. (1967) Light microscopy of gestational trophoblastic disease. In Transcript of 4th Rochester Trophoblast Conference. Ed. Lund, C.W. and Choate, J.W. pp. 6-24. New York: Rochester.

34 Hertig, A.T. (1968) Human Trophoblast. Springfield: C.C. Thomas.

35 Fox, H. (1978) The Pathology of the Placenta. Holt-Saunders, Philadelphia and London.

36 Greene, R.R. (1959) Chorioadenoma destruens. Annals of the New York Academy of Sciences, 80, 143.

37 Ober, W.B. (1965) Clinical and pathological aspects of abnormal trophoblast: discussion. In The Early Conceptus, Normal and Abnormal. Ed. Park, W.W. pp. 141-144. London: Livingstone.

38 Hsu, C.T., Huang, I.C. and Chen, T.Y. (1962) Metastases in benign hydatidiform mole and chorioadenoma destruens. American Journal of Obstetrics and Gynecology, 84, 1412.

39 Ishizuka, N. (1967) Chemotherapy of chorionic tumours. In Choriocarcinoma: Transactions of a conference of the International Union against Cancer. Ed. Holland, J.F. and Hreshchyshyn, M.M. pp. 116-118. Berlin, Heidelberg and New York: Springer Verlag.

40 Chun, D. and Braga, C.A. (1967) Choriocarcinoma in Hong Kong. In Proceedings of the 5th World Congress of Gynaecology and Obstetrics. Ed. Wood, C. pp. 398-405. Chatswood, New South Wales: Butterworths.

41 Boyd, J.D. and Hughes, A.F.W. (1954) Observations on human chorionic villi using the electron microscope. Journal of Anatomy, 88, 356.

42 Wislocki, G.B. and Dempsey, E.W. (1955) Electron microscopy of the human placenta. Anatomical Record, 123, 133.

43 Rhodin, J.A.G. and Terzakis, J. (1962) The Ultrastructure of the human full-term placenta. Journal of Ultrastructure Research, 6, 88.

44 Terzakis, J.A. (1963) The ultrastructure of normal human first trimester placenta. Journal of Ultrastructure Research, 9, 268.

45 Lister, U.M. (1964) Ultrastructure of the early human placenta. Journal of Obstetrics and Gynaecology of the British Commonwealth, 71, 21-32.

46 Knoth, M. (1968) Ultrastructure of chorionic villi from a four-somite human embryo. Journal of Ultrastructure Research, 25, 423.

47 Wynn, R.W. (1972) Cytotrophoblastic specializations: an ultrastructural study of the human placenta. American Journal of Obstetrics and Gynecology, 144, 339

48 Wynn, R.W. (1975) Fine structure of the placenta. In The Placenta and its Maternal Supply Line. Ed. Gruenwald, P. pp. 56-79. Lancaster: Medical and Technical Publishing.

49 Wynn, R.W. (1975) Development and ultrastructural adaptations of the human placenta. European Journal of Obstetrics, Gynecology and Reproductive Biology, 5, 3.

50 Wakitani, T. (1962) Electron microscopic observations on the chorionic villi of the normal human placenta and chorioepithelioma malignum. Part II. Electron microscopic observations on the chorio-epithelioma malignum. Mie Medical Journal, 12, 43.

51 Inferrera, C., Pulle, C., Rigano, A. and Palmara, D. (1967) Aspetti ultra strutturali e citochimici del coriocarcinoma uterino. Archivio di Ostetricia e Ginecologia, 72, 707.

52 Knoth, M., Pattilo, R.A., Garancis, J.C., Gey, G.O., Ruckert, A.C.F. and Mattingly, R.F. (1969) Ultrastructure and hormone synthesis of choriocarcinoma in vitro. American Journal of Pathology, 54, 479.

53 Larsen, J.F. (1973) Ultrastructure of the abnormal human trophoblast. Acta Anatomica, 86, Supplement 1, 47.

54 Larsen, J.F., Ehrmann, R.L. and Bierring, F. (1967) Electron microscopy of human choriocarcinoma transplanted into hamster liver. American Journal of Obstetrics and Gynecology, 99, 1109.

55 Brosens, I., Robertson, W.B. and Dixon, H.G. (1967) The physiological response of the vessels of the placental bed to normal pregnancy. Journal of Pathology and Bacteriology. 93, 569.

56 Robertson, W.B. (1976) Uteroplacental vasculature. Journal of Clinical Pathology, 29, Supplement (Royal College of Pathologists) 10, 9

57 Harris, J.W.S. and Ramsey, E.M. (1976) The morphology of human uteroplacental vasculature. Contributions to Embryology. Carnegie Institution of Washington, 38, 43.

58 Robertson, W.B., Brosens, I. and Dixon, G. (1975) Uteroplacental vascular pathology. European J. Obstetrics Gynecology & Reprod. Biology, 5, 47.

59 Robertson, W.B. and Warner, B. (1974) The ultrastructure of the human placental bed. Journal of Pathology, 112, 203.

60 Marchard, F. (1898) Uber das maligne Chorion-Epitheliom, nebst Mittheilung von 2 neuen Fällen. Zeitschrift für Geburtshilfe und Gynäkologie, 39,173.

61 Elston, C.W. (1976) The histopathology of trophoblastic tumours. Journal of Clinical Pathology, 29, Supplement (Royal College of Pathologists) 10, 111.

62 Novak, E. and Seah, C.S. (1954) Benign trophoblastic lesions in Mathieu Chorionepithelioma Registry (hydatidiform mole, syncytial endometritis). American Journal of Obstetrics and Gynecology, 68, 376.

63 Elston, C.W. and Bagshawe, K.D. (1972) The diagnosis of trophoblastic tumours from uterine curettings. Journal of Clinical Pathology, 25, 111.

64 Kurman, R.J., Scully, R.E. and Norris, H.J. (1976) Trophoblastic pseudotumor of the uterus: an exaggerated form of 'syncytial endometritis' simulating a malignant tumor. Cancer, 38, 1214-1226.

65 Schmorl, G. (1893) Pathologisch-anatomische Untersuchungen über Puerperal-eklampsie. Leipzig: Vogel.

66 Veit, J. (1901) Uber deportation von Chorionzotten. Zeitschrift für Geburtshilfe und Gynäkologie, 44, 466

67 Bardawil, W.A. and Toy, B.L. (1959) The natural history of choriocarcinoma: problems of immunity and spontaneous regression. Annals of the New York Academy of Sciences 80, 197.

68 Attwood, H.D. and Park, W.W. (1961) Embolism to the lungs by trophoblast. Journal of Obstetrics & Gynaecology of the British Commonwealth, 68, 611.

69 Park, W.W. (1957) The occurrence of sex chromatin in chorionepitheliomas and hydatidiform moles. Journal of Pathology and Bacteriology, 74, 197.

70 Wagner, D. (1958) Zur Frage der chromosomalen Geschlechtsbestimmung bei Frühaborten und Tubargraviditäten. Geburtshilfe und Frauenheilkunde, 18,1460.

71 Marquez-Monter, H. (1963) El sexo de la mola hidatidiforme. Revista Latinoamericana de Anatomia Patologica, 7, 57

72 Atkin, N.B. (1965) Sex chromosome studies in trophoblast. In The Early Conceptus, Normal and Abnormal. Ed. Park, W.W. pp. 130-134. London: Livingstone.

73 Tominaga, T. and Page, E.W. (1966) Sex chromatin of trophoblastic tumors. American Journal of Obstetrics and Gynecology, 96, 305.

74 Beischer, N.A. and Fortune, D.W. (1968) Significance of chromatin patterns in cases of hydatidiform mole with an associated fetus. American Journal of Obstetrics and Gynecology, 100, 276.

75 Stolte, L.A.M., von Kessel, H.I.A.M., Seelan, J.C. and Tijdink, G.A.J. (1960) Chromosomes in hydatidiform mole. Lancet, ii, 1221.

76 Harden, D.G. (1961) Congenital abnormalities with an apparently normal chromosome complement. In Human Chromosomal Abnormalities. (Ed.) Davidson, W.M. and Smith, D.R. pp. 123-130. London: Staples.

77 Sasaki, M., Fukuschima, T. and Makino, S. (1962) Some aspects of the chromosome constitution of hydatidiform moles and normal chorionic villi. Gann, 53, 101.

78 Makino, S., Sasaki, M.S. and Fukuschima, T. (1963) Preliminary notes on the chromosomes of human chorionic lesions. Proceedings of the Japanese Academy 39, 54.

79 Makino, S., Sasaki, M.S. and Fukuschima, T. (1964) Triploid chromosome constitution in human chorionic lesions. Lancet, ii, 1273.

80 Schlegal, R.J., Nen, R., Leao, J.C., Farias, E., Lewczak, P. and Gardner, L.I. (1966) Arborizing amniotic polyps in triploid conceptuses: a diagnostic anatomic lesion? American Journal of Obstetrics and Gynecology, 96, 357.

81 Carr, D.H. (1969) Cytogenetics and the pathology of hydatidiform degeneration. Obstetrics and Gynecology, 33, 333.

82 Honore, L.H., Dill, F.J. and Poland, B.J. (1974) The association of hydatidiform mole and trisomy 2. Obstetrics and Gynecology, 43, 232.

83 Bourgoin, P., Baylet, R., Ballon, C. and Grattepanche, H. (1965) Exploration d'une hypothese sur l'etiopathogenie des mole hydatiformes. Etude chromosomique. Revue Française de Gyncologie et d'Obstetrique, 60, 673

84 Ross, G.T. (1974) Human chorionic gonadotrophin in vivo and in vitro. In The Placenta, Biological and Clinical Aspects. Ed. Moghissi, K.S. and Hafez, E.S.E. pp. 258-274. Charles C. Thomas, Ill.

85 Siiteri, P.K., Gant, N.F. and MacDonald, P.C. (1974) Synthesis of steroid hormones by the placenta. In The Placenta, Biological and Clinical Aspects. Ed. Moghissi, K.S. and Hafez, E.S.E. pp. 238-257. Charles C. Thomas, Ill.

86 Thau, R.B. and Lanman, J.T. (1975) Endocrinological aspects of placental function. In The Placenta and its Maternal Supply Line. Ed. Gruenwald, P. pp. 125-144. Lancaster: Medical and Technical Publishing.

87 Frandsen, V.A. and Stakemann, G. (1964) The excretion of hormones in cases of hydatidiform mole and chorionepithelioma. Acta Endocrinologia Supplement 190, 81.

88 Zondek, B. and Finkelstein, M. (1967) Urinary excretion of gonadotrophin and the estrogens in hydatidiform mole and choriocarcinoma. In Choriocarcinoma: transactions of a conference of the International Union against Cancer, Ed. Holland, J. F. and Hreshelyshyn M.M., pp. 84-93. Springer-Verlag, Berlin.

89 Godden, J.D., Garnett, E.S., Sommerville, I.F. and Bagshawe, K.D. (1967) The effect of choriocarcinoma on serum thyroid hormone-binding capacity. Journal of Endocrinology, 39, 21.

90 Brinck-Johnsen, T., Solc, J. and Galton, V.A. (1970) Urinary excretion of estrogens in women with hydatidiform mole and choriocarcinoma. Obstetrics and Gynecology, 36, 671.

91 Kaufmann, C. and Zander, J. (1954) Progesteron und Chorionepitheliom. Acta Acta Endocrinologia (Kbh) 17, 216

92 Dawood, M.Y. (1975) Evaluation of serum progesterone during treatment of malignant trophoblastic disease. American Journal of Obstetrics and Gynecology, 123, 291.

93 Aschheim, S. and Zondek, B. (1928) Die schwangerschafts diagnose ans dem harn durch nachweis des hypophysenvorderlappenhormons. Klin. Wochenschrift 7, 1404.

94 Friedman, M.H. (1929) Mechanism of ovulation in rabbit; ovulation produced by injection of urine from pregnant women. American Journal of Physiology, 90, 617.

95 Delfs, E. (1941) Assay method for human chorionic gonadotrophin. Endocrinology, 28, 196.

96 Wilde, C.E., Orr, A.H. and Bagshawe, K.D. (1965) A radio-immunoassay for human chorionic gonadotrophin. Nature 205, 191.

97 Wilde, C.E., Orr, A.H. and Bagshawe, K.D. (1967) A sensitive radio-immunoassay for human chorionic gonadotrophins and luteinising hormone. Journal of Endocrinology, 37, 23.

98 Kardana, A. and Bagshawe, K.D. (1976) A rapid sensitive and specific radioimmunoassay for human chorionic gonadotrophin. Journal of Immunological Methods, 9,297.

99 Edwards, R.G., Howe, C.W.S. and Johnson, M.H. (Editors) (1975) Immunobiology of Trophoblast. London: Cambridge University Press.

100 Medawar, P. (1944) Behaviour and fate of skin autografts and skin homografts in rabbits (report to War Wounds Committee of Medical Research Council). Journal of Anatomy, 78, 176.

101 Waksman, B.H. (1960) A comparative histopathological study of delayed hypersensitivity reactions. In Ciba Foundation Symposium on Cellular Aspects of Immunity. Ed. Wolstenholme, G.E.W. and O'Conor, M. pp. 280-329. London: Churchill Livingstone.

102 Gowans, J.L. (1965) The role of lymphocytes in the destruction of homografts. British Medical Bulletin, 21, 106.

103 Elston, C.W. (1969) Cellular reaction to choriocarcinoma. Journal of Pathology, 97, 261.

104 Elston, C.W. and Bagshawe, K.D. (1973) Cellular reaction in trophoblastic tumours. British Journal of Cancer, 28, 245.

105 Mogensen, B. and Olsen, S. (1973) Cellular reaction to geational choriocarcinoma and invasive mole. Acta Pathologica et Microbiologica Scandinavica, A 81, 453.

106 Junaid, T.A., Hendrickse, J.P. de V., Williams, A.O. and Osunhoya, B.O. (1976) Choriocarcinoma in Ibadan: Clinicopathologic studies. Human Pathology, 7, 215.

107 Golding, P.G., Elston, C.W., Levison, V.B. and Bagshawe, K.D. (1968) The diagnosis of trophoblastic tumours of testis. British Journal of Surgery, 55, 508.

108 Pugh, R.C.B. and Cameron, K.M. (1976) In Pathology of the Testis Ed., Pugh, R.C.B. Blackwell, London. pp. 199-244.

109 Lawler, S.D. (1976) Immunogenetics of trophoblastic tumours. Journal of Clinical Pathology, 29, Supplement (Royal College of Pathologists) 10, 132.

110 Rudolph, R.H. and Thomas, E.D. (1970) Histocompatibility studies in patients with trophoblastic tumors. American Journal of Obstetrics and Gynecology, 108, 1126.

111 Lawler, S.D., Kouda, P.T. and Bagshawe, K.D. (1971) The HL-A system in trophoblastic neoplasia. Lancet, ii, 834.

112 Lewis, J.L., Jr. and Terasaki, P.T. (1971) HL-A leukocyte antigen studies in women with gestational trophoblastic neoplasms. American Journal of Obstetrics and Gynecology, 111, 547.

113 Mogensen, B. and Kissmeyer-Nielson, F. (1971) Current data on HL-A and ABO typing in gestational choriocarcinoma and invasive mole. Transplantation Proceedings, 3, 1267.

114 Lewis J.L., Jr. (1973) Human leukocyte antigens and ABO blood groups in gestational trophoblastic neoplasms. Proceedings National Cancer Conference, 7, 205.

115 Dawood, M.Y., Tech, E.S. and Ratnam, S.S. (1971) ABO blood group in trophoblastic disease. Journal of Obstetrics and Gynaecology of the British Commonwealth, 78, 918.

116 Bagshawe, K.D. (1973) Recent observations related to the chemotherapy and immunology of gestational choriocarcinoma. Advances in Cancer Research, 18, 231.

117 Bagshawe, K.D. (1976) Risk and prognostic factors in trophoblastic neoplasia. Cancer, 38, 1373.

118 Acosta-Sison, H. (1955) Can the implanting trophoblasts of the fertilized ovum develop immediately into chorionepithelioma? American Journal of Obstetrics and Gynecology, 69, 442.

119 Schiffer, M.A., Pomerance, W. and Mackles, A. (1960) Hydatidiform mole in relation to malignant disease of the trophoblast. American Journal of Obstetrics and Gynecology, 90, 516.

120 Douglas, G.W. (1962) Malignant change in trophoblastic tumours. American Journal of Obstetrics and Gynecology, 84, 884.

121 Hunt, W., Dockerty, M.B. and Randall, L.M. (1953) Hydatidiform mole: clinicopathologic study involving 'grading' as a measure of possible malignant change. Obstetrics and Gynecology, 1, 593.

122 Tow, W.S.H. and Yung, R.H. (1967) The value of histological grading in prognostication of hydatidiform mole. Journal of Obstetrics and Gynaecology of the British Commonwealth, 74, 292.

123 Elston, C.W. and Bagshawe, K.D. (1972) The value of histological grading in the management of hydatidiform mole. Journal of Obstetrics and Gynaecology of the British Commonwealth, 79, 717.

124 Hutchinson, J.R., Peterson, E.P., Zimmermann, E.A. (1968) Coexisting metastatic choriocarcinoma and normal pregnancy. Therapy during gestation with maternal remission and fetal survival. Obstetrics and Gynecology, 31, 331.

125 Brewer, J.I. and Gerbie, A.B. (1966) Early development of choriocarcinoma. American Journal of Obstetrics and Gynecology, 94, 692.

126 Driscoll, S.G. (1963) Choriocarcinoma: an 'incidental finding' within a term placenta. Obstetrics and Gynecology, 21, 96.

127 Bagshawe, K.D., Klouda, P.T. and Lawler, S.D. (1976) The relationship between HLA antibodies and the causal pregnancy in choriocarcinoma. British Journal of Obstetrics and Gynaecology, 83, 651.

128 Greene, H.S.N. (1952) The significance of the heterologous transplant ability of human cancer. Cancer, 5, 24.

129 Hertz, R. (1959) Choriocarcinoma of women maintained in serial passage in hamster and rat. Proceedings of the Society of Experimental Biology and Medicine, 102, 77.

130 Hertz, R. (1960) Suppression of Human choriocarcinoma maintained in the hamster cheek pouch by extracts and alkaloids of vinca rosea. Proceedings of the Society of Experimental Biology and Medicine, 105, 281.

131 Lewis, J.L., Jr., Davis, R.C. and Ross, G.T. (1969) Hormonal, immunologic and chemotherapeutic studies of transplantable human choriocarcinoma. American Journal of Obstetrics and Gynecology, 104, 472.

132 Pattillo, R.A. and Gey, G.O. (1968) The establishment of a cell line of human hormone-synthesising trophoblastic cells in vitro. Cancer Research, 28,1231.

133 Knoth, M., Pattillo, R.A., Garancis, J.C., Gey, G.O., Ruckert, A.C.F. and Mattingly, R.F. (1969) Ultrastructure and hormone synthesis of choriocarcinoma in vitro. American Journal of Pathology, 54, 479.

134 Garancis, J.C., Pattillo, R.A., Hussa, R.O., Schultz, J. and Mattingly, R.F. (1970) Electron microscopic and biochemical patterns of the normal and malignant trophoblast. American Journal of Obstetrics and Gynecology, 108,1257.

135 Pattillo, R.A., Gey, G.O., Delfs, E., Huang, W.Y., Hause, L., Garancis, D.J., Knoth, M., Amatruda, J., Bertino, J., Friesen, H.G. and Mattingly, R.F. (1971) The hormone-synthesising trophoblastic cell in vitro: a model for cancer research and placental hormone synthesis. Annals of the New York Academy of Sciences, 172, 288.

136 Kim, W., Takahashi, T., Nisselbaum, J.S. and Lewis, J.L., Jr. (1978) Heterotransplantation of human choriocarcinoma in nude mice. 1. Morphologic and biologic characteristics. Gynecologic Oncology, 6, 165.

137 Lindsey, J.R., Wharton, L.R., Woodruff, J.D., Baker, H.J. (1969) Intrauterine choriocarcinoma in a rhesus monkey. Pathologia Veterinaria, 6, 378.

138 Stein-Werblowsky, R. (1960) Induction of chorionepitheliomatous tumour in the rat. Nature 186,980.

139 Marin-Padilla, M. and Benirschke, K. (1963) Thalidomide-induced alterations in the blastocyst and placenta of the armadillo, dasypus novemcintus mezicanus, including a choriocarcinoma. American Journal of Pathology, 43,999.

140 Kushima, K., Noda, K. and Makita, M. (1967) Experimental production of chorionic tumour in rabbits. Tohuku. Journal of Experimental Medicine, 91, 209.

141 Shintani, S., Glass, L.E. and Page, E.W. (1966) Studies of induced malignant tumors of placental and uterine origin in the rat. 1. Survival of placental tissue following fetectomy. 2. Induced tumors and their pathogenesis with special reference to choriocarcinoma. 3. Identification of experimentally induced choriocarcinoma by detection of placental hormone. American Journal of Obstetrics and Gynecology, 95, 542.

142 Miyamoto, M., Nilsuwarn, N. and Angsubhakorn, S. (1972) The morphology of experimental chorionic tumours in rats. Acta Pathologica Japonica, 22, 343.

143 Komuro, N. (1976) Experimental induction of choriocarcinoma in pregnant rats. Acta Obstetricia et Gynaecologica Japonica, 23, 32

144 Tanaka, T. (1976) Studies on histogenesis of experimentally induced chorio-epithelioma in rats. Acta Obstetricia et Gynaecologica Japonica, 23, 43

145 Acosta-Sison, H. (1967) Trophoblastic or chorionic tumors as observed in the Philippines. In Choriocarcinoma: Transactions of a Conference of the International Union against Cancer. (Ed.) Holland, J.F. and Hreshchyshyn, M.M. pp 35-36. Berlin, Heidelberg & New York: Springer Verlag.

146 Reynolds, S.R., (1976) Hydatidiform mole: a vascular congenital abnormality. Obstetrics and Gynecology, 47, 244

CHARACTERISTICS OF THE MALIGNANT CELL AND THE CELL CYCLE IN TUMOURS

P. P. Dendy and R. A. Meldrum

1 Tubiana, M. and Malaise, E. (1976) Comparison of cell proliferation kinetics in human and experimental tumours: Response to Irradiation. Cancer Treatment Report, 60, 1887.

2 Cleaver, J.E. (1967) Thymidine metabolism and cell kinetics. Elsevier, Amsterdam.

3 Ashley, D.J.B. (1978). Evans' histological appearances of tumours. 3rd edn. Churchill-Livingstone.

4 Difruscio, D. and Desa, D.J. (1977) Application of the Papanicolaou stain to routine histological examination of the placenta, J. Clin. Path 30, 682.

5 Koss, L.G. (1968) Diagnostic cytology and its histopathologic bases. 2nd edn. Lippincott, Philadelphia.

6 Lerch, V.L., Todd, J., Lattimer, J.K. and Tannenbaum, M. (1970) A technique for the study of human prostatic ephithelial cells in vitro by time-lapse cinematography, J. Urol, 104, 564.

7 Wright, J.E.M. and Dendy, P.P. (1976) Human tumour cell identification in short term monolayer culture.in Human tumours in short term culture-techniques and clinical applications. Acad. Press, London and New York, 88, 96.

8 Morasca, L., Balconi, G. And Erba, E. (1976) Advances in morphological identification of cell types in primary culture, in Human tumours in short term culture-techniques and clinical applications Ed. Dendy, P.P. Academic Press, London and New York, 78, 84.

9 Bean, M.A. and Hajdu, S.I. (1975) Cytological characterisation of human tumour cells from monolayer cultures, in Human tumour cells in vitro. Ed. Fogh, J., Plenum Press, New York, 333.

10 Hajdu, S.I., Bean, M.A., Fogh, J., Hajdu, E.O. and Ricci, A. (1974) Papanicolaou smear for cultured human tumour cells. Acta Cytol. 18, 327.

11 Qizilbash, A.H., Liao, S.K. and Dent, P.B. (1977) Characterisation of human malignant melanoma cell lines IV Cytologic and histochemical characteristics. Acta Cytol. 21, 147.

12 Hayat, M.A. (ed.) (1972) Principles and techniques of electron microscopy - Biological Applications (Vol. 2), Van Norstrand Reinhold Co., New York.

13 Weinstein, R.S., Merk, F.B. and Alroy, F. (1976) The structure and function of intercellular junctions in cancer Adv. in Cancer Research. 23, 23.

14 Wiernik, G., Bradbury, S., Plant, M., Cowdell, R.H. and Williams, E.A. (1973) A quantitative comparison between normal and carcinomatous squamous epithelia of the uterine cervix. Brit.J. Cancer, 28, 488.

15 Hayat, M.A. (ed.) (1974-1976) Principles and techniques of scanning electron microscopy-biological applications. Vols 1-5, Van Norstrand Reinhold Co., New York.

16 Porter, K.R., Fonte, V., Weiss, G. (1974) A scanning microscope study of the topography of Hela Cells. Cancer Res. 34, 1385.

17 Spring-Mills, E. and Elias, J.J. (1975) Cell surface differences in ducts from cancerous and non cancerous human breasts. Science 188, 947.

18 Ambrose, E., Mistry, D.H., Stephen, J. and Tchao (1976) Opical and scanning electron microscopy of human carcinomas. J. Microscopic Biol. Cell, 25, 173.

19 Springer, E.L., Hackett, A.J., Nelson-Rees, W.A. (1976) Alteration of the cell membrane architecture during suspension and monolayer culturing. Int. J. Cancer, 17, 407.

20 Gonda, M.A., Aaronson, S.A., Ellmore, N., Zeve, V.H., Nagashima, K. (1976) Ultrastructural studies of surfact features of human normal and tumour cells in tissue culture by scanning and transmission electron microscopy. J. Nat. Cancer Inst. 56- 245.

21 Miles, C.P. (1967) Chromosome analysis of solid tumours. I Twenty-eight nonepithelial tumours. Cancer, 20, 1253.

22 Miles, C.P. (1967) Chromosome analysis of solid tumours.II Twenty-six epithelial tumours. Cancer, 20, 1274.

23 Miles, C.P. and Wolinska, W. (1973) A comparative analysis of chromosomes and diagnostic cytology in effusions from 58 cancer patients. Cancer, 32, 1458.

24 Youis, J.J. (ed.) (1974) Human chromosome methodology, 2nd edn Academic Press, New York.

25 Sonta, S.J. and Sandberg, A.A. (1978) Chromosomes and causation of human cancer and leukaemia XXX Banding studies of primary intestinal tumours. Cancer, 41, 164.

26 Mark, J. (1977) Chromosomal abnormalities and their specificity in human neoplasms. An assessment of recent observations by banding techniques. Adv. in Cancer Res. 24, 165.

27 Jones, K.W. (1974) Chromosomes and malignancy Nature, 252,525

28 Codish, S.D. and Paul, B. (1974) Reversible appearance of a specific chromosome which suppresses malignancy Nature, 252, 610.

29 Biedler, J.L. (1975) Chromosome abnormalities in human tumour cells in culture in Human tumour cells in vitro. Ed. Fogh, J. Plenum Press, New York, 359.

30 Gohde, W., Schumann, J. and Buchner, T.L. (eds), (1976) 2nd International Symposium on Pulse Cytophotometry - applications in cancer research and haematology with special reference to cell kinetics. European Press, Ghent, Belgium.

31 James, J. (1973) Extinction effects in Feulgen-DNA scanning photometry of human lymphocytes. Acta cytol, 17, 15.

32 Atkin, N.B., Mattinson, G., Becak, W., Ohno, S. (1965) The comparative DNA content of 19 species of placental mammals, reptiles and birds. Chromosoma, 17, 1.

33 Atkin, N.B., Richards, B.M. and Ross, A. (1959) The DNA content of carcinoma of the uterus. An assessment of its possible significance in relation to histopathology and clinical course based on data from 165 cases. Brit. J. Cancer, 13, 773.

34 Reid, B.L. and Singh, S. (1960) Deoxyribonucleic acid values (Feulgen micro-spectrophotometry) in epithelium of human ectocervix,normal and cancerous. J. Nat. Cancer Inst. 25, 129.

35 Wied, G.L., Messina, A.M. and Rosenthal, E. (1966) Comparative quantitative measurements on Feulgen-stained cervical epithelial cells. Acta Cytol. 10, 31.

36 Bohm, N, and Sandritter, W. (1975) DNA in human tumours - a cytophotometric study. Current topics in Pathology, 60, 151.

37 Muller, W. (1972) DNA estimations in cerebral tumours in man. Neuropath. Pol. 10, 121.

38 Atkin, N.B., Mattinson, G., Baker, M.C. (1966) A comparison of DNA content and chromosome number of fifty human tumours. Brit.J.Cancer, 20, 84.

39 Frederiksen, P., Reske-Nielsen, E. and Bichel, P. (1978) Flow cytophotometry in tumours of the brain. Acta Neuropath (Berl) 41, 179.

40 Tribukait, B. and Esposti, P. (1976) in 2nd International Symposium on Pulse Cytophotometry - applications in cancer research and haematology with special reference to cell kinetics Ed. Gohde, W., Schuman, J. and Butchner, T.L. European Press, Ghent, Belgium 176

41 Fossa, S.D., Kaalhus, O. and Scott-Knudsen, O. (1977) The clinical and histopathological significance of Feulgen DNA values in transitional cell carconoma of the human urinary bladder. Europ. J. Cancer, 13, 1155.

42 Atkin, N.B. (1971) Modal DNA value and chromosome number in ovarian neoplasia. Cancer 27, 1064.

43 Granberg, I., Gupta, S., Joelsson, I., Sprenger, E. (1974) Chromosome and nuclear DNA study of a uterine adenocarcinoma and its metastases. Acta Path. Microbiol Scand 82, Sect A, 1.

44 Sandberg, A.A. and Sakurai, M. (1974) Chromosomes in the causation and progression of cancer and leukaemia. in The Molecular Biology of Cancer Ed. Busch, H. Academic Press, New York and London, 81.

45 Atkin, N.B. (1976) Cytogenetic aspects of malignant transformation. Exptl. Biol. and Med. Vol. 6.

46 Sprenger, E., Sandritter, W., Naujoks, H., Hilgarth, M., Wagner, D. and Vogt-Schaden, M. (1977) Routine use of flow-through photometric prescreening in the detection of cervical carcinoma. Acta Cytol. 21, 435.

47 Johannisson, M.D., Landgren, B.M. and Hagenfeldt, M.D. (1977) The effect of interuterine progesterone on the DNA content in isolated human endometrial cells. Acta Cytol. 21, 441.

48 Hainau, B. and Dombernowsky, P. (1974) Histology and cell proliferation in human bladder tumours. An autoradiographic study. Cancer 33, 115.

49 Lederer, B. and Autengruber, M. (1976) Statistical analysis of cytophotometric DNA measurements demonstrated on malignant testicular teratoma. Acta Cytol. 20, 5.

50 Wied, G.L. (ed) (1966) Introduction to quantitative cytochemistry. Academic Press London and New York.

51 Wied, G.L. and Bahr, G.F. (eds) (1970) Introduction to quantitative cytochemistry II. Academic Press London and New York.

52 Fishman, W.H. and Ghosh, N.K. (1967) Isoenzymes of human alkaline phosphatase. Adv. in Clin. Chem. 10, 255.

53 Miki, K., Oda, T., Suzuki, H., Iino, S., Niwa, H. (1976) Alkaline phosphatase izoenzymes in intestinal metaplasia and carcinoma of the stomach. Cancer Res. 36, 4266.

54 Fishman, L., Miyama, H., Driscoll, S.G. and Fishman, W.H. (1976) Developmental phase-specific alkaline phosphatase isoenzymes of human placenta and their occurrence in human cancer. Cancer Research, 36, 2268.

55 Fishman, W.H. (1976) Activation of developmental genes in neoplastic transformation. Cancer Research 36, 3423.

56 Schwartz, M.K. (1977) Enzyme patterns in cancer. Ann. Clin. Lab. Sci. 7/2, 99.

57 Weber, G. (1974) Molecular correlation concept in The Molecular biology of cancer. Ed. Busch, H. Academic Press, London & New York, 487.

58 Salih, H., Flax, H. and Hobbs, J.R. (1972) In vitro oestrogen sensitivity of breast cancer tissue as a possible screening method for hormonal treatment. Lancet i, 1198.

59 Salih, H., Flax, H., Brander, W. and Hobbs, J.R. (1972) Prolactin dependence in human breast cancers. Lancet ii, 1103.

60 Beeby, D.I., Easty, G.C., Cazet, J.C., Grigor, K. and Neville, A.M. (1975) An assessment of the effects of hormones on short term organ cultures of human breast carcinomata. Brit.J Cancer, 31, 317.

61 Masters, J.R.W., Sangster, K., Smith, I.I. and Forrest, A.P.M. (1976) Human breast carcinomata in organ culture. The effects of hormones. Brit.J.Cancer 33, 564.

62 Woods, K.L., Cove, D.H. and Howell, A. (1977) Predictive classification of human breast carcinomas based on lactalbumen synthesis, Lancet ii, 14.

63 Horne, C.H.W., Reid, I.N. and Milne, G.D. (1976) Prognostic significance of inappropriate production of pregnancy proteins by breast cancers. Lancet ii, 279.

64 Trempe, G.L. (1976) Human breast cancer in culture, in Breast Cancer - a multidisciplinary approach. Recent Results in Cancer Research Vol. 57 Ed. Arneault G.St., Band, P. and Israel, L. Springer Verlag, Berlin, Heidelberg, New York, pp. 33.

65 Laing, L., Leake, R.E. and Freshney, R.I. The growth of mammary tumour epithelial cells on feeder layers. Proceedings of the 26th Annual Meeting of the European Tissue Culture Society, Glasgow, July 1978.

66 Burger, M.A. (1969) A difference in the architecture of the surface membrane of normal and virally transformed cells. Proc. Nat. Acad. Sci. (Wash), 62, 994.

67 Buck, C.A., Glick, M.C. and Warren, L. (1970) A comparative study of glycoproteins from the surface of control and Rous sarcoma virus transformed hamster cells. Biochemistry 9, 4567.

68 Van Beek, W.P., Smets, L.A. and Emmelot, P. (1975) Changed surface glycoprotein as a marker of malignancy in human leukaemic cells. Nature 253, 457.

69 Smets, L.A., Van Beek, W.P. and Van Roij, H. (1976) Surface glycoproteins and concanavalin - A mediated agglutinability of clonal variants and tumour cells derived from SV 40 virus transformed mouse 3T3 cells. Int. J. Cancer 18, 462.

70 Ambrose, E.J. and Easty, D. (1976) Cellular dynamics of human breast carcinoma in Human Tumours in Short Term Culture. Techniques and Clinical Applications, Ed. Dendy, P.P., Academic Press, London and New York.

71 Ambrose, E.J. (1967) Surface properties of mammalian cells in culture, in The Proliferation and Spread of Neoplastic Cells - 21st Annual Symp. on Fundamental Cancer Research. The Williams & Wilkins Co. Baltimore.

72 Abercrombie, M. (1975) The contact behaviour of invading cells in cellular membranes and tumour cell behaviour. 28th Annual symp. of Fundamental Cancer Research. The Williams and Wilkins Co. Baltimore.

73 Bell, P.B. (1972) Criss-crossing contact inhibition and cell movement in cultures of normal and transformed 3T3 cells (abstract) J. Cell Biol. 55, No.2, 16A.

74 Projan, A. and Tanneberger, S. (1973) Some findings on movement and contact of human normal and tumour cells in vitro. Europ. J. of Cancer, 9. 703.

75 Turbitt, M. and Curtis, A.S.G. (1974) Are there differences in contact inhibition of movement between normal and malignant cells. Nature 249, 453.

76 Westermark, B. (1973) The deficient density-dependent growth control of human malignant glioma cells and virus transformed glia-like cells in culture. Int. J. Cancer 12, 438.

77 Marcel, M. Is invasiveness in vitro characteristic of malignant cells? Proceedings of the 24th annual meeting of the European Tissue Culture Society, Glasgow, July 1978.

78 De Ridder, L., Mareel, M. and Vahaet, L. (1975) Adhesion of malignant and non-malignant cells to cultured embryonic substrates. Cancer Res. 35, 3164.

79 Coman, D.R. (1944) Decreased mutual adhesiveness, a property of cells from squamous cell carcinomas, Cancer Res. 4, 625.

80 McCutcheon, M., Coman, D.R. and Fontaine, B.M. (1948) Studies on invasiveness of cancer. Cancer, 1, 460.

81 Tjernberg, B. and Najicik, J. (1965) Cannulation of lymphatics leaving cancerous nodes in studies on tumour spread. Acta Cytol. 9, 197.

82 Easty, G.C. and Mercer, E.H. (1960) An electron microscopy study of the surfaces of normal and malignant cells in culture. Cancer Res. 20, 1608.

83 Easty, D.M. and Easty, G.C. (1974) Measurement of the ability of cells to infiltrate normal tissues in vitro. Brit.J.Cancer, 29, 36.

84 Santesson, L. (1935) Characteristics of epithelial mouse tumour cells in vitro and tumour structures in vivo - a comparative study. Acta path. microbiol. Scand.Suppl. 24, 1.

85 Willbanks, G.B. and Rickart, R.M. (1966) The in vitro interaction of intra epithelial neoplasia, normal epithelium, and fibroblasts from the adult human uterine cervix. Cancer Res., 26, 1641.

86 Schleich, A.B., Frick, M. and Mayer, A. (1976) Patterns of invasive growth in vitro. Human decidua graviditatis confronted with established human cell lines and primary human explants. J. Nat . Cancer Inst. 56, 221.

87 Kruse, P.F. and Patterson M.K. (1975) in Tissue Culture: Methods and Applications. Academic Press.

88 Mareel, M., Vakaet, L., De Ridder, L., Debrabander, M., Bozzi, A. and Deman, J. (1974) Possibility of distinction between malignant and non malignant cells by transplantation into chick blastoderms; further evidence from animal and human biopsy specimens. J. Nat. Cancer Inst. 53, 1351.

89 Dubois, R., Cunninge, D. and Smith, J. (1976) Interpretation of some recent results in experimental embryology and the problem of the germ line, in 'Organ culture and biomedical research , Ed. Balls and Monnickendam, Cambridge University Press, p.61.

90 Le Douarin, N. (1976) Cell migration in early vertebrate development studied in interspecific chimeras, in Embryogenesis in Mammals. North Holland, Amsterdam, p.71.

91 Courtney, V.D. and Mills, J. (1978) An in vitro colony assay for human tumours grown in immune suppressed mice and treated in vivo with cytotoxic agents. Brit.J. Cancer, 37, 261.

92 Easty, G. (1976) in Human Tumours in Short Term Culture, Ed. Dendy, P. P., Academic Press, London and New York.

93 Houghton, J.A. and Taylor, D.M. (1978) Maintenance of biological and biochemical characteristics of human colorectal tumours during serial passage in immune-deprived mice. Brit.J.Cancer 37, 199.

94 Houghton, J.A. and Taylor, D.M. (1978) Growth characteristics of human colorectal tumours during serial passage in immune deprived mice, Brit. J. Cancer, 37, 213.

95 Damadian, R. (1971) Tumour Detection by NMR. Science, 171, 1151.

96 Hollis, D.P., Economou, J.S., Parks, L.C., Eggleston, J.C. and Saryon, L.A. (1973) NMR studies of several experimental and human malignant tumours. Cancer Res., 33, 2156.

97 Goldsmith, M., Koutcher, J.A. and Damadian, R., (1977) NMR in Cancer XII. Application of NMR malignancy index to human lung tumours. Brit.J.Cancer, 36, 235.

98 Koutcher, J.A., Goldsmith, M. and Damadian, R. (1978) NMR in cancer X - A malignancy index to discriminate normal and cancerous tissue. Cancer, 41,174.

99 Slater, T.F. and Cook, J.W.R. (1968) in Proceedings of the Second Tenovus Symposium Cardiff. Ed. Evans, D.M.D., pp. 108, Livingstone.

100 Dodd, N.J.F. and Silcock, J.M. (1976) ESR study of changes during the development of a Yoshida tumour, II Paramagnetic metal ions. Brit.J.Cancer 34, 556.

101 Cercek, L. and Cercek, B. (1977) Application of the phenomenon of the structuredness of cytoplasmic matrix (SCM) in the diagnosis of malignant disorders - a review. Europ. J. Cancer 13, 903.

102 Straus, M.J., Straus, S.E., Baltista, L. and Krezoski, S. (1977) The uptake, excretion and radiation hazards of tritiated thymidine in humans. Cancer Res, 37, 610.

103 Chang, T.H., Liebeskind, D., Hsu, K.C., Elequin, F., Janis, M. and Bases, R. (1978) Labelling index in clinical specimens estimated by the antinucleoside antibody technique. Cancer Res., 38, 1012.

104 Tubiana, H. (1971) The kinetics of tumour cell proliferation and radiotherapy. Brit.J.Radiology, 44, 325.

105 Lamerton, L.F. (1972) Cell proliferation and the differential response of normal and malignant tissues. Brit.J.Radiol. 45, 161.

106 Tubiana, M. and Malaise, E.P. (1973) Cinétique de proliferation cellulaire des tumeurs et traitement des cancers. Pathol. Biol., 21, 647.

107 Seed, J. (1966) The synthesis of DNA, RNA and nuclear protein in normal and tumour strain cells. J. Cell Biol., 28, 233.

108 Nias, A.H. and Fox, M. (1971) Synchronisation of mammalian cells with respect to the mitotic cycle. Cell Tiss. Kinet., 4, 357.

109 Hoshino, T., Barker, M. and Wilson, C.B. (1975) The kinetics of human glioma cells. Autoradiographic studies. Acta neuropath, 32, 235.

110 Hoshino, T. (1972) Cell kinetics of human gliomas. J. Neurosurg., 37, 15.

111 Lepont, A., (1977) Selection of Ehrlich tumour cells in different phases of the cell cycle by Ficoll Gradient Centrifugation. Virchow Arch.B Cell Path, 25, 53.

112 Mendelsohn, M.L. (1962) Autoradiographic Analysis of Cell Proliferation in Spontaneous Breast Cancer of CsH Mouse. III The Growth Fraction. J. Nat. Cancer Inst., 28, 1015.

113 Baserga, R. and Kisieleski, W.E. (1962) Comparative study of the kinetics of cellular proliferation of normal and tumorous tissues with the use of tritiated thymidine. J. Nat. Cancer Inst., 28, 331.

114 Steel, G.G., Adams, K. and Barrett, J.C. (1966) Analysis of the cell population kinetics of transplanted tumours of widely-differing growth rate. Brit. J. Cancer, 20, 784.

115 Frindel, E., Malaise, E., Alpen, E. (1967) Kinetics of cell proliferation of an experimental tumour. Cancer Res., 27, 122.

116 Clarkson, B.D., Fried, J. and Ogawa, M. (1969) in Normal and Malignant Growth p. 175, Springer-Verlag, Berlin, Heidelberg, New York.

117 Bennington, J.L. (1969) Cellular kinetics of invasive squamous carcinoma of the human cervix. Cancer Res., 29, 1082.

118 Steel, G.G. (1967) Cell loss as a factor in the growth rate of human tumours Europ.J.Cancer, 3, 381.

119 Iverson, O.H. (1967) Kinetics of cellular proliferation and cell loss in human carcinomas. Europ. J. Cancer, 3, 389.

120 Nervi, C., Arcangeli, G., Badaracco, G., Cortese, M., Morelli, M. and Starace, G. (1978) The relevance of tumour size and cell kinetics as predictors of radiation response in head and neck cancer. Cancer, 41, 900.

121 Price, L.A., Hill, B.T., Calvert, A.H., Shaw, H.J. and Hughes, K.B. (1975) Kinetically based multiple drug treatment for advanced head and neck cancer. Brit. Med. J. 3,10.

122 Stathopoulos, G., Wiltshaw, E. and Price L.A. (1976) Quadruple chemotherapy in advanced squamous cell carcinoma of the head and neck. Brit.J.Clin. Practice, 30, 188.

123 Hillen, H., Wessels, J. and Haanen, C. (1975). Bone marrow proliferation patterns in acute myeloblastic leukaemia determined by pulse cytophotometry Lancet, i, 609.

124 Smets, L.A., Mulder, E., Waal, F.C. de, Cleton, F.J. and Bloh, J. (1976) Early responses to chemotherapy detected by pulse cytophotometry, Brit.J. Cancer, 34, 153.

125 Billiau, A., Cassiman, J.J., Willems, D., Verhelst H. & Heremans, H. (1975) In vitro cultivation of human tumour biopsies, Oncology 31, 257

126 Smith, H.S., Owens, R.B., Hiller, A.J., Nelson-Rees, W.A. and Johnston, J.O. (1976) The biology of human cells in tissue culture, I Characterisation of cells derived from osteogenic sarcomas. Int. J. Cancer, 17, 219.

127 Pontén, J. (1978) The deficient growth control of human glioma. Proceedings of the 26th annual meeting of the European Tissue Culture Society, Glasgow, July, 1978.

128 Dendy, P.P. (ed.) (1976) Human tumours in short term culture - techniques and clinical applications. Academic Press London and New York.

129 Azzarone, B. (1977) Differences in vitro between skin fibroblasts derived from human embryos, normal donors and neoplastic patients. Annual report of the cell, tissue and organ culture study group of the Co-ordinating Committee for Human Tumour Investigation.

130 Azzarone, B., Billard, C. and Macieira-Coelho, A. (1978) Essay of characterisation of skin fibroblasts derived from patients with mammary tumours. Annual report of the cell tissue and organ culture study group of the Co-ordinating Committee for Human Tumour Investigation.

SECTION III

IMMUNOLOGY

'NATURE'S ALLOGRAFT'

Editors' note: Immunological interest in the placenta centres on its role in protecting 'nature's allograft' - David Billington's evocative term for the conceptus - from rejection during the second and third trimesters.

But what protects the pre-placental stages of insemination, fertilisation, implantation, and embryonic development from immunological attack?

And what can the immunological process at work in pregnancy teach us about the contrasting problems of graft rejection and the body's apparent tolerance of malignant tumours?

Most of the third session was taken up with detailed discussion related to these questions, in the light of placental and pre-placental research. Much has already been learned, as the following review papers show. But many promising avenues for future immunological study remain to be explored and new ones are still opening up. Perhaps more than any other contemporary field of basic biological research, placental studies hold out bright prospects for practical application.

The main benefits seem likely to accrue from better understanding of the mechanisms of immunoprotection. Once we know how rejection of 'nature's allograft' is prevented, it may not prove too difficult to manipulate the underlying mechanisms:

- to promote acceptance of tissue and organ transplants
- to treat (or even prevent) autoimmune disorders, and - the greatest prize of all -
- to provoke immune rejection of malignant tumours.

In the opening paper, David Billington discusses fetal/maternal histocompatibility and immunoregulatory mechanisms, the evidence for the uterus being an 'immunologically privileged' site, immune tolerance during fertilisation and implantation, and the antigenic status of trophoblast - which for all its invasiveness into maternal tissue may also constitute an immune barrier. Finally, he compares immunological 'escape mechanisms' in tumours with those in the placenta - and considers the possible immunological initiation of labour.

That the mother reacts immunologically to fetal antigens is now certain. Yet rejection is somehow prevented. In the second paper, Guy Voisin seeks to solve this conundrum by reference to the 'facilitation reaction' - which appears to counterbalance rejection and thus protect the conceptual allograft. There also apears to be a balance between suppressor cells and enhancing antibodies, and possible protection from maternal attack by placental filtration. This leads naturally into the third paper in which W. Page Faulk considers the role of major histocompatibility complex (MHC) antigens in the innumobiology of trophoblast - the 'operational interface' between mother and conceptus, where blocking factors appear to play an important part in immunoprotection.

Finally, a complete change. The mechanisms by which maternal antibody crosses the placenta in late pregnancy to protect the newborn from infection, were described by Arthur Wild. How do these antibodies pass undamaged through the very tissues that protect the conceptus from immunological attack? By a highly selective, active transport mechanism, in chorio-allantoic primate placentae, which may conceivably be exploited as a means of targeting drug therapy. Other prospects for practical application include the fields of tumour enhancement, immunosuppression, and antigen receptors - all subjects of discussion here that also promise to become important leads in the study of graft rejection and cancer.

SECTION III

IMMUNOLOGY

Chairman: Albert Neuberger

THE PLACENTA AND THE TUMOUR: VARIATIONS ON AN IMMUNOLOGICAL ENIGMA

W. D. Billington

The aim of this paper is to introduce the placenta as an organ of immunological interest, for discussion of its relevance in pregnancy and of its potential as a model for studying malignancy. A prerequisite for this, especially in relation to the more specific aspects covered in the following papers, is to know something of the early events in the reproductive process and of the development programme of the placenta, viewed against the background of the mother's immunological reactions as host to this natural but genetically alien graft. It must be stated at the outset that there are many unknowns in this field of enquiry, with hypothesis and controversy as much in evidence as established fact. While this is stimulating for the researcher, any information should be regarded with suspicion until it can be confirmed and set in context. Hypothesis is perhaps the most interesting pathway to fact, and it here takes precedence over the recording of unsubstantiated or conflicting findings. The words of Wilfred Trotter[1] will also be borne in mind: In Science the primary duty of ideas is to be useful and interesting even more than to be 'true'.

THE EARLIEST EVENTS

Insemination

Under normal conditions pregnancy is initiated by the deposition into the female's reproductive tract of many millions of spermatozoa suspended in a rich proteinaceous seminal fluid, and it has been suggested that this may elicit maternal immunological reactions of relevance to the development of the subsequently formed zygote.[2] Seminal plasma is undoubtedly immunogenic, and spermatozoa possess a variety of cell surface antigenic molecules, either of intrinsic origin or adsorbed from the seminal plasma, which are capable of triggering a wide range of immunological responses under experimental conditions.[3] Evidence for an essential role for such responses - in the form of maternal immunological conditioning for successful pregnancy - is, however, very scarce. There are reports that in rodents the uterus affords a highly effective route for induction of maternal transplantation immunity by both naturally inseminated and innoculated allogeneic spermatozoa, and that prior local sensitisation of the uterus by experimental means improves its subsequent reproductive performance, with more embryos of greater size implanting and developing to term.[4,5] It has also recently been suggested that repeated natural insemination by way of regular sexual intercourse prior to the establishment of a first pregnancy may significantly reduce the incidence of pre-eclampsia in women by eliciting some form of protective immunological state, perhaps involving 'blocking' antibody[6] (further discussed below). Pregnancy following limited coital experience in young women is certainly reputed to carry an increased risk of pre-eclampsia.

Whether or not there is any beneficial immunological effect of insemination it is quite clear that the normal female is in a general sense relatively unresponsive to this natural innoculation of seminal antigens. The possible reasons have recently been reviewed in detail.[7] Much more attention has been paid to the possibility that the normal processes involved in this unresponsiveness may be disrupted and lead to pathological sensitisation responsible for some forms of infertility in women. This belief has provoked innumerable attempts to demonstrate a casual relationship between elevated responses to spermatozoal antigens and otherwise unexplained infertility, but final proof is still awaited.[8]

Fertilisation

Immunological factors have for long been thought to play a role in fertilisation, although here again there is no wholly compelling evidence. The fusion of spermatozoon and oocyte undoubtedly involves a complex and apparently highly-specific interaction of genetically dissimilar cells that can be inhibited both *in vitro* and *in vivo* by immunological procedures in a variety of species,[9] but the relevance of this to an understanding of the normal fertilisation process is still unclear. Perhaps the most important aspect of these investigations lies in the hope that they give for the development of an effective and specific method for human fertility control.

Implantation

Implantation of the fertilized egg into the wall of the hormonally prepared uterus constitutes a naturally occurring instance of tissue transplantation, and its continued development and survival as an intrauterine allograft represents an apparent infringement of one of the fundamental laws of transplantation immunology. The paternally inherited histocompatibility genes of the embryo should endow it with a range of cell-surface antigenic determinants sufficient to elicit effective immunological rejection reactions in the maternal organism. The duration of pregnancy is, however, well beyond the time necessary for the rejection of any surgically constructed allograft, and there is little evidence for deleterious maternal-fetal incompatibility reactions, except in the case of a few clinical disorders - notably rhesus incompatibility. There clearly must be significant immunoregulatory mechanisms for the female host to sustain her histo-incompatible offspring during the period of their intimate parabiotic relationship. Elucidation of the nature of these mechanisms is occupying the efforts of an ever increasing number of investigators, since it is central to an understanding not only of normal and pathological conditions of pregnancy but also of those other biological situations in which the host fails to effect the rejection of rather less desirable foreign 'grafts', especially in the cases of tumour development and virus infection. Novel approaches to organ transplantation and to immunological manipulation of reproduction are other goals that may result from better understanding of the maternal-fetal immunological relationships.

EVALUATION OF NATURE'S ALLOGRAFT

The basis of graft rejection has been explored in minutest detail since the foundations of transplantation immunology were established some 30 years ago. In briefest outline, primary allograft rejection follows:

1. The presentation of alien histocompatibility antigens by the graft, in sufficient quantity and strength and in a suitable exposed form on the cell surface, for

2. Recognition via an established vascular pathway and effective response by immunocompetent cells of the host, and

3. Access to the antigenic target sites by agents of the rejection reaction, largely cellular in nature.

In principle, any element missing from this rejection process, either intrinsically or by interference, could prevent the initiation or execution of a destructive immune attack on the fetal allograft. The situation is in fact very much more delicately balanced than this simple statement of the phenomenon suggests, since it is becoming increasingly obvious that exceeding complex interactions regulate host immunological responsiveness and cytotoxic effector mechanisms.

Before examining the various hypotheses that have been proposed to explain the survival of the intrauterine fetal allograft, two important features distinguishing it from surgically constructed grafts and from the great majority of tumours need to be stressed. First, the fetus is a continuously changing entity, undergoing not only simple physical growth but marked morphogenesis and differentiation, with differing tissue relationships being established with the maternal host at various stages of their association. At the initial phase of implantation the embryo consists of a hollow ball of cells, perhaps 200 or less in number, with a relatively undifferentiated unilaminar outer layer of trophectoderm enclosing a small group of cells attached to one side of the wall which are destined to form the fetus and certain fetal membranes. The trophectoderm subsequently undergoes proliferation and differentiation into a highly invasive tissue that erodes the uterine stroma and gives rise to a number of biologically different forms of trophoblast that eventually become incorporated into the structurally complex fetal-maternal composite organ known as the placenta. The developing fetal membranes should also be recognised as providing an additional interface for maternal immunological interactions.

Second, at no time during the entire course of their association is the fetus <u>directly</u> attached to the maternal tissue, but only through its initial surrounding envelope of trophoblast or its later definitive placenta. Although there is great variation between mammals in the precise tissue relationships at the placental site, there is never any ingrowth of maternal vessels, the circulatory systems remaining entirely independent. The placenta is thus not vascularised in the manner of a conventional organ graft and the fetal components of the placenta are, at most, simply bathed in maternal blood. By comparison, the tumour, following an early phase when the emerging tiny nodule is avascular, shows ingrowth of new capillary vessels from the host that provide an extensive blood supply to promote its very rapid further development. The immune response of the host almost certainly varies very considerably in the avascular and vascular phases since it is only in this latter phase that the extensive antigen shedding believed to play a fundamental role in tumour-host interaction occurs.[10]

The lack of vascularity of the fetal-placental unit (the conceptus) could therefore impair or delay the primary recongnition process by the maternal host. This cannot, however, provide a complete answer to the invulnerability of the conceptus because maternal sensitisation to paternally-derived histocompatibility antigens occurs at some stage in at least a proportion of primiparous human pregnancies,[11] and non-vascularised grafts can undergo rejection in an already immune host.[12] However, pre-immunisation does not prejudice the outcome of pregnancy in experimental animals and many other factors need to be taken into account(as detailed below).

Consideration of the requirements for experimental allograft rejection leads to several possible explanations for maternal acceptance of the fetal allograft. Many of these have been based upon the ideas of Medawar,[13] embodied in a philosophical appraisal of some of the problems raised by the evolution of viviparity. For the reasons stated previously it is not strictly relevant to question the survival of the fetus itself since it is only the placenta and the outermost of the fetal membranes that are in direct and continuous contact with the maternal host. Earlier claims[14] that the agents of immune destruction, primarily lymphocytes, are able to traverse the placenta and gain access to the fetal environment in large numbers are not now accepted.[15,16] Since there is no information on the immunological status of the human chorion, even though this membrane provides an extensive covering for the conceptus and is potentially vulnerable to immune attack because of its position of intimate apposition to the maternal decidua, the trophoblastic surface of the placenta is of major concern. This is still largely true of other animal species, since the only reliable information available on the antigenicity of any fetal membranes comes from a few isolated experiments on the yolk sac and amnion of the mouse.[17]

Expression of histocompatibility antigens

One of the earliest attempts to explain the privileged position of the conceptus came from Little[18] in 1924 when he commented that this would be possible 'under a condition in which the embryo has no definite physiological characteristics which are individual enough to be recognised as foreign by the mother, until well along in its ontogeny'. In modern immunological terms this can be translated into the suggestion that histocompatibility antigens may not be expressed on the surface of the embryo until the later stages of differentiation - which would have the effect of preventing either the induction of effective maternal rejection response or the destruction of the tissues by any pre-existing immunity. Although many elegant studies on the mouse embryo have demonstrated that these antigens in fact appear during the first cleavage stages in the pre-implantation period of development,[19-21] the picture is not a simple one. There is evidence of differential expression of both the important major and the, apparently less important, minor histocompatibility antigens on different tissues of the embryo following its implantation and subsequent development.[22,23] The critical factor is the antigenic status of the trophoblastic components in direct contact with the maternal host; this is further considered below and also in Faulk's paper on trophoblast antigens.

Immunoregulatory mechanisms in the pregnant female

Although the changing physiological state of pregnancy does not grossly impair the ability of the female to respond immunologically to such challenges as skin grafts or a wide range of injected antigens, there is growing evidence of more subtle regulation of the immune response during this period. Contrary to widespread earlier belief, it is now clear that both humoral and cell-mediated responses elicited by antigens of fetal origin can be detected in the pregnant female.[24] There appears to be considerable variability in these responses between individual females, especially in antibody production, but it is not known whether this is due to genetic factors or kinetic changes within the individual or simply reflects the sensitivity of the measurement techniques currently employed. Nevertheless, it now seems reasonable to assume that there is an adequate maternal cellular immune response to the paternally derived fetal transplantation antigens and that the survival of the fetus must therefore be related to a failure of the effector mechanisms. This could result from the involvement of a number of factors, operating in an antigen-specific or non-specific manner.

Non-specific regulators: Any of the variety of protein or steroid hormones or macromolecular factors found in pregnancy serum might be capable of interfering with the effector cell attack on the fetal target. Most of the studies implicating these factors have in fact been concerned with assessing their ability to suppress lymphocyte transformation in vitro. This form of suppressive ability has now been ascribed to the placental protein hormones HCG (human chorionic gonadotrophin) and HPL (human placental lactogen), to prolactin, the steroid hormones cortisone, progesterone and the naturally-occurring oestrogens, and to various pregnancy-specific or pregnancy-associated serum proteins and glycoproteins, including alpha-fetoprotein.[25,26] Whilst an explanation can be devised for the mode of action of all these diverse factors, it also requires belief that interference with lymphocyte transformation in vitro is indicative of potential for inhibiting the effector-target cell level of an immune response - and that this is possible in the circumstances pertaining in vivo. There are reports of immunosuppressive activity of some of these factors in different in vivo models in laboratory animals,[27] but a clear demonstration of their precise role in pregnancy is still awaited.

In addition to the suggested general suppressive effect of these various factors a more direct local role has been postulated for HCG in the protection of the placenta.[28] Very high concentrations of this hormone on the trophoblast surface may prevent maternal lymphocytes from attacking either by inhibiting their approach or by physical masking of the target antigens, assuming that these are in fact present.

It should perhaps also be noted that an HCG-like hormone has so far been demonstrated in rather few mammalian species.

Specific regulators: Exposure to fetal antigen may provide not only the stimulus for a female to initiate a rejection response but also a means for averting its destructive effect. There is accumulating evidence to support the notion that efferent immunological enhancement may be operating in pregnancy in a manner similar to that described for tumour survival in immune hosts.[25,29] Although earlier believed to involve antibody, acting by binding to the target antigenic determinants in a non-cytotoxic way and preventing recognition by the host's immunocompetent lymphocytes, current views are largely in favour of the blocking of either lymphocyte receptors or target antigens (or both) by free antigen or antigen-antibody complexes.[30] A prolonged low dose release of relatively weak antigen provides the most favourable conditions for the elicitation of immunological enhancement - and the developing conceptus would seem likely to offer this form of stimulus.

For completeness, it should also be mentioned that one of the earlier hypotheses to account for fetal allograft survival was that pregnancy might lead to the induction of a state of classical specific immunological tolerance in the mother. This preceded an appreciation of the more subtle mechanisms recognised in 'high zone' and 'low zone' tolerance and there is now little support for this form of maternal unresponsiveness.

Suppressor cells: Unravelling the complex mechanisms involved in the regulation of the immune response has revealed subpopulations of lymphocytes with a variety of interacting roles. Among those is a T-lymphocyte subset that has been shown by numerous *in vitro* and *in vivo* model systems to have a suppressive effect on immune reactions; these lymphocytes have hence been termed suppressor T-cells (Ts).[31] Their presence and activity in the maternal-fetal relationship is currently being evaluated in a number of laboratories. From published experimental and human data it would appear at present that Ts cells are detectable in late-stage fetal spleen and liver and in neonatal umbilical cord blood.[32,33] Whether the suppressive effect of these fetal Ts cells is specific or non-specific *in vivo* has yet to be established, as also has their precise role. It is possible that they could be responsible for the 'inactivation' of any primed maternal lymphocytes that may occasionally breach the placental barrier in small numbers, thus acting as a final line of defence against these potentially aggressive maternal cells, or their role may be restricted solely to involvement in regulatory processes during the development of fetal immunocompetence, perhaps in the control of potential autoimmunity to newly emerging self antigens.

Data are also now available indicating the presence of Ts cells in the pregnant female. Maternal spleen and lymph node cells have been shown to suppress an *in* vitro mouse mixed lymphocyte reaction,[34,35] and survival of skin and tumour allografts is prolonged following transfer of cells from pregnant or post-partum female mice.[36-38] In most of these assays evidence was obtained for the involvement of a T-lymphocyte population. Since Ts cells have been demonstrated under a number of conditions of experimentally induced tolerance to skin grafts, they probably have some significance in the immunoregulatory processes occurring in the maternal-fetal relationship. A more detailed consideration of their activity and specificity in this situation is presented in the next paper. Surprisingly, there are as yet rather few reports of the presence of Ts cells in tumour bearing animals.[39] However, in view of their widespread involvement in the regulation of immune responsiveness, it seems likely that future studies will demonstrate that they have some role in the response to tumour antigens. If this should prove so, then attempts to remove or inactivate them might provide another avenue of approach to tumour immunotherapy.

Macrophages: Increased production and functional activity of macrophages takes place during the growth of transplanted tumours, although their precise role in this situation is not clear.[40] It seems reasonable, however, to presume that they are somehow involved in the host-tumour immunological relationship, and they have now been shown to undergo considerable change in activity during murine pregnancy.[41]

In pregnancy and in the tumour-host relationship it is likely that immunoregulatory processes of both specific and non-specific nature are in operation, probably with varying degrees of suppression at different stages in the development of both embryos and tumours.

The uterus as an immunologically privileged site

There are a number of sites in the body, principally the anterior chamber of the eye, the brain and cartilagenous areas, where transplanted tissues enjoy an extended survival, largely because of deficiencies in vascular supply or lymphatic drainage that delay either the recognition of foreign antigen or access of the agents of immune destruction.[42] The possibility that fetal allograft survival may at least in part result from such a protection within the uterine environment has stimulated considerable investigation. Although it is now clear that transplantation immunity can be elicited via the uterine route and that tissue graft rejection may in certain circumstances take place in utero,[2] it is apparent that experimentally immunised female mice reject alien embryos transplanted ectopically, yet cannot prevent the normal development of similar embyros transplanted at the same time into the uterus.[43] There are grounds for believing that the decidual tissue, composed of large, tightly-packed, transformed uterine stromal cells, induced at the time of implantation, may constitute a form of protective barrier exerting an immunological 'quarantining' effect on the fetal allograft, especially during its early, and probably most vulnerable, stages of development prior to formation of the definitive placenta. Decidual transformation of the uterus effectively cuts off the lymphatic drainage from the organ and this would appear to be an important factor in any explanation of its privileged nature in pregnancy. The absence of any extensive ingrowth of host blood vessels would also contribute to this property.

Invasive activity of trophoblast

In order to fulfil its role in the establishment of a successful attachment of the embryo to the maternal uterine tissues, the trophoblast commonly exhibits some degree of invasive activity, ranging from simple erosion of the uterine epithelium in a few species to the large scale destruction of the stroma and maternal blood vessels seen in the haemochorial placenta of man and many laboratory animals. Although the mechanism and control of this invasiveness is poorly understood, it has some possible immunological implications. The phagocytic ability of trophoblast might, for instance, allow it to ingest sensitised maternal lymphocytes before they could mount an immune attack.[44] There is, however, no direct evidence for this, and such a mechanism could only be operative during the very early stages of pregnancy since the invasiveness of the trophoblast by means of phagocytosis is limited to the period before definitive formation of the placenta.

The extent to which trophoblast development and invasion in normal, pathological and experimental circumstances is controlled by genetic and immunological factors is a contentious issue. Although the growth of trophoblast is a highly variable phenomenon, as evidenced by the ultimate size of the placenta, and by its propensity in man both for occasional excessive erosion of the uterine wall and for spontaneous malignant transformation (particularly in the form of choriocarcinoma) the underlying reasons for this variability are unknown. While the immunological status of the mother appears to be an important determinant of placental size in a number of rodent species,[45-47] this conclusion has not gone unchallenged.[48-50] The development of choriocarcinoma is associated with the ABO blood group, but apparently not the HLA relationship between patient and husband, although there is frequently some degree of host cellular immune response to this tumour, and this correlates strongly with susceptibility to chemotherapy.[51] Immunotherapeutic approaches based on the assumption that antigens of paternal origin are likely to be expressed by the choriocarcinoma have not proved rewarding.

ANTIGENIC STATUS OF TROPHOBLAST

One of the most crucial questions in reproductive immunology is whether or not the fetal trophoblast expresses upon its cell surface antigenic determinants that are capable of eliciting maternal immune responses and acting as targets for the effector mechanisms of a rejection reaction. The question is not as simple as it may at first appear, and the answer has proved unexpectedly elusive. The reasons are manifold but lie in three general directions. First, trophoblast is not a uniform tissue but occurs in a number of biologically different forms that arise from the trophectodermal layer of the blastocyst and come to assume various anatomical positions during placental ontogeny, not all at the feto-maternal interface: Second with few exceptions it has not so far been possible to isolate trophoblastic material, free from contaminating maternal or other fetal elements, in a form suitable for analysis: Third, there can be difficulty in determining the specificity of an immunological reaction, especially when several different antigen systems may be involved (see below). To these difficulties must be added the problems that arise when material from different sources is put together and when attempts are made to extrapolate findings from one species to another.

Mouse trophoblast

Most of the available information on the antigenic properties of trophoblast has been derived from studies on rodent and human tissue and concerns the antigens of the histocompatibility system (H-antigens) that are pertinent to allograft rejection.[52] The lack of readily available human material earlier than that from first trimester therapeutic abortions has meant that all the data on the early stages of trophoblast development has come from laboratory animals, mainly the mouse. In this species, the trophectoderm of the pre-implantation stage blastocyst expresses both major and minor histocompatibility antigens.[53-55] Most significantly, however, these are lost from the cell surface during the implantation process,[53,54] preventing recognition by the maternal immunological system at the critical time of initial tissue contact. During the subsequent early proliferation and differentiation of the trophoblast, the outer population, at least, seems to maintain its antigenic deficiency, providing an inert covering barrier for the developing fetus.[55,56]

At the time of placental formation, when trophoblastic diversity and anatomical complexity are reaching a maximum, the antigenic status of the tissue becomes much more difficult to define. Current evidence indicates that populations of trophoblastic cells are present in the placenta which express paternally-derived histocompatibility antigens.[56] While the precise identity of these populations has not yet been fully established, some, at least, must have direct contact with maternal uterine cells or blood. The reason for their apparent insusceptibility to maternal immune destruction in vivo has therefore to be explained. Many suggestions have been put forward, most of them related to the possible inaccessibility, by topographical features of the membrane or by surface masking materials or sparse distribution, of the antigenic determinants. These hypotheses are considered in more detail below.

Possible role of histocompatibility antigens

The expression of H-antigens by trophoblast cells may not only not be prejudicial but actually be a necessary element in the survival of the placental allograft. These antigens could be responsible, in whole or in part, for the presence of the enhancing or 'blocking' maternal serum factors, antigen or antigen-antibody complexes, or even for the induction of suppressor T-cells, that have been considered as immunoregulatory factors in pregnancy. Their expression might also provide a means of allowing the placenta to act as a selective filter,[57-59] preventing access to the fetus of potentially deleterious antibody by specific binding, whilst allowing transmission of beneficial molecules, especially the maternal immunoglobulins involved in the endowment of passive immunity to the fetus, to protect it during early neonatal life before it can develop its own full immunocompetence. This latter aspect of placental immunobiology is by Arthur Wild, in his paper on immunological protection at the end of this section.

Human trophoblast

Histocompatibility antigen expression on the human trophoblast is also an unresolved issue. Many of the earlier studies claiming positive findings can be criticised for the reasons given above,[52] and more recent evidence suggests that there may be deficiency of these antigens. It has been reported that HLA determinants are present on human full-term placental membrane preparations but only at about 5% of the levels found on spleen lymphocytes.[60] This could reflect the presence of normal quantities of HLA on a small population of non-trophoblastic elements in the placenta, with the outer syncytiotrophoblast being completely antigen deficient. This interpretation is supported by immunofluorescence studies on cryostat sections of first trimester and term placentae showing that anti-HLA antisera do not bind to the trophoblastic surface or trophoblast basement membrane but react strongly with cells in the mesenchymal stroma.[61]

Although the results of studies in man and in the mouse are conflicting, the possibility of a low level of HLA antigen expression on human trophoblast cannot yet be completely discounted since immunofluorescence techniques are not always sufficiently sensitive to detect determinants that are widely spaced. In any case, the current findings relate only to the chorionic villous region of the human placenta which is bathed in maternal blood and not to the trophoblast of the basal plate which is in direct cellular contact with maternal uterine tissue. Recent information on the mouse placenta indicates that it is the spongiotrophoblast cell population, having direct maternal tissue contact, not the labyrinthine trophoblast percolated by maternal blood, that is primarily responsible for its antigenic nature.[62] The preferential and specific binding of maternal anti-fetal immunoglobulin to the spongiotrophoblast demonstrated by immunofluorescence[63] may also be indicative of H-antigen presence.

Trophoblast as an immunological barrier

In terms of the mechanisms allowing placental allograft survival it is noteworthy that the trophoblast appears to act as a barrier tissue by virtue of its insusceptibility to immune destruction not only in vivo but even under extreme conditions in vitro. This privileged position may result from one or other of the following factors, which have been considered in detail in an earlier review:[52]

1. Failure to express cell surface products of the major histocompatibility gene complex
2. Ineffective antigen expression, which may arise from (i) low antigen density, with determinants too widely spaced for linkage with lymphocytes, antibody or complement, (ii) cell surface antigen masking by such agents as mucoprotein, HCG or other hormones, (iii) antigen aggregation in membrane convolutions, (iv) rapid shedding (or even internalisation) of antigens, and/or (v) 'modulation' of antigens by the presence of antibody directed against them
3. Efficient cellular repair processes, allowing recovery from the early stages of the immune lytic process.

In summary, the most recently available evidence points firmly to the conclusion that there is absence of antigen expression in the early stages of trophoblast development. From the beginnings of placental formation, which heralds the main period of gestation, the picture is rather less clear, but there is probably either a continuing absence or only a very low level of antigen expression on the main mass of trophoblast tissue in direct contact with the maternal blood. However, at least in the mouse, there is a very appreciable degree of antigen expression on the trophoblast in direct confrontation with uterine tissues - which implies a need for effective mechanisms to protect the trophoblast against immune attack. The unique immunological properties of the trophoblast and the diverse maternal immunoregulatory processes apparently contrive together, under the conditions of a special anatomical relationship between the conceptus and uterine tissues, to avert the anticipated rejection reactions resulting from feto-maternal tissue incompatibility.

This complex immunological equilibrium in pregnancy must have arisen independently on a number of occasions during the multifocal evolution of viviparity. The extent to which any one particular mechanism is in evidence, or operative at a given stage of gestation, may therefore vary from one species to another.

IS LABOUR AN IMMUNOLOGICALLY MEDIATED EVENT ?

There have been sporadic suggestions that despite the general invulnerability of the fetus to maternal immune attack there may be a gradual tissue incompatibility reaction, culminating in the eventual rejection of the placental allograft and the concomitant initiation of labour. While the full-term human placenta bears histological hallmarks of immune conflict not unlike those seen in organ allograft rejection,[64] it is not clear to what extent this may simply be a secondary effect of tissue degeneration in an ageing organ. Immunological rejection reactions tend to be rather conservative in their temporal development and it would be difficult to explain on this basis the extreme variation in the duration of gestation in different eutherian mammals, from as little as 16 days in the golden hamster to 22 months or more in the African elephant. In addition, it is clear that parturition occurs normally in inbred strains (where there is little or no histoincompatibility between mother and offspring), in female rodents that have been rendered immunologically tolerant to the histocompatibility antigens of the mating male, and in women suffering from a variety of immunological deficiency diseases. Although it may not yet be possible wholly to discount the involvement of non-histocompatibility antigens, such as those of an organ or tissue specific nature, there is no evidence to support this thesis, and it seems rational to conclude that the induction of labour is largely, if not entirely, a hormone-controlled event initiated by signals emanating from the fetus.[65]

THE PLACENTA-TUMOUR PARALLEL

Apart from its own intrinsic interest the placenta is clearly worthy of consideration as a potential model for the study of tumour development and survival. There are many similarities from a general biological as well as an immunological viewpoint and it is relevant to examine these in a wider context.

Antigen systems

The placenta has been considered as an intra-uterine allograft which may express paternally-derived histocompatibility antigens, to which the maternal immune system may produce specific responses. Although histocompatibility antigens are probably present on most tumours, these will in the great majority of cases be identical with those of the host. Other distinctive antigens must therefore be involved in immunological responses to the autochthonous tumour. Indeed, much of the early work on tumour immunity in experimental animals is now disregarded, because only when inbred mouse strains were introduced was it possible to use syngeneic tumours and transplantation techniques to produce evidence of tumour-specific antigenicity. A more directly relevant comparison with the placenta would thus concern information on any non-histocompatibility antigen systems of this organ. Such information is as yet rather limited and not well established.[52] It is clear that the trophoblast surface membrane is not completely devoid of antigenic determinants since there is evidence for the presence of both xenogeneic, (species-specific)[66] and tissue-specific antigens.[52-67] Although the possible existence of the latter type of determinants has been suggested for many years, the evidence was rather unsatisfactory until more recent studies employed well-defined reagents and experimental conditions. The most convincing reports to date have concerned the production of anti-trophoblast antisera and attempts to demonstrate their specificity by in vivo[68] and, especially, in vitro[69] assays.

A specific non-cross-reacting antibody against trophoblastic tissues would have immense clinical value. It could provide an effective agent both for the induction of abortion from the early post-implantation stages of pregnancy and for the immunotherapy of trophoblastic neoplasms, always assuming that these tumours also express the tissue-specific antigen(s). Choriocarcinoma, at least, appears susceptible to immune attack in vitro.

Tumour cells, like normal cells, express a diversity of antigens. Their precise number and nature is defined only by the techniques so far applied to their detection, and the extent to which they can act as transplantation rejection antigens is not clear in all cases. Although classification schemes vary, there are generally considered to be three main types of antigen systems in tumours:

1. Tumour specific antigens (TSA) are expressed only by tumours.

2. Tumour associated antigens (TAA) are present on tumours but may also under special circumstances be detectable on other tissues. This term should be used in preference to TSA unless it can be demonstrated quite unequivocally that the antigen is not present elsewhere, which is always a difficult task. This category includes the embryonic or phase-specific antigens believed to be expressed otherwise only at certain stages of embryonic development[71,72] - though very low levels of such antigens may be found on normal adult tissues. The use of high-sensitivity techniques may thus lead to reconsideration of one of the basic hypotheses of tumour development - derepression of the embryonic genome,[73] in favour of the acceptance of a mechanism causing simple quantitative change in cell surface components.

3. Tumour associated transplantation antigens (TATA) are capable of inducing immunity and resistance to tumour transplantation, either in the autochthonous

host or in syngeneic recipients. These are also referred to as tumour rejection antigens (TRA) since this is indicative of their functional involvement. TATAs share many features in common with the histocompatibility antigens, especially in their cell surface location, high degree of polymorphism, biochemical composition and capacity to induce both cellular and humoral immune responses.[74] There is in fact a reasonable possibility that TATAs on chemically induced tumours may be rearranged histocompatibility specificities rather than neoantigens.[74] These certainly have a much greater individuality than virally-induced TATAs, which show considerable cross-reactivity between different tumours.

It is notable that most experimental studies on tumour immunity have employed tumours of high immunogenicity, and the relevance of these findings to 'spontaneously' arising human tumours of apparently rather low or undetectable immunogenicity might be questioned. Moore[74] has recently gone so far as to state that 'there are now substantial grounds for concluding that immunogenicity may be an artefact of the laboratory and largely restricted to neoplasms appearing in a high incidence after induction by artificial means'. However, this is undoubtedly an overstatement of the situation, since some human tumours clearly do evoke host immune responses,[75] and the apparent failure of others to do so may merely reflect the inadequacy of the techniques so far employed for their detection. In addition, the relatively small amount of information on human tumour antigens has come largely from approaches using cell-mediated immunity, and it seems likely that the application of suitable serological assays will eventually lead to a better understanding of their variety and identity and of the immune responses to them.

Immunological escape mechanisms

It is undeniable that malignant tumours arise in both man and other animals and that they can grow progressively to kill their hosts. If it is accepted that most, if not all, of these tumours are likely to express an array of antigenic determinants and that these are capable of provoking apparently adequate cytocidal immune responses, then how is it that the abberant cells survive? This central paradox of tumour immunology closely parallels the situation in reproductive immunology. (The continued presence of virus in the face of a host immune response is another comparable problem). From the above account of the mechanisms proposed to explain the trophoblast survival, it plainly has many features in common with the tumour-host immunological relationship. The fetal antigen systems shown to elicit significant maternal immune responses have been almost entirely of the histocompatibility category, although there is some evidence for both cellular and humoral immunity to phase-specific embryonic antigens, which show cross-reactivity with certain tumour antigens, in multiparous syngeneically-mated rats.[76] This aspect of maternal reactivity is worthy of further investigation since it may afford a more direct comparison with host responses to tumours.

In the general nature of their immune responses, the pregnant female and the tumour host show a similar reaction to the alien cells within them, and the value of examining one in order to gain understanding of the other has frequently been emphasised. The essential difference lies in the fact that the conceptus, or more specifically, the trophoblast, normally has a limited life-span with a programmed restriction on its growth and invasiveness, whereas the tumour in its malignant form does not. The immunological escape mechanisms in pregnancy therefore do not need to be sustained at the same level over such a prolonged period. One of the simplest explanations for the survival of tumours in the very early stages of their development is the 'sneaking through' hypothesis.[77] This presumes that a small nodule of cells, not yet vascularised by host vessels, presents too low an antigenic profile for recognition and rejection reaction by the host. By the time an effective response is generated the tumour mass is too large to be eliminated. Although this would explain why tumours escape the host's immunological surveillance mechanisms (always presuming that they really exist) in the first place, it is still necessary to explain the failure of the full immune response to deal with a well-established tumour. It cannot be that the replicative power of the tumour is so great that it outpaces the proliferation of the host lymphoid tissue, since it is now apparent that the mean doubling time for most human tumours is - perhaps rather surprisingly - no greater, and often less, than that of their normal tissue counterparts.[78,79] Various immunoregulatory processes of the kind described earlier for placental trophoblast survival have therefore to be considered. In addition to the possibilities of antigen modulation, non-specific depression of host immune responses, suppressor cells and blocking factors, the antigen 'smokescreen'[80] hypothesis has been given much attention. Tumours may shed their surface components more extensively and more rapidly than normal cells, and this would very likely confer a significant degree of immunoresistance, not only through a lack of stability of target antigen on the tumour, but by diverting the host effector-cell attack. It could also lead to the ready formation of 'blocking' immune complexes. Since the more weakly immunogenic tumours appear to exhibit the greater degree of shedding,[81] this may also be a possible mechanism for the escape of trophoblast.

CONCLUSION

It is clearly possible to envisage a number of different mechanisms for the apparently paradoxical survival of both the placenta and the tumour. However, the extent to which any of the mechanisms so far proposed are actually involved in vivo remains to be established, and others yet to be discovered may have an equal or greater role. It is still difficult to ascertain whether the identifiable immune responses in the pregnant female and the tumour host are in fact protective or simply ineffectual. The sceptic's view that they are merely irrelevant 'epiphenomena' provoked by the presence of the polymorphic antigen systems of embryo and neoplasm is becoming increasingly less acceptable but cannot yet be firmly refuted.

There is continuing belief that a full understanding of the factors involved in the induction and maintenance of tumours will depend to a substantial degree upon recognition of the controlling regulating mechanisms in normal embryonic development and differentiation. In this context, an examination of the immunological events surrounding the growth of the trophoblast and the formation and survival of the placenta is clearly of considerable value. It is of course of particular relevance to tumours of trophoblastic origin. Although John Beard's provocative trophoblastic or unitarian thesis of cancer proposed at the beginning of the century[82] - with its assertion that there is no property possessed by the cancer cell that is not shared by the trophoblast cell - is manifestly untenable, there nevertheless remains much of interest in this comparison.

For discussion of this paper, see end of section

IMMUNE AGENTS OF THE FACILITATION REACTION. THEIR POSSIBLE ROLE IN PROTECTION OF THE PLACENTAL ALLOGRAFT*

G. A. Voisin

Studies of allograft rejection provide an important means of investigating the mechanisms of the immunological privilege enjoyed by the conceptus. In a normal host, alloantigen-bearing cells induce a complex immune reaction with opposing features and consequences:[1-3] a rejection reaction involving specific killer T cells and specific antibodies, able to fix complement or activate K cells, and a facilit-

* work partially supported by DRGST

ation reaction consisting of enhancing antibodies and suppressor cells. The main consequence of the latter is to antagonise the former both at the induction and at the effector level. The final fate of the antigen-bearing target cells depends on the relative intensity of those two competing reactions. In allo-transplanted organs or tissues, the rejection reaction usually predominates to the point that the facilitation reaction goes unnoticed. In indigenous tumours, either of the two reactions may apparently predominate, determining the fate of the tumour. As regards embryonic and fetal graft, we think that the main problems are: whether or not these two types of reaction are present, whether or not a facilitation reaction may play an effective part in protecting the conceptus, and whether the placenta and trophoblast are concerned in directing the immune response of the mother toward facilitation rather than rejection. These three problems will be considered in succession.

MATERNAL REJECTION AND FACILITATION REACTIONS

That the mother reacts immunologically against the conceptus is now amply demonstrated, the reaction being directed toward antigens borne by the conceptus and absent in the mother. These are of two kinds: inherited paternal antigens and placento-embryonal or differentiation antigens. Antigens of paternal origin induce immune reactions in the mother, as attested by the presence of anti-H-2 or anti-HLA (and apparently also anti-Ia or Ia-like) antibodies in the sera of pregnant - especially multiparous - females, and inherited antigens of paternal origin also include minor histocompatibility and H-Y sex-linked antigens. Placento-embryonal antigens include early trophoblastic and carcino-embryonic or carcino-placental antigens, against which the mother presumably reacts, as evidenced by murine studies. Growth of sarcoma Sa 1 (indigenous in the A/J strain) grafted on A/J individuals is enhanced by preimmunisation of the recipient with syngeneic (A/J x A/J) placenta,[4] and tumour resistance to isogeneic tumour can be induced in C57BL/6 females inocculated with irradiated C75BL/6 fetal cells.[5]

In order to analyse the components of the maternal anti-conceptus immune reaction and to compare it to those of an allotransplantation reaction, it is desirable to chose the mother and father from two different inbred strains and to study the anti-MHC reactions of the mother. When spleen cells from post-delivery allogeneically mated mothers are injected to young hybrid mice (mother x father strain F1), this gives a higher spleen index than spleen cells from isogeneically mated or virgin mice,[6] demonstrating a cellular component in the maternal anti-paternal antigen reaction. Hellstrom et al,[7] using a sensitive colony inhibition test and a 250:1 cell ratio, saw that lymph node cells from allogeneically pregnant mothers (but not from isogeneically pregnant ones) were active against isolated embryonic cells of paternal strain. Furthermore, adding serum from allogeneically pregnant mothers (but not from isogeneically pregnant ones) to the culture could prevent this action. This suggested the possibility of two opposing reactions being present in the mother during gestation and directed toward the conceptus antigens of paternal origin.

We worked on this problem with G. Chaouat in three areas of study, concerned with: the presence and localisation of enhancing maternal anti-paternal antibodies, the presence of maternal anti-paternal suppressor cells, and the presence of maternal anti-paternal immune cells. In addition, the phylogenetic emergence of the double (aggressive and protective) reaction have been studied in salamanders with Pierrette Chateaureynaud and Marie-Thérèse Badet in Bordeaux.

Maternal anti-paternal enhancing antibodies in allogeneically pregnant mothers

Maternal antibodies directed against paternal antigens of the conceptus should be absorbed *in vivo* on the placenta, the first part of the conceptus to be met by maternal agents (humoral and cellular), provided the relevant antigens are present on the placenta. This hypothesis was shown to be correct in a murine model where CBA ($H-2^k$) or C57BL/Ks ($H-2^d$) females were mated with A/J males (or isogeneic ones, as controls). It was first shown that transplantation antigens are present on 14-day placentae, but their nature (H-2, Ia or minor, non H-2) was not determined.[8] Secondly, a large amount of immunoglobulins was revealed by immunofluorescence to be present on the placentae. Part cannot be removed by careful perfusion, sectioning (5 µm) and several washes of the sections. That part is definitely more important in hybrid placentae than in homozygous, control ones. It consists mainly of IgG1, with less IgG2, only traces of IgA, and no IgM, Thirdly, it is specific to paternal antigens since it specifically binds to cells or structures that possess them, i.e. paternal strain thymocytes or previously eluted placentae that contain antigens of the corresponding paternal strain. Finally, injecting these eluted antibodies into normal mice of the maternal strain made them unable to reject allografted tumours from the paternal strain as they normally would.[8,9]

It follows that allopregnant mothers make enhancing antibodies directed towards conceptus transplantation antigens inherited from the father, and that these antibodies are specifically fixed on the placenta.

Specific suppressor cells in spleens of allogeneically pregnant mice

We have found evidence for T suppressor cells in spleens of allogeneically pregnant mice by both *in vivo* and *in vitro* methods. The same strain combinations were used as in the preceding experiments. *In vivo*, injection of spleen cells from 16 day allopregnant mice (but not from virgin or even isopregnant ones) in high doses (10^8 to 2×10^8) to non-pregnant mice of the maternal strain rendered them less able to reject tumour allografts of the paternal strain. This required the presence of anti-theta sensitive (T) cells but not B cells or macrophages.[9,10]

In vitro spleen cells from 16 day allopregnant mice (but not from virgin or even isopregnant ones) exhibited an important suppressive capacity (up to 90%) when added to a MLR of normal spleen cells from the maternal strain versus mitomycin-treated spleen cells from the paternal strain. This suppressive capacity was abrogated by anti-theta and C' complement treatment of the added regulatory cell populations. Two populations of regulatory cells were found: an early acting one, presumably at (or close to) the recognition phase (added, after mitomycin treatment, at day 0 of the MLR) and a late acting one, presumably at the proliferation phase (added, without mitomycin treatment, at day 2 of the MLR). The early acting regulatory cells were inhibited by an appropriate anti-idiotypic serum (directed against maternal strain immunoglobulins directed against paternal strain spleen cells). The minimum histocompatibility requirements for this activity and the phenotypes of the responsible cells are currently under study using various recombinant strains.[10]

It follows that allopregnant mothers elaborate suppressor cells specific to the maternal reaction against the paternal antigens of the conceptus. These suppressor cell populations are unable, when injected to mice isogeneic with the mother, to diminish their rejection reaction to tumour allografts of paternal strain. They can also suppress a maternal strain cell MLR versus father strain cells.

Immune cells specific to paternal antigens in the spleens of allopregnant mothers.

The evidence for this was given by in vivo experiments similar to the ones designed to reveal suppressor cells. Injection of spleen cells from allopregnant mothers (but not from virgin or isopregnant ones) in relatively low doses (3×10^7 to 5×10^7) to non-pregnant mice isogeneic to the mother rendered them able to reject a tumour allograft of paternal strain faster (in a second set manner).[9,11] This rejection reaction is not easily detected in the mother, because it requires unbalancing of the ratio between donor spleen cells and recipient spleen cells. (It is known that a great number of cells favour the expression of the suppressor cell population while a small number favour the expression of the immune, helper or amplifier cell populations.)

It follows that allopregnant mothers can elaborate cells immune to the paternal antigens of the conceptus and able to participate in a rejection reaction against cells that bear these antigens.

Phylogenetic emergence of maternal/fetal rejection and facilitation reactions

Salamandra salamandra Lin represents one of the first attempts at viviparity in tetrapods. Salamanders of this type reject skin grafts against which they mount a double (specific) immune reaction, both cellular (killer cells) and humoral (antibodies).[12] Their gestation period lasts from four to twelve months with varying success. Embryos are kept in the mother and 'rejected' at various times from very immature (sometimes dead) larvae to more mature states, sometimes even after metamorphosis. Pregnant *Salamandra salamandra* make an immune reaction against their embryos which is detectable *in vitro*. Mothers' spleen cells incubated with dissociated epidermal embryo cells (readily recognisable) kill up to 90% of the latter in 48 hours. The proportion killed depends on the relative numbers of maternal and embryo cells, and on the number of embryos borne by the mother. This cytotoxicity is specific for the embryos of a given mother, although weak degree of killing may be seen with embryos of other mothers, presumably due to some cross-reactivity. When serum from the same mother is added to the mixed culture of embyronic and maternal cells, the former are protected against the aggression of the latter.[13,14] This protective capacity of maternal serum is a function of the number of embryos borne by the mother. The maternal serum apparently acts in two different ways, as shown by pre-incubation studies, by exerting:

- a protective action on the embryonic cells, which is quite specific for the mother's embryo (and thought to be antibody-mediated) and

- an inhibitory action on the mother's spleen cells, which is also active on other mothers' spleen cells (and thought to be mediated by an immune complex or a non-immunological substance.

An increase in beta protein peaks is noted in pregnant *Salamandra salamandra*, as seen after allografting. The embryos are surrounded in the uterine cavity by a small amount of fluid, containing numerous cells morphologically similar to those seen in the maternal blood but different from the embryo's blood cells. They might play a part in the *in utero* death of a small proportion of embryos.[15]

It follows that *allopregnant mothers are able to elaborate immune agents of the rejection reaction toward paternal antigens. At the same time, they elaborate immune agents of the facilitation reaction (enhancing antibodies and suppressor cells) that are able to inhibit the induction and/or the expression of the rejection reaction. This dual expression of a maternal reaction directed toward the paternal antigens of the embyro can be detected at the very dawn of viviparity as well as in highly evolved mammals*.

EFFECTS OF REJECTION AND FACILITATION REACTIONS ON THE CONCEPTUS

Could all these complex and specific actions and interactions have been selected and retained in the course of evolution without having a biological and physiological purpose? This question was explored in the next set of experiments done with Janine Voisin and Paulette Mannot.

Studies on newborn mice of paternal strain

Since it is extremely difficult to work in vivo on embyros and fetuses, these studies were performed on newborn mice less than 20 hours old, which are immunologically (and even physiologically) close to fetuses. We wanted to find out if the immune cells, suppressor cells and enhancing antibodies elaborated by allopregnant mothers towards paternal antigens of the conceptus could have a physiological and pathological influence on newborns of the paternal strain. Two H-2 compatible strains, BALB/C and DBA2, both H-2k, were chosen for two purposes: first, to study the possible role of non-H-2 transplantation antigens in feto-maternal relations and, second, to ensure that spleen cells from a non-immunised mouse would not (or would only very weakly) react against the allogeneic newborn mice in a graft versus host assay. Spleen cells from BALB/c mice fertilised by DBA 2 males were taken after delivery (3 to 18 days) and injected intravenously to DBA 2 newborn mice. Suppressor cells had first been eliminated from some specimens, but not from others by simple short-term (6-20 hour) culture of the maternal spleen cells. Similarly, some DBA 2 mice received injections of serum from the same mothers, but others did not. Spleen cells and sera from isopregnant BALB/C mice were used as controls.

The results of the first experiments, intended to test the presence of immune cells and enhancing antibodies, showed that 25% of the DBA 2 newborn mice which received allopregnant maternal spleen cells were lethally runted with typical GVH disease. Addition of serum from the same mother reduced the runting to 3%, identical to the control level of newborn DBA 2 mice which received spleen cells from isopregnant BALB/C mice and serum from isopregnant or allopregnant ones.

The next experiments showed a difference between cells from primiparous and multiparous mice; elimination of suppressor cells was necessary for spleen cells from multiparous mice to show a clear GVH reactivity. This seems to imply that repeated gestations result in an increase of both sensitised and suppressor cells, with an advantage for the latter. This may be the expression of a suppressor cell memory phenomenon.[16]

It follows that mother cells become naturally sensitised against allogeneic (H-2 compatible) paternal antigens and able lethally to runt new-born mice of the paternal strain, while both suppressor cells and enhancing antibodies elaborated by the same mothers are able to antagonise the preceding rejection reaction and to protect the newborn mice.

These results suggest that a defect in the facilitation reaction might lead to maternal immunological aggression against the fetus, especially in view of Beer and Billingham's finding[17] that preimmunisation of mother rats differing from the father at the AgB locus led to postnatal runting - presumably through colostrum transmission of sensitised maternal lymphocytes.

Possible mechanisms of the antagonistic interactions

What are (or may be) the mechanisms by which the immune agents of the facilitation reaction mounted by the mother counter or prevent the rejection reaction that the same mother is able to make against her conceptus? They are still hypothetical. However, from the converging and complementary results of the preceeding experiments, added to what we know from transplantation and tumour immunology a tentative general scheme can now be drawn up:

Enhancing antibodies made by the mother toward paternal antigens of the conceptus, and active *in vivo* as well as *in vitro*, act according to two mechanisms. One is 'peripheral' and protects the target by masking (or modulating or 'interiorising') the paternal antigens on accessible cells of the conceptus. This mechanism is of the type in which pre-incubation of *Salamandra* embyronic cells with maternal serum protects them against *in vitro* cytolysis by maternal spleen cells. The other, 'central' mechanism acts by inhibiting the maternal lymphocytes, presumably through immune complexes. It is of the type in which pre-incubation of *Salamandra* maternal spleen cells in maternal serum inhibits their capacity to kill their embryonic cells *in vitro*.

Suppressor cells have also shown activity *in vivo* and *in vitro*. Their mechanism of action is more doubtful although the results obtained *in vitro* (MLR suppression) suggest that they act at two or more levels:

- On the induction of the reaction (recognition?) e.g. with mitomycin-treated cells from allopregnant mice added on day 0 of a relevant MLR.
- At a later stage (proliferation), e.g. when untreated cells from allopregnant mice are added on day 2 of the relevant MLR.
- A third level of action, on the effector phase, is conceivable and suggested by a recent report.[18]

Relations between suppressor cells and enhancing antibodies; it would be satisfying to know that these two agents of the facilitation reaction do not act completely independently from each other. Transplantation experiments suggest cooperation between them that might apply during gestation. A MLR can be inhibited by adding enhancing-antibody-containing immune sera isogeneic to the reactor cell strain and directed against the stimulator cell strain. This inhibitory power was found to be reduced by a mean of 51% when suppressor cells were eliminated (either by adult thymectomy of the prospective reactor cell donors or by passing the cell population through an isolubulised histamine column).[19] Suppressor cells therefore appear to be necessary for enhancing (or blocking) antibodies to exert their inhibitory activity on MLR. The interaction is probably attributable to stimulation of the suppressor cells by the antibodies complexed to their corresponding antigens through their Fc region. As for the part (49%) of the inhibitory power of the antibodies that remained intact, it may reflect incomplete elimination of the suppressor cells or, more probably, a direct, peripheral action of the antibodies on the target (stimulator) cells.

Paternal antigens as model for maternal immune behaviour

Conceptus antigens of paternal origin (H-2, non-H-2, and H-Y) provide a well-defined model with strong antigenicity and much in common with transplant immunity. Although likely to play the major role in all natural situations (especially in man) these paternal antigens are unlikely to be the only ones inducing both a rejection and a facilitation reaction during gestation. Differentiation antigens of the conceptus (placenta as well as embryo) and early trophoblastic antigens might also play definite parts, especially during second and later pregnancies. This can be tested in isopregnant mice of inbred strain.[4,5]

AN IMMUNOLOGICAL ROLE FOR TROPHOBLAST AND PLACENTA

What are the roles of the placenta and trophoblast in the immune reactions and interactions that take place during gestation? The trophoblastic cells of the ectoplacental cone and of the more mature placenta are certainly among the most important tissues, physiologically speaking. They are likely to have the major role in immunological relations between mother and fetus, since the placenta (which separates the fetus from the mother) is the first hybrid (i.e. paternal-antigen-containing) anatomical structure to be met by the cells and molecules of the mother. This immunological role may be of three main types, acting through:

- altered antigenic solicitation of the mother's lymphoid system
- immunological filtration, and
- immunodepression and immunodeviation.

Altered antigenic solicitation of maternal lymphoid system

The evolution of H-2 antigens at the surface of the conceptus during development from fertilised egg to placenta and embryo seems to have been designed to prevent the occurrence of a transplantation rejection reaction. First (if present) they are partially shielded behind the zona pellucida. Then low levels of H-2 antigens, undetected by several researchers, appear on the blastocyst.[20] At the time of implantation they increase in the embryonic sac while becoming barely detectable on the peripheral part, the ectoplacental cone trophoblast. At that time, through their phagocytic and enzymatic (plasminogen activator) capacities, the trophoblast cells enter the uterus wall and its decidua and are exposed to maternal immunoglobulins.[21] The non-H-2 transplantation antigens are more consistently present. Whether the disappearance of peripheral H-2 at the time of implantation results from repression of their synthesis or from an antigenic modulation (or masking) brought by maternal immunoglobulins remains to be determined. The latter mechanism is more likely to be operative in the later stages on both the placenta and the umbilical cord lymphocytes.[22] However transplantation antigens (presumably H-2 as well as non-H-2) seem to be expressed on mature placenta, although this has been denied for H-2 and may concern cells other than the trophoblast.

Whatever the mechanism (shedding of soluble antigen, direct contact with the blood without macrophage treatment, presentation in the form of immune complexes or other), the result is that the immune system of the mother is led to react to the transplantation antigens of the conceptus and that this reaction is not quite the same as after an allograft (or even a semi-allograft). Its rejection components (the only ones to be detected in the case of a graft) are not strongly activated, while its facilitation components (enhancing antibodies and suppressor cells) are relatively more activated. This decreased aggressive reaction towards paternal antigens does not usually go to the point of acceptance of paternal skin allograft (although that may sometimes be the case immediately post-partum[23]). But it may be revealed by the specific take of tumours of the paternal strain[8] and even of cardiac allografts of paternal strain.[24] In spite of fetal blood cells passing into the mother during the late stage of pregnancy, her previous immunisation is likely to have been due to the part of the conceptus in direct contact with her, i.e. the placenta, which would also be responsible for the form taken by the immune reaction.

This view is supported by the active enhancement toward syngeneic tumour grafts obtained by preinjecting the recipient with syngeneic fetal cells.[4]

Immunological filtration

Clearly, the immunological buffer role of the placenta is partly exerted through its immunological filtration capacity. This capacity is actually two-fold, being addressed both to the two immunoglobulin extremities, Fab and Fc, as well as to the antigen-specific receptors of the lymphocytes. Immunoglobulins with no specificities for antigenic determinants borne by the placenta are selectively filtered through it since only IgG can be transferred to the fetus. Strongly C'-fixing and cytotoxic Igms are not allowed through. Furthermore, IgG is the class for which corresponding Fc receptors exist on placenta and trophoblast cells.[25] This is in agreement with Brambell's proposed mechanism of Ig passage through placenta.[26] Antibodies to antigenic determinants borne by the placenta (including histocompatibility antigens) get fixed to it, possibly leading to redistribution, interiorisation and antigenic modulation. But its main effect is to produce heavy Ig deposition and formation of specific immune complexes (others may also get trapped here through their Fcs), as well as antigen-antibody shedding in the form of soluble complexes or metastatic, antibody-coated trophoblast cells. This heavy local immunoglobulin and antibody coating should prevent specific and sensitised lymphocytes from attaching themselves to placental structures and acting cytotoxically, thanks to the blocking action of these complexes. To this, one should add the possible protective role of the fibrinoid deposit and the sialomucin coat, together with a conceivable non-specfic inactivation of the sensitised lymphocytes by anti-inflammatory substance(s). It would not be easy to imagine another system of specific immunological filtration that would be as efficient as this one for protecting the fetus.

Immunodepression and immunodeviation

A satisfactory explanation for a number of immunological events observed during gestation could be offered on the assumption that some substance or mechanism inherent in the placenta would have the capacity to interfere with the intensity and quality of the immune response triggered in its presence. Immune deviation may be considered to consist of selective immunodepression of the agents of the rejection reaction (especially C'-fixing antibodies, beginning with IgM and cell-mediated immunity), with conservation or even increase of the agents considered to be active in the facilitation reaction (murine IgG_1 antibodies, enhancing and suppressor cells). In classical experiments, deviation is induced by injecting the antigen in a soluble intravenous or subcutaneous form, sometimes with aluminium hydroxide; sometimes in the form of immune complexes.[27,28] The conditions for natural occurrence of this type of phenomenon seem to be favourable in the placenta, especially if certain substances contribute.

Immunodepressive and immunodeviating effects of placental extracts or substances have been, or are currently being looked for by the following techniques, either in vitro: MLR, lymphoblastogenesis to mitogens and PPD, CML, ADCMC, EA rosette formation and antibody synthesis (Mishell-Dutton) or, in vivo: antibody synthesis (SRBC); allotransplantation of skin, organ or tumour.

The substances that have been studied from this viewpoint are not all well defined, neither has their placental origin been ascertained in all cases. In addition to their role as immune complexes released from the placenta, they may be classified as defined hormones, pregnancy-associated proteins and enzymes.

Among defined hormones, steroids (especially corticosteroids) must be mentioned and also HCG, although its immunosuppressive action might be due to some impurity.[29]

Pregnancy-associated proteins include many undefined ones, especially of beta or alpha 2 mobility, known under different names by different workers, such as pregnancy inhibitory macroglobulin (PIM), pregnancy associated macroglobulin (PAM), A B C and D proteins, SP 1 etc. One that has been well defined and studied, alpha-fetoprotein (alpha-FP), is not of placental origin.

Amongst enzymes, one, a plasminogen activator secreted by the trophoblast during the invasive phase, is of particular interest in view of the immunological activities ascribed to plasmine. In our laboratory, we found that plasmine can increase antibody production through B cell activation, without having such an effect on T cells; furthermore it has been shown to be inhibitory and even lymphotoxic at high doses,[30] though some of the findings have yet to be published.

Another factor of possible interest is the one described by Fauve, Hevin et al[31] and common to placenta and tumours. It would prevent macrophages from migrating towards and reaching trophoblastic and tumour cells. In our laboratory, we are working with G. Chaouat in collaboration with S. Chaffeaux and M. Duchet-Suchaux on the immunological properties of placental extracts and, more especially, of an antigen detected through extensively absorbed duck immune sera. The mechanisms of action of these substances and placental constituents resulting in immunodepression and immunodeviation are still hypothetical.

A factor preventing macrophage access to antigens might result in a direct contact between the antigen and the lymphocytes, with stimulation of suppressor cells. Actually suppressor T cells have been induced <u>in vitro</u> by alpha-FP extracted from mouse amniotic fluid.[32] These suppressor cells are non-specific. Their target is not B cells but rather T helper cells (therefore the formation of protective antibodies against pathogenic germ polysaccharides is not interfered with). Immune complexes present in high quantity on placenta might result in an immunodeviating type of stimulus.

Substances present at an immunologically inefficient level in the serum or even in the lymphoid system of the mother will be sufficiently concentrated to be efficient at their site of production (placenta or trophoblast). Furthermore, immunomodifying substances acting non-specifically (in the immunological sense) but at the very same site where the antigen is located (i.e. the placenta or an ectopic cell), may be expected to modify the only reaction against this precise antigen and thus act as a specific agent.

This would decrease the maternal anti-fetal reactions without impairing the immune defence system of the mother or the fetus - showing how good Nature may be as an immunologist. Through the immunological reactions of pregnancy, she already shows us the way for immunological manipulations. She might well teach us to understand the reasons why, and the mechanisms through which, an antigen induces this or that type of immune reaction.[33]

In conclusion, the placenta may be considered a naturally allografted tissue which, through the selective evolution process has discovered how to exist, how to become accepted, and how to make the fetus accepted over a period long enough for fetal development, whereas tumours may be regarded as pathological tissues that have 'understood' and utilised some of the placenta's tricks.

For discussion of this paper, see end of section

ROLE OF THE MAJOR HISTOCOMPATIBILITY COMPLEX IN THE IMMUNOBIOLOGY OF TROPHOBLAST ANTIGENS

John A. McIntyre
W. Page Faulk (Speaker)

Pregnant human mothers normally produce antibodies to allotypically incompatible antigens from the fetus. The specificity of such antibodies can be easily determined and have, indeed, been used to define and expand several useful and important immunogenetic systems such as Rh, ABO, HLA,[1] B-cell alloantigens, Gm,[2] Am and Inv.[3] The production of these highly selective antibodies is a normal maternal response to paternal antigens inherited by the fetus, but whether the trophoblast plays a role in maternal immunisation is still unclear. A central theme of many materno-fetal studies has been the immunobiology of trophoblast associated antigens. Trophoblasts lie at the operational interface of the materno-fetal relationship,[4] and it has been known for many years that they normally break away from the placenta and eventually pass into the maternal lung[5,6] where they remain silently undisturbed.[7]

Park[8] demonstrated a similar lack of inflammation in mice following the intravenous injection of suspensions of autologous trophoblast, but mice given intravenous injections of homologous renal or hepatic tissues mount inflammatory reactions around the embolism sites. On the other hand, Basdawil and Toy[9] found that rabbits given human trophoblast intravenously displayed histological evidence of inflammation at sites of pulmonary emboli. These early observations suggested that trophoblasts have species-specific antigens, probably without allotypic variation.

Although studies using heterologous anti-trophoblast sera have been useful in fitting together the puzzle of trophoblast antigens, caution is nonetheless required in interpreting results obtained with these reagents, because the antigens used to raise such antisera usually contain placental constituents in addition to trophoblasts. Seegal and Loeb[10] showed, for instance, that rabbit anti-rat placental serum is as potent as rabbit anti-rat kidney serum in producing glomerulonephritis in rats, and Pressman and Korngold,[11] using radiolabelled IgG from immunised rabbits, showed that anti-placental antibodies localised in the livers and kidneys of virgin rats, and that anti-rat kidney sera localised in the placentae of pregnant rats as well as in their kidneys. Boss and Craig[12] produced immunohistological data which suggest that basement membranes are largely responsible for kidney-placental cross-reactivity, and Boss[13] was later able to show, using placental tissue fractions obtained by differential ultracentrifugation, that mitochondria and microsomes, epithelium, and several unidentified soluble antigens were also shared by kidney and placenta. Gaugas, Wright and Curzen[14] have also shown that rabbit antisera to an ultracentrifuge prepared, solubilised and fractionated, placental microsomal fraction contain antibodies which cross-react with a similarly prepared microsomal fraction from kidney, but they also produced data suggestive of trophoblast-specific antigens. Indeed, using the ultracentrifugation technique of Smith, Brush and Luckett[15] which selectively harvests syncytiotrophoblast microvilli, Faulk ,Lovins, Yeager et al[16] have been able to prepare human trophoblast membranes which - following extraction with chaotrope, solubilisation in deoxycholate, and fractionation through columns of polyacrylamide - generate heterologous anti-trophoblast sera that do not cross-react with normal adult tissues. However, even these reagents, before solid-phase immunoabsorption according to the technique of Galbraith et al,[17] contain antibodies to human IgG, transferrin, alpha-2-macroglobulin and albumin.[18] It thus appears that specific anti-trophoblast sera can be raised in hetrologous species, if careful attention is paid to the chemistry of antigen preparation as well as to appropriate immunoabsorption with certain serum proteins. These reagents can be very helpful in studies of the localisation and distribution of major histocompatibility complex (MHC) antigens in normal placentae.

STUDIES IN EXPERIMENTAL ANIMALS

A certain degree of species-specificity for trophoblast antigens has been shown using heterologous anti-trophoblast sera. In 1903, Dobrowatski found that antisera raised to guinea pig or rabbit placentae caused abortion when administered to the respective pregnant species.[19] Cohen and Nedzel[20] also showed this effect in pregnant guinea pigs injected with rabbit anti-guinea pig placenta serum. These antisera retained their abortifacient properties following several absorptions with guinea-pig liver and kidney, suggesting that the antibodies were organ-specific as well as species-specific. Seegal and Loeb[21] achieved a similar result when they gave rabbit anti-rat placenta serum to pregnant rats. Beer, Billingham and Yang[22] confirmed and extended the concept of organ-specific trophoblast antigens by showing that lymphocyte-absorbed rabbit anti-rat trophoblast serum, which has potent abortifacient effects in pregnant rats, lost its activity when absorbed with rat trophoblasts.

Trophoblast antigens have also been studied using a variety of transplantation models. Fawcett and his coworkers [23] set an early theme for these models by their descriptions of normal proliferation and development of trophoblast tissues when fertilised mouse ova were explanted to the anterior chamber of the eye, the abdominal cavity, or under the renal capsule, but noted very little if any differentiation of the inner-cell-mass. Kirby[24] later reported that trophoblast giant cells differentiated from fertilised mouse ova, regardless of their cleavage stage at explant. Simmons and Russell[25,26] in a now classical series of experiments were able to show that seven-day mouse embryos were rapidly rejected when implanted beneath the maternal kidney capsules, and that such implants sensitised mothers to reject skin grafts from the father more rapidly. On the other hand, they also found that allogenic trophoblasts prepared from seven-day embryos were accepted for much longer than embryo transplants, and that trophoblast explants did not sensitise mothers to subsequent paternal skin transplants. Simmons and Russell[27] also provided evidence that protrophoblastic tissue expressed transplantation antigens since explanted allogeneic fertilised eggs were rejected in an accelerated fashion by immune recipients. They suggested that the trophoblast represents a differentiated form of embryonic cell which is incapable of either manufacturing or expressing histocompatibility antigens. They did however show quite clearly, again using transplants of ectoplacental cone cells to extrauterine sites, that mouse trophoblasts were immunologically recognised by rats that had previously rejected a mouse skin graft.[28]

Cryptic antigens

In 1968, Currie et al[29] introduced the idea of cryptic antigens into reproduction research when they demonstrated that transplantation of ectoplacental cone cells, following treatment with neuraminidase, resulted in accelerated rejection of donor skin. This led them to speculate that transplantation antigens present on trophoblasts were protected or masked by a coat of sialomucin; this concept also attracted considerable attention in the area of cancer research.[30-32] Attempts by Simmons et al[33] to confirm this observation were unsuccessful, and the concept of masked antigens on trophoblasts or tumour cells has now lost credibility. Finally, Kaneko and Nishimura[34] have re-examined the effect of genetic dissimilarity between trophoblast and host on trophoblast growth in extrauterine sites and found some suppression of trophoblast growth in recipients sensitised by two previous skin grafts. Their experimental model employed the implantation of either blastocysts or ectoplacental cone (i.e. trophoblast) cells from ddN mice to the kidney or testis of C57BL/6 mice, some of which had been pre-sensitised. Sensitised recipients were found to mount a vigorous round-cell infiltrate into their grafts, suggesting the presence of transplantation antigens on the trophoblast. It is unfortunate that ddN mice were chosen to presensitise C57BL/6, because Furuya and Hirao[35] have shown that 50% of adult ddN mice retain an infant red cell antigen, designated MO(+), which is absent from adult C57BL mice. This curious circumstance introduces the possibility that ddN trophoblast and skin share the MO(+) antigen. Preimmunising C57BL with ddN skin grafts could therefore generate a C57BL immune response to the ddN embryonic antigen, but this might have nothing whatsoever to do with the problem of H-2 antigens on trophoblast.

Unique trophoblast antigens

That the trophoblast may express unique embryonic antigen(s) was indicated when Kirby[36] and Hulka and Mohr[37] showed that repeated grafting of allogeneic blastocytes or trophoblast tissue to extra-uterine sites in the mouse resulted in progressive suppression of trophoblast growth. Furthermore, subsequent skin grafts from blastocyst donors to previous trophoblast recipients were not rejected as second set grafts. Kirby[38] later reported that extrauterine grafts of allogeneic blastocytes specifically prolonged survival of grafts of the skin taken from the blastocyst donors but had no effect on the longevity of grafts of skin taken from third-party donors. Vandeputte and Sobis[39] confirmed that preimmunisation did not interfere with the growth of allogeneic ectoplacental cone cells transplanted under the host kidney capsule. They also extended contemporary knowledge of MHC-antigens, or the lack thereof, on trophoblasts by demonstrating that primed lymphoid or peritoneal effector cells added to cultures of trophoblast giant cells or embryonic fibroblasts showed cytotoxicity only for fetal fibroblasts. Another in vitro study by Jenkinson and Billington[40] showed that mouse ectoplacental cone cells are not lysed by killer lymphocytes generated from spleens of their original donors, thus providing additional data for the lack of histocompatibility antigens on trophoblast cell membranes. Clearly, resistance of trophoblast to immune lysis by host cells is an important biological property for a tissue responsible for providing the interface of materno-fetal contact for mammals having haemochorial placentae. Additional evidence from Billington's group[41] confirms, by mixed haemagglutination, that trophoblast giant cells lack both major and minor H-2 antigens; and they have also shown that epithelioid outgrowths of placental cells in monolayer culture exhibit both the major and minor histocompatibility alloantigens. A role for these epitheloid cells, and their relationship to trophoblasts, remains to be established.

The use of xenogeneic antisera to mouse trophoblasts has suggested the presence of unique antigens on these cells. Johnson[42] has for instance shown that rabbit anti-mouse trophoblast sera identify candidate trophoblast antigens, which seem to be neither passively absorbed nor loosely membrane-bound (by virtue of their cytotoxic activity and lateral membrane mobility upon warming). Subsequent immunofluorescence studies by Muggalton-Harris and Johnson[43] have shown that hyperimmune allogeneic antisera can detect incompletely defined so-called non-H-2 alloantigens on most cleavage stages of mouse embyros, including cells of the inner-cell-mass and trophoblast. They have thus confirmed and extended earlier observations[44] that H-3 and H-6 were found concentrated on the surface of two-cell blastomeres; this also provides an immunological basis for the observation[45] that presensitisation to non-H-2 antigens is associated with the failure of mouse eggs to develop in extra-uterine sites. Searle et al[46] have extended their serological findings by using immuno-electron-microscopical techniques to search for transplantation antigens on cleavage-stage mouse embryos. They were able to substantiate their previous findings, showing a lack of H-2 antigens on eight-cell embryos but noted its presence on 3.5-day blastocysts. To investigate this further, the authors experimentally induced a ten-day delay of blastocyst implantation by hormone treatment, and found both non-H-2 and H-2 antigens on blastocysts recovered from oestrogen-treated uteri. The trophectoderm, often being devoid of identifiable histocompatibility antigens, suggests a selective loss of transplantation antigens as the time for blastocyst implantation approaches. These observations are consistent with Heyner's indirect immunofluorescence finding[47] that H-2 antigens are present on 6.5-day embryo cells but not on trophoblasts.

Maternal and paternal antigens in trophoblast

That mouse trophoblast cells express both maternal and paternal antigens was shown in vitro for the first time by Carter[48] using a mixed immune haemabsorption technique, but whether the antigens were of major or minor H-2 type was not determined. Whatever their precise genetic identity, the density of maternal antigens on trophoblast membranes was greater than that found for paternal antigens. Sellens[49] also used the same technique to study antisera raised between mouse strains congenic for H-2 and found that these reagents were negative on early trophoblast membranes, indicating that only non-H-2 antigens are expressed on blastocyst outgrowths. Webb et al[50] confirmed and extended much of the earlier mouse data using a sensitive immune precipitation reaction in vitro to show that H-2 antigens are first expressed at the last blastocyst stage by cells of the inner-cell-mass, and that H-2 antigens are never present on trophoblasts. Moreover, they were unable to detect H-2 antigens at any time between the two-cell blastomere stage and formation of the late (4.5-day) blastocyst.

STUDIES USING HUMAN TISSUES

Monospecific heterologous antisera to human beta-2-microglobulin (B_2M), a plasma protein which is invariably associated with the HLA molecule,[51] has been used by Faulk and Temple[52] in immunohistological studies employing traditional immunofluorescence techniques and antibody peroxidase methods with electron microscopy to map the distribution of B_2M in human chorionic villi. The results of this investigation showed, for the first time, that B_2M was not present on trophoblast, and exposure of cryostat sections of placenta to several different enzymes, including neuraminidase, failed to reveal B_2M, again suggesting that former concepts of masked MHC antigens on trophoblasts were probably incorrect. However, cells in the mesenchymal stroma of chorionic villi, including fibroblasts, pericytes, endothelium and Hofbauer cells were brilliantly positive for B_2M. The localisation of B_2M to stromal cells and absence of trophoblast reactivity were confirmed in another immunohistological study[53] of the distribution of a large number of proteins in mature and immature[54] chorionic villi. In addition, Faulk et al[55] were able to show that both rabbit and monkey anti-HLA sera followed the same distribution of B_2M in chorionic villi, indicating that neither B_2M nor HLA are found on either mature or immature human trophoblasts. These observations are consistent with the subsequent report[56] that small amounts of B_2M as well as A and B locus antigens of both parents could be extracted from term placenta, the amounts being less than 5% of that found on splenic lymphocytes, which suggests that the MHC antigens they identified in placentae were in fact representative of MHC-positive cells within chorionic villi.

MHC antigen synthesis

The studies of Lawler[57] indicate that human pregnancy with a hydatiform mole often stimulates the mother to produce antibodies specific for paternal histo-incompatible antigens, raising the interesting possibility that trophoblasts contain the genetic potential necessary for MHC antigen synthesis, and that normal pregnancy represses these genes. If MHC antigens are indeed not found on human normal trophoblasts, this puts forward a possible mechanism which could be instrumental in protecting the blastocyst from an onslaught of cell-mediated immunity by the mother. In several systems, most notably those involving virus-infected cells, cytotoxic reactions depend on the presence of HLA antigens on target cells;[58] absence of these antigens from trophoblasts would tend to frustrate maternal cellular efforts to immunologically cast-out the implanted blastocyst. This is of course based on the concept that maternal surveillance of self-antigens is mediated by way of the same genetic information that determines her ability to recognise allogeneic cells; a good deal of evidence has, however, accumulated to support this hypothesis.[59] Another possible mechanism which could frustrate maternal efforts to recognise blastocyst antigens immunologically is one evolved by invertebrates apparently to escape analogous systems of surveillance in the host-parasite relationship. This involves the synthesis of a receptor by the parasite for a host protein, as for instance is done by schistosomes. We have recently shown[60] that human syncytiotrophoblast (the 'parasite') normally produces a receptor which binds maternal ('host') transferrin, thus providing a dense matrix of host protein at the materno-fetal interface - which further frustrates maternal immunosurveillance.

HLA antigens in human trophoblast

Evidence for the presence of HLA antigens on human trophoblasts was reported by Loke et al[61] in their cytotoxicity studies of cultured human trophoblast cells using what they referred to as a polyspecific HLA antiserum that was cytotoxic for trophoblasts. These results obviously differ from a large number of other studies in humans and experimental animals which tend to support the growing concept that MHC antigens are absent from trophoblasts. In this regard it is important to point out that the multispecific anti-HLA serum they employed was produced in a human volunteer immunised by four reciprocal skin-grafts plus an intradermal injection of leucocytes from the skin-donor. The antibody seems to have broad specificity for an antigen designated variously as 4b,[62] or what is currently known as Bw6.[63] The genetic implications of Bw6 and its associated antigens are not clear even using several better-defined typing sera from parous women - which further complicates the possibility of obtaining complete specificity data for human antisera raised by skin-graft and intradermal immunisation. Another problem with the use of polyspecific homograft-stimulated antisera is the possible presence of cold-reactive lymphocytotoxins. These 19S antibodies can be stimulated by organ grafting;[64] they are polyspecific on a non-HLA basis, and we have recently shown that they manifest specificity both for lymphocytes and trophoblasts.[65] Such antibodies would of course be cytotoxic for trophoblasts, so until the Loke group's experiments are confirmed using monospecific reagents, it is perhaps best to view their results with circumspection.

MHC antigens on trophoblast

Heterologous anti-trophoblast sera have been used to study the possibility of MHC antigens being present on trophoblasts. We have recently shown[55] that rabbits immunised with ultracentrifuge-prepared syncytiotrophoblast microvilli from a large number of different placentae failed to produce anti-B_2M, as measured by a sensitive radioimmunoassay. In addition, we have studied these antisera to MHC specificity using the standard micro-cytotoxicity assay with a panel of lymphocytes of known HLA-type and, although all sera were cytotoxic at high dilution, none of the rabbits could be shown to manifest HLA specificity.[18] Although these anti-trophoblast sera were initially raised to study the possible presence of MHC antigens on human trophoblasts, these reagents could be used as a valuable probe to study other trophoblast antigens which might be important in the materno-fetal relationship. For instance, we know from that ABO blood-group antigens are not found on trophoblasts,[66] and that Rh-antigens are also absent,[67] but antigens of human erythrocytes, such as Chido or Rogers, which are known to be present on lymphocyte membranes, [68,69] have not been studied on placental membranes. This should be done, particularly in view of the fact that mouse embryos are reactive to the murine blood group antigen H-6.[44] The PP_1P^k complex is another blood group which could be important in the materno-fetal relationship, especially in view of the high incidence of abortions in women of genotype pp.[70] It is, however, not yet known whether P-antigen is found on trophoblasts. This antigen is of additional interest because it has caught the attention of cancer researchers due to its presence in certain tumours, and to the apparent benefit of P immunisation to pp patients having P-containing tumours.[71] One final note concerning a possible role for P-antigen in human transplantation biology comes from the report of Oliver[72] that P-negative (i.e. pp) recipients of renal transplants tend to reject their grafts rapidly. Of course, most people are P-positive,[70] so the chances of receiving a P-positive kidney would be very great, unless this antigen was specifically studied in screening for kidney donors. Finally, it would be useful to examine several HLA-C locus antigens, since they are weakly antigenic[73] and may functionally resemble some of the mouse minor histocompatibility antigens and especially because mouse trophoblasts tend to manifest antigens of the minor histocompatibility complex.[49] Another relatively weak histocompatibility antigen is the male marker H-Y. Evidence from laboratory animals has indicated that zygotes which are antigenically dissimilar from the mother are favoured at implantation, and H-Y antigens of the zygote may play a role in sex determination through their obvious difference with maternal cells.[74] Kirby later proposed[75] that H-Y should be present on the blastocyst, but there are as yet no data on whether trophoblasts manifest H-Y antigen. Galbraith et al[17] have recently published an immunohistological technique especially for the localisation of H-Y antigen, and this should be a useful approach towards gathering such data.

Teratoma associated antigens

Anti-trophoblast sera have been used to explore the possibility of teratoma-associated antigens being represented on trophoblast membranes. Teratocarcinomas contain embryo-like cells which display embryonic antigens that appear to be related to the T-locus system.[76] These have been reported independently in mice.[77-79] Their biological function is unknown, but they seem not to be species-specific. Rabbit antisera to mouse teratoma antigens react with three heteroantigens found on fertilised ova but not on any adult tissues.[78] Of these, antigen II, a surface antigen, first appears in the development of trophectoderm cells just prior to implantation. Jacob[79] has also identified teratoma-associated antigens, of which only the antigen F-9 appears on trophectoderm. F-9 is also found on the sperm and spermatogonia of several mammals and has been identified in the early cleavage stage of mouse embryos, but cannot be easily identified on fertile eggs which simultaneously manifest H-2 antigens during preimplantation. Interestingly, F-9 and H-2 antigens have similar molecular weights and subunit composition[80] although rabbit antisera to papainsolubilised H-2 fail to react with cells which carry F-9 antigen.[81] It should be stressed that very little is known about F-9 antigen on human tissues, and whether this antigen is expressed by human trophoblasts is at present not clear. One might speculate that F-9 is involved in very early embryonic cell recognition events; this is at least reasonable in light of contemporary evidence that histocompatibility antigens seem not to play a role in this important process.[82]

Blocking factors

A more difficult antigeneic system to define, yet one which appears to be characteristic of trophoblasts, has emerged from studies of maternal sera, placental eluates, and maternal lymphocytes. Blocking factors in serum to cell-mediated immunity reactions have been identified in maternal[83,84] and neonatal[85] plasma as well as in extracts of certain placental glycoproteins,[86] but their direct relevance to trophoblast antigens has yet to be established. Rather closer to direct incrimination of trophoblasts are observations[87,88] showing that lymphocytes from post-partum women react to pooled placental antigens as measured in a lymphocyte assay employing measures of macrophage-inhibition-factor (MIF). Further experiments showed that antigens from a single placenta were recognised only by lymphocytes from the mother, suggesting a degree of specificity. Rocklin et al[89] have shown that this reaction is indeed specific, since only autologous plasma could block the suppression. Pence et al[90] then confirmed earlier reports of specificity by showing that multigravid women produce MIF when presented with paternal alloantigens, and they have extended their original observation by experiments which indicate that autologous sera or plasma from normal multigravid patients contain a factor that specifically blocks their lymphocytes from producing MIF in response to incubation with paternal lymphocytes. In addition, Rocklin and his colleagues[91] showed that chronic aborters normally produce MIF in response to allogeneic stimulation, but they lack the ability to produce MIF blocking factor: the factor is maternal IgG which can be absorbed out with paternal lymphocytes but not with pooled platelets, suggesting that its specificity is not based on classical HLA genetics.

Trophoblast in maternal immunisation

That trophoblasts play a part in maternal immunisation was indicated by the elegant *in vitro* experiments of Taylor and Hancock[92] when they demonstrated that maternal lymphocytes recognise trophoblasts and become cytotoxic for them if cultured together for 72 hours. Such cytotoxicity could however be completely blocked by the presence of maternal serum, suggesting the presence of maternal antibodies with anti-trophoblast specificity. Finally, blocking antibodies with placental specificity do seem to be generated during normal pregnancy. We have been able to elute IgG immuno-chemically from placentae,[93] and these immunoglobulins, which have been shown by genetic markers to be of maternal origin, are potent inhibitors of the mixed lymphocyte culture reaction.[94] Voisin and Chaouat[95] have produced very similar results from studies of mouse placentae, but nobody else who has studied the specificity of placental eluates has been able to ascribe HLA specificity for lymphocyte membrane antigens which are shared with trophoblasts.[96]

In an attempt to define the trophoblast antigens to which mothers might respond, we have raised rabbit antisera to both intact and fractionated trophoblast membranes.[18] Following absorption with normal human sera, red blood cells, liver powder and peripheral blood lymphocytes, these antisera do not recognise unstimulated lymphocytes using either immunohistological or cytotoxicity techniques, yet they are potent inhibitors of MLC reactions, without effect on lymphocyte responses to lectin stimulation.[97] Our present interpretation of these results is that specific activation of lymphocytes by alloantigens makes available a recognition-product or antigen on lymphocyte membranes which cross-reacts with trophoblast antigens. Another interesting observation about the specificity of heterologous anti-trophoblast sera is the ability of these reagents to recognise the cell membranes of certain human tumour and transformed cell-lines. The nature of these cross-reactive oncofetal and trophoblast antigens is currently a major point of investigation in our laboratory.

Maternal antibodies to placental components

In human pregnancy, maternal antibodies to several placental components have been identified. Kaku[98] first isolated a placental polysaccharide ans showed that a proportion of mothers with pre-eclampic toxaemia produced antibodies to these sugars; and this has since been confirmed.[99] Others have reported[100-102] an exciting observation of anti-trophoblast antibodies in post-partum sera, demonstrated by immunofluorescence, but these reports have never been confirmed. It is not an unlikely hypothesis that mothers would react immunologically to trophoblasts, since many investigators have observed that these cells stream into the maternal circulation during normal pregnancy[5,6] but confirmatory reports of anti-trophoblast antibodies have not been forthcoming. Gaugas and Curzen[103] have however isolated a placental glycoprotein, thought to be trophoblastic, against which many mothers have antibodies. At this point it might be stressed that thereis no evidence that the Gaugas-Curzen glycoprotein is related to either the Kaku polysaccharide or the Hulka antigen. Transformed and human tumour cells from another group of antigens against which pregnant humans have been found to manifest antibodies. Tal[104] reported that HeLa cell agglutinins could be identified in pregnancy sera and in blood samples from patients with certain tumours, and Hersey et al[105] found antibodies in pregnancy sera which were cytotoxic for melanoma cells. Finally, Hirsch et al[106] have identified antibodies to primate C-type oncoviruses in normal pregnant women. Neither the effect of these immunoglobulins on the fetus nor their relationship to trophoblast antigens is yet altogether clear.

Maternal immunity and the fetus

In view of the punitive presence of maternal immunity to oncofetal antigens, we must consider its effect upon the fetus. Biochemical studies of anti-tumour antibodies in multiparous mouse sera have indicated that they are IgG,[107] thus introducing the possibility of transport across haemochorial placentae into the fetal circulation.[108] It should however be appreciated that it is extremely unlikely that such antibodies will ever reach the fetus. For example, in the case of maternal anti-Gm,[109] and anti-GKAm[96] we have previously shown that fetal Gm and HLA antigens within chorionic villi serve as immuno-absorbents; trophoblast Fc-receptors thus allow maternal IgG anti-allotype to enter but never leave the placenta. Indeed, fetal pathology may only occur in those circumstances, such as Rh and ABO, where antigen is not avialable within the placenta. Maternal anti-oncogetal antibody probably never even enters the chorionic villous, because of its shared specificity with trophoblasts.[110] The natural history of these cells is to enter the maternal circulation, perhaps accounting for the observation of immune complexes in maternal sera during normal pregnancy.[111]

CONCLUSION

These findings may help to explain the puzzling epidemiological data that pregnancy seems to protect from mortality in breast cancer.[112] Pregnancy only protects if it occurs before age 20 and seems to augment mortality when the first pregnancy occurs after the 33rd year.[113] In view of our observation that trophoblast antigens are present on breast tumour cells and trophoblasts, it is likely that pregnancy early in life generates sufficient anti-trophoblast immunity to disallow the establishment of malignant cells with cross-reactive trophoblast antigens, but that anti-trophoblast immunity generated later in life would tend to block cell-mediated immunity to an already established tumour, thus making possible its continued growth and eventual clinical presentation. A possible final conclusion from these studies is that trophoblasts - so as to maintain an efficient immunoabsorption capacity for maternal antibodies to oncofetal antigens throughout evolution - contain an antigenic configuration which is common to several tumours. This theoretical speculation is not without precedence, since hybridisation experiments of normal cells with several different lines of transformed cells have shown the appearance of the same glycoprotein.[114] Our results coupled with epidemiological reports of the protective effect of pregnancy in certain tumours suggest that trophoblast membrane oncofetal antigens may be a candidate in future considerations of antigens to be used in well-defined conditions of immunotherapy for certain forms of human cancer.

For discussion of this paper, see end of section

PLACENTAL ANTIBODY TRANSPORT AND IMMUNOLOGICAL PROTECTION — THEIR CELLULAR MECHANISMS

Arthur E. Wild

Selective transport of antibodies from the maternal to the fetal circulation is an important immunological function of the choroc-allantoic placenta, at least in primates. It confers passive immunity upon the fetus and newborn infant. The immunological experience of the mother, encapsulated in her antibodies, thus provides a ready-made protective screen, beneath which the newborn infant's own immunological education can take place when it first encounters pathogens and other antigenic stimuli. Much has been learned about the protective effects, specificity and class of transported antibody,[1-3] but this review is more concerned with the cellular transport mechanisms operating within the placenta. After many years of neglect we now have some insight into these mechanisms, and further studies could contribute much to our understanding of selective protein uptake by cells. The placenta or, specifically, its trophoblastic component has come to be looked upon more as a filter than as the barrier it was once thought to be. Whilst I do not believe filtration to be a particularly apt description for the mechanism of antibody transport, it has been used to convey the idea that certain potentially cytotoxic antibodies (and cells) directed against 'paternal' antigens inherited by the fetus might possibly be trapped during transport and have their effects neutralised.[4] The mechanisms by which this might be effected are also considered below.

EVIDENCE OF ANTIBODY TRANSPORT

The human placenta was for long simply assumed to be a site of antibody transport. There was no direct evidence, but the Grosser classification of placental types classed it as haemochorial and therefore presenting the thinnest possible barrier to maternal blood constituents. This contrasted with the supposedly thicker epitheliochorial and syndesmochorial placentae of mammals like pigs and cows which were known not to transport antibodies.[5] Antibody transport in them was thought to take place only after birth, via absorption from colostrum. However, the more recent work of Brambell and his associates[2] focused attention on the greater importance of antibody transport before birth, via the fetal membranes (in particular the yolk-sac splanchnopleur), in mammals such as the rabbit and rat. They also suggested[6] that human placental transport might be via the chorion laeve into the amniotic fluid, followed by intestinal absorption of antibody from swallowed amniotic fluid. Although this route has proved not to be of significance, the suggestion at least stimulated more direct investigation in primates. Studies on humans[7,8] and monkeys[9,10] in which I^{131}-labelled homologous immunoglobulins and other proteins were injected into the maternal blood, demonstrated much greater transport of IgG to the fetal blood than to the amniotic fluid. Moreover, injection of immunoglobulins and other serum proteins directly into the amniotic sac did not result in significant transport to the fetal blood. These findings, together with the fact that newborn babies with oesophageal atresia have blood levels of diptheria antitoxin equal to or higher than the mother's,[11] point strongly to the placental route.

In vitro studies[12] of transport across the perfused human placenta have now shown that immunoglobulins of the antibody class, IgG, are the only ones to pass through; those of classes IgA and IgM do not. Such class selection is in agreement with in vivo observations on transport of labelled immunoglobulins from maternal to fetal blood[8] and on the distribution of specific antibodies in cord serum.[2] The in vitro findings obtained by placental perfusion provide us with the most direct evidence of immunoglobulin transport in humans, and it seems surprising that greater use has not been made of this technique. Besides the ethical considerations, in vivo studies are bedevilled by the fact that equilibration with the various compartments of the conceptus makes absolute levels of protein transport difficult to estimate - a problem compounded by the varied size and half lives[8] of the different immunoglobulins and their fragments.

Selective events during placental transport

Both prenatal transport of immunoglobulins across the rabbit yolk-sac splanchnopleur and postnatal transport across the gut of suckling rats and mice involve selective events which are independent of molecular size but related to immunoglobulin class, structure, and species of origin. Immunoglobulin transport in these species is also associated with considerable proteolysis, only about 12% of experimentally administered IgG actually reaching the circulation of the fetal or newborn animal.[13] At least some of these features apply to transport across the human placenta where they have to be accounted for at cellular level. Since there is little if any transport of albumin or IgA to the fetal blood after injection into the maternal circulation[8] although their molecular masses (60,000 and 170,000 respectively) are well below or only slightly above that of IgG (150,000), it follows that molecular size, and therefore diffusion processes, cannot be limiting factors. Although IgM is frequently stated not to be transported because of its very large molecule (900,000), a more likely explanation, as for IgA, is that appropriate receptor sites are lacking from the syncytiotrophoblast. Evidence for this is considered later.

An important conclusion drawn from laboratory studies of the mammals referred to above is that the Fc region of the IgG molecule carries the configuration necessary for the whole molecule to be recognised and transported. That the Fc fragment may be more readily transported from human mother to fetus than Fab fragments was demonstrated by Gitlin and co-workers[8] in 1964, but they also expressed doubts about the significance of this finding. In maternal blood, the Fab fragment was found to have a much shorter half-life than the Fc fragment, and if such a difference took place in fetal blood, this could have seriously affected the results. However, no such differences between rabbit Fc and Fab pieces are found in fetal rabbit blood.[14] Moreover, the demonstration of receptors specific for the Fc region of IgG on syncytiotrophoblast, yolk-sac endoderm and proximal enterocytes of suckling-rat gut (referred to later) confirms the importance of the Fc region for transport across these cellular barriers.

Some organisms (i.e. Bordetella pertussis, streptococci, staphylococci and Escherichia coli) evoke continuing IgM rather than IgG responses, with the result that selective placental transport prevents the newborn infant from receiving much immunological protection in these instances.[3] This appears to be the price of preventing the passage of naturally occurring maternal anti-A and anti-B iso-agglutinins and possibly other cytotoxic antibodies of the IgM class to the fetal blood, where they might otherwise cause disastrous haemolytic and cytolytic effects.

Since antibodies of certain specificities may sometimes be restricted to one or more subclasses of IgG, some interest has centred on whether or not subclass selection takes place in the placenta. All four subclasses are in fact transported to the human fetus, perhaps with some preference for IgG_1.[15-17] In the mouse, however, IgG_3 has been estimated to reach the fetus some 20 to 50 times more readily than IgG_1 and IgG_2.[18]

Mechanism of selective transport

Application of erythrocyte-antibody adherence and rosette techniques to human placental tissue sections[20-23] and to isolated cells[24] has confirmed the presence of Fc receptors on syncytiotrophoblast. These findings suggest a single class of receptor specific for IgG, since IgA and IgM do not compete for binding of IgG-sensitised erythrocytes[20] or for binding to placental cell-membrane preparations.[25] Similarly, application of erythrocyte-antibody rosette techniques to isolated mouse[26] and rabbit[27] yolk-sac endoderm has shown that these cells too have IgG-specific Fc receptors on their surfaces. A relationship between Fc attachment and selective transmission of IgG from different species across rabbit yolk-sac endoderm has also been clearly demonstrated. Bovine IgG, for example, is non-selectively endocytosed, not bound to Fc receptors and not transported significantly to the fetal blood, whereas human IgG, which competes most effectively with rabbit IgG for Fc receptor attachment, is bound and transported.[27] Receptors specific for IgG are also present on the proximal enterocytes of suckling-rat gut,[28,29] and it is across the proximal region of the small intestine that most selective transport of antibody appears to take place.[30]

Brambell[2,19] has attempted to explain how immunoglobulin could be selectively transported across rabbit yolk-sac endoderm and gut enterocytes of suckling rodents (and, by implication, across human syncytiotrophoblast), by suggesting that receptors specific for the Fc region of IgG might be present on the limiting membrane of endocytic vesicles formed in these cells. According to this concept, such receptors would provide selective protection against proteolysis during transport of endocytic vesicles, in which non-selectively endocytosed proteins fused with lysosomes. Exocytosis was thought to be the mechanism by which the selectively protected immunoglobulin left the cells, when it would become free to diffuse across the basement membrane, mesenchymal and endothelial layers, to reach the underlying fetal circulation.

Although there is now no doubt about the presence of Fc receptors on immunoglobulin transporting cells, it is highly unlikely that they function in the way that Brambell envisaged. Multivesiculate bodies positive for acid phosphatase have been detected in human syncytiotrophoblast and these might possibly represent phagolysosomes carrying out selective degradation of proteins,[31] but there is no indication that these bodies ever exocytose their contents. The same is true of phagolysosomes in yolk-sac endoderm, and such evidence as we have indicates that proteolysis and selection are not intimately related during transport.[32] For these reasons, I have postulated a different role for the Fc receptors,[33] suggesting that they become associated with coated vesicles forming from the apical cell surface and thus serve to segregate the IgG selected for transport from the immunoglobulins (and other proteins) destined for proteolysis within phagolysosomes. Selection would therefore be a cell surface event and independent of proteolysis, since the transporting vesicles would not be fused with lysosomes. Ultrastructural studies of protein transport across rabbit yolk-sac endoderm have lent support to this concept. Coated vesicles containing rabbit or human IgG, but not bovine IgG, have been observed apparently forming from the apical cell surface and apparently exocytosing their contents at the lateral and basal plasmalemma.[34] Coated vesicles are also the vehicle for selective transport of immunoglobulin across proximal enterocytes of suckling-rat gut.[35,36] And both coated vesicles and specific cell-surface receptors have been implicated in other cell types where there is a need to either store, break down or transport specific proteins present in the external medium.[37]

In view of this evidence it would be surprising if coated vesicles were not in some way involved in selective transport of IgG across human syncytiotrophoblast, and there is some supporting evidence. In guinea-pig placenta, which has a syncytiotrophoblast layer not unlike that of human placenta, a low level of ferritin transport appears to take place across it in coated vesicles.[38] That coated pits and vesicles are abundant at the more microvillous surfaces of human syncytiotrophoblast is well established,[39,40] and one brief report[41] indicates that human IgG-HRP conjugates become localised in coated vesicles in syncytiotrophoblast when human placental villi are cultured _in vitro_. While immunofluorescence studies have consistently failed to show much evidence of endogenous IgG in human syncytiotrophoblast, other than in basement membrane, IgG has been readily detected in the placental villous core.[42-46] This would not be surprising if transport were mediated by coated vesicles, because their submicroscopic size might not permit penetration with labelled antiserum - and thus prevent their subsequent visualisation. Homologous and heterologous immunoglobulins and other proteins are, on the other hand, readily detected by immunofluorescence in yolk-sac endoderm.[47,48,32] However, protein detected in this way appears to be resident in phagolysosomes and not destined for transport but for supplying the growing fetus with essential amino-acids.

It may well be that little if any non-selective uptake of proteins takes place in human syncytiotrophoblast and that the placenta is functionally much less significant as a source of amino-acids. Although haemoglobin is degraded by human 'trophoblast' cells cultured _in vitro_,[49] the presence of macrophages in these cultures makes interpretation with respect to syncytiotrophoblast very difficult. The multivesiculate bodies described by Martin and Spicer[31] have the appearance of being formed from coated vesicles that have lost their clathrin coats, and it is possible that much of the IgG selectively endocytosed through mediation of Fc receptors may be rapidly broken down. Ockleford and Whyte[40] found coated vesicles in syncytiotrophoblast to be largely restricted to the cell surface region, and accounted for this by suggesting that loss of coat material took place. Clearly this is an area requiring much further study.

Techniques have, however, been developed for isolation of coated vesicles from various organs[50] and successfully applied to human placenta.[40] It ought not to be too difficult to analyse the contents of coated vesicles isolated from human placenta, and thus determine more directly whether or not they have selectively endocytosed IgG. The bulk of material available makes human placenta a more practical choice than yolk-sac or gut for study of coated vesicle function. Applied to perfused placentae, such an approach might elucidate the discriminatory endocytic functions of coated vesicles, since it would facilitate study of labelled immunoglobulins and their fragments derived from different species. Placental coated vesicles ought also to provide a useful source of Fc receptor molecules for biochemical characterisation, assuming their role in selective immunoglobulin transport is substantiated. Two differences between the Fc receptors concerned in IgG transport and those present on macrophages and B lymphocytes have already emerged. Placental Fc receptors are distinguished by high affinity for native IgG, as shown by the ease with which relatively low concentrations block erythrocyte-antibody adherence and rosette formation in rabbit and human placentae,[20,27] and by the failure of human placental Fc receptors to bind C gamma 3 antibody fragments due to lack of affinity for them.

IMMUNOLOGICAL PROTECTION IN THE PLACENTA

That the pregnant female can respond to her non-histocompatible fetus by production of specific humoral and cell-mediated immunity now seems well established. However, there is no good evidence that this response causes the feto-placental unit to be rejected like other allografts - for reasons that appear to be multifactorial.[51,52] Considered in the context of antibody transport across the placenta, so-called efferent enhancement has come to be regarded as one possible means of feto-placental protection. There are now numerous reports of 'blocking antibody' being found in the serum of normal multigravid women.[53] Blocking antibody also appears to be present in both multiparous[54] and hybrid mated[55] mice. Indeed, it has been suggested that failure to produce blocking antibody may contribute to chronic abortion in some women.[53] Efferent enhancement might be mediated by specific blocking antibody, directed against placental and paternally-inherited antigens, combining with these antigenic sites in the feto-placental unit - and thus protecting them from more injurious attack by cytotoxic IgM and cell-mediated immune responses. As already noted, mouse IgG_3 is preferred to other IgG subclasses during transport to the fetus, and the fact that it does not bind complement could mean that it contains blocking antibodies (for which its non-complement binding properties would be appropriate) in addition to those conferring passive immunity.

Antibody capable of bringing about tumour enhancement (presumably by protective blocking) has been demonstrated by immunofluorescence to be fixed on trophoblast in placentae of hybrid mouse matings, but this was reported to be mainly IgG_1.[55] Much of the IgG detected in (or close to) the basement membrane of human syncytiotrophoblast by immunofluorescence has been shown by Faulk and co-workers[56,57] to be somehow fixed there yet extractable with acid buffer - suggesting that it is complexed with antigen. These workers have also shown that the eluted IgG is maternal in origin and inhibits certain lymphocyte responses in vitro. They could not, however, attribute this to anti-HLA activity but suggest that the fixed IgG represents blocking antibody with specificity directed against 'trophoblast antigen'shared by lymphocytes. Presumably blocking antibody recognises such antigen at the cell surface and then somehow transports it to the basement membrane (possibly in coated vesicles) where the immune complexes remain because their large size restricts their passage. The effect at the cell surface, however, would be to block cell-mediated immunity.

Besides effecting IgG transport for the purposes of passive immunity, Fc receptors on syncytiotrophoblast might also subtly confer protection against IgG antibodies with specifity for trophoblast antigen. As Ockleford[58] has pointed out the effector function for target-cell elimination operate through Fc adjunctive mechanisms when Fab portions of the antibody molecule are bound to the cell surface, but antibodies are actually bound by their Fc receptors in order to be transported, with the result that they are wrongly orientated for target-cell elimination. Greater affinity for Fc than for Fab binding might therefore be expected to act as a protective mechanism; coupled with rapid micropinocytosis, it might keep potentially injurious antibody to a low level. This idea might usefully be tested in mouse yolk-sac cells, since they contain histocompatibility antigens[59] and Fc receptors,[26] and can also be isolated in pure preparation. As regards the light that such mechanisms protecting the feto-placental unit might throw on tumour development, Fc receptors have also been detected on human malignant tissues,[60,61] and the role of enhancing factors in maintenance of tumours is well established.[62]

Further clearance mechanisms may operate should the syncytiotrophoblast be traversed by immune complexes, antibodies with specificity directed against histocompatibility antigens,[63] fetal incompatible immunoglobulin allotypes[64] and possibly other antigens present in the villous core. Fc receptors have been demonstrated[65] on endothelial cells of fetal stem vessels with specificity and high affinity for all subclasses of heat-aggregated IgG, but with little or no affinity for native IgG. Such receptors are ideally suited, and situated, to prevent immune complexes entering the fetal circulation. Macrophages (Hofbauer cells) present within the villous core have also been shown to possess Fc[24,66] and C3 receptors[66] - and may also remove immune complexes. In addition, they may remove antibodies that have become denatured during the transport process. In rabbit yolk-sac splanchnopleur, where macrophages underlie the basement membrane of the endodermal layer, and in the exocoel, where they are most abundant, they readily endocytose FITC-conjugated (but not un-conjugated) rabbit and human IgG.[47] They must therefore be sensitive to relatively minor changes in the IgG molecule.

Although the question has sometimes been raised whether the placenta is immunologically competent in its own right, the evidence for this is scant.[51] Human placental tissue cultured in vitro does not appear to synthesise immunoglobulins,[67-8]

Adinolfi and Wood[69] stating that 'There is nothing in the morphology of the normal human placenta that would suggest that this tissue is capable of immunological function'. Claims that trophoblast cells in the mouse placenta might be pluripotential and effect reactions of graft-versus-host type[70] have not apparently been corroborated.[52] It therefore seems unlikely that more fundamental immunological processes than the ones described here modulate what is, or is not, transported across the placenta.

CONCLUSIONS AND PROSPECTS

That the chorio-allantoic placenta in primates provides antibody transport from mother to fetus can now be regarded as an established fact. Highly selective processes must be involved since only antibodies of type IgG and its subclasses are transported. Selective transport of antibodies across the chorio-allantoic placenta of primates has much in common with what is known about selective transport across rabbit yolk sac and the gut of suckling rodents. It would therefore be surprising if the same (or very similar) mechanisms did not underlie selective transport at the cellular level.

Older ideas of antibody transport by diffusion, with the stress they placed on the thickness of the so-called 'placental barrier', are no longer of importance. That was succeeded by the 'Brambell hypothesis', which provided the most plausible explanation of selective antibody transport at cellular level until further research failed to confirm its validity. However, one basic tenet of that hypothesis, namely that the cells involved (yolk-sac endoderm, gut enterocytes and syncytiotrophoblast) possessed specific receptors for the Fc region of theimmunoglobulin molecule, has been proved correct. These receptors are well adapted for antibody transport since, unlike their counterparts on macrophages and B cells, they have high affinity for native IgG. It is of interest that porcine placenta, which is epitheliochorial in nature and does not allow antibody transport, has been reported not to contain Fc receptors.[20] Although this finding needs confirmation by techniques employing homologous IgG, and not the rabbit IgG used to date, it further supports the concept of specialised protein transporting mechanisms, rather than the thickness of the placental barrier, as the determinants of antibody transport.

Brambell considered antibody selection to be an intracellular event taking place in transporting phagolysosomes, with the Fc receptor providing protection against proteolysis. I have subsequently favoured the idea that selection takes place at the cell surface through the mediation of Fc receptors associated with coated micropinocytic vesicle formation. The modus operandi of the Fc receptors would therefore not be to protect against proteolysis, but to direct a proportion of the available IgG into specialised transporting endocytic vesicles, segregated from the lysosomal system. There is good evidence for such a mechanism in rabbit yolk-sac endoderm and in the proximal enterocytes of suckling-rat gut - and reason to think this may be the means of selective antibody transport across human syncytiotrophoblast.

While selectivity can be looked upon as a method for lessening the chances of potentially harmful antibodies in other immunoglobulin classes from reaching the fetal-placental unit, antibodies of the IgG class with specificity directed against parternally-coded antigens are themselves potentially damaging, and they appear to be covertly transported. Paradoxically, these antibodies might be beneficial if their binding with target antigens on the trophoblast surface (i.e. at the maternal interface) blocked the interaction of more cytotoxic IgM antibodies and lymphocytes. Cytotoxic IgG antibodies might also find it difficult to interact with antigen if they had greater affinity for Fc receptors. A combination of high Fc receptor affinity and low paternal antigen affinity would clearly favour this effect, and there are indications that such a relationship exists in theplacenta. While these concepts of interactions at the trophoblast-maternal interface are still largely hypothetical, it seems increasingly likely that any antigen-antibody complexes formed during transport across the placenta could be eliminated through the mediation of further Fc receptors present on endothelial cells of fetal stem vessels and on macrophages in the villous core. Transfer of passive immunity is still ensured, because these receptors have little or no affinity for native antibody.

I have already suggested that the use of perfused placental preparations could do much to further understanding of antibody transport across the placenta. All too often, studies have been made on fetal and maternal blood alone; conclusions are then drawn about transport and protection - without the placental function itself having been examined in a physiological situation. Placental insufficiency for example, has been reported to reduce the endowment of IgG to the fetus,[17] and this could be related to defects in the mechanism of transport. Paucity of receptor molecules would produce such an effect, as could the mismatching of specific receptor molecules and transmembrane proteins needed for incorporation into coated vesicles[71] (and postulated to occur in defective fibroblasts engaged in uptake of low-density lipoprotein).

It may well be that transported IgG could be used to direct drugs (otherwise unable to cross the placenta) to a sick fetus. Similarly, it might be possible to supply the fetus with other macromolecules it lacked through genetic defects. The idea of targeting therapy is not new in itself,[72] but taking advantage of a normal transcellular transport mechanism in the initial phases of targeting would be novel. Some means of attaching the therapeutic agent to the Fab ends of IgG molecules would most probably be required, in order to leave the Fc component to bind to its receptor free from steric hindrance. In this respect, it is noteworthy that human IgG is prevented from being transported across rabbit yolk-sac endoderm by conjugation with ferritin[48] and that it can then no longer be detected in coated vesicles.[34] The placenta might also provide more general insights into drug targeting, but this could only be explored in a perfused placental system and would be dependent upon more complete understanding of the normal transport mechanism. Finally, there are situations (notably rhesus incompatibility and maternal autoimmune diseases such as thrombocytopenia) in which it may become possible to prevent the fetus from acquiring passive immunity in the form of harmful covertly-transported antibodies. When more is understood about the placental Fc receptor biochemically, competing innocuous compounds capable of binding specifically to Fc receptors might be tailored to produce such a blocking effect.

DISCUSSION

What are the specific characteristics of the placenta, or of pregnancy, which modify or fundamentally change normal immunological responses? That was the sweeping question with which Albert Neuberger opened discussion from the chair. And although it cannot as yet be adequately answered - as Peter Beaconsfield and others pointed out - several aspects of antigenicity and immune responses in pregnancy were further illuminated during discussion, and outstanding problems more precisely defined. Contributions on enhancing antibodies, immunoprotection and immune suppression led to discussion of the immunological features of neoplastic and placental tissue, the porosity of the placental 'barrier', and the transmission of immunological information between mother and fetus. Finally, speakers considered the placenta as an experimental model, with particular reference to its value in immunology - for investigation of tumour growth and graft rejection, to elucidate habitual abortion and toxaemia, and for the possible exploitation of immunological mechanisms as a means of 'targeting' drug therapy. But first, by way of introduction, John Maxwell Anderson amplified and commented on the foregoing papers in the light of his own work and cast an eye to the future.

Problems and prospects

As regards the immunological relationship between mother and fetus, his group's earlier work had shown that skin experimentally transplanted between offspring and mother enjoyed some protection from rejection. Graft survival within a species was always specific to the partners in the pregnancy. Control grafts from other mothers did not survive in the fetus, and control grafts from other offspring did not survive in the mother. Although its features varied from species to species, the specific state in which maternal/fetal grafts were partially protected was always temporary. This phenomenon might be associated with cell transfer during pregnancy (a subject further discussed below - see subheading 'Porosity of placenta'). In man, for example, many millions of trophoblast cells are probably transported to the mother daily. But how long they stay in the human maternal lung, or what their eventual fate may be, is entirely unknown. Maxwell Anderson suggested that more work on this should prove of interest. The specific mechanism underlying absence of rejection might be partially attributed to the activity of T-suppressor cells described by Guy Voisin. As regards non-specific mechanisms of immunoprotection, a pregnancy-associated macroglobulin (described as SP_3 or $alpha_2PAG$) has been found in the serum of pregnant women at about ten times the levels in non-pregnant women. Its level also rises in some cancers. For instance, Maxwell Anderson's group have shown that the serum concentration of this pregnancy-associated macroglobulin remain close to the baseline during a year in which 60 women with breast cancer remained clinically well, whereas levels rose in women who developed metastases. Other factors found to be common to the developing fetus and some cancers include chorionic gonadotrophin, the alkaline phosphotases and the pregnancy proteins. Such parallels strongly suggest the relevance of placental immunology to cancer research.

Commenting on Guy Voisin's reported findings of suppressor lymphocytes and blocking IgG, Maxwell Anderson outlined studies of the responsivity of primiparae to the membrane antigen prepared from their own placentas. The direct leucocyte migration inhibition test was employed because it is applicable to primiparae,unlike the indirect macrophage migration inhibition test which works only with multiparae. Moreover the new direct leucocyte preparation may be more sensitive. Although some cross-reactivity was observed, inhibition of leucocyte migration was generally specific to the mother's own placenta. In normal pregnancy, autologous plasma produced total blocking of the migration. But plasma from women subject to spontaneous abortion, of so far unknown aetiology, produced no blocking. The blocking factor appears to be IgG; it cannot be absorbed out with the platelets, but (on affinity chromatography) it can be absorbed with anti-IgG, though not with normal rabbit serum. The absence of platelet specificity indicates that the blocking factor is not HLA of types A, B, or C. Some other antigenic system appears to be responsible, as suggested by Page Faulk's findings presented earlier.

What of the future? Maxwell Anderson felt that immunological negation, or interaction, between mother and fetus during pregnancy should be conceived as a constantly changing, dynamic, multimodal system - without unduly emphasising any one mechanism as if it operated throughout pregnancy. There are several possible mechanisms of immune suppression, as noted in the foregoing papers. Some may be operative and essential at one stage of pregnancy, some at another. Localised immunosuppression produced by HCG acts at the morula and blastocyst stage and at implantation, while the interaction of different forms of T-cells and blocking factors takes over later - once an exchange of appropriate information has taken place between mother and conceptus. Future studies should seek to follow the whole course of these and other processes through pregnancy. The findings of necessarily isolated research studies need to be brought together in a synthesis. Similarly, Maxwell Anderson regretted the polarisation of studies that tended to concentrate on either morphological or functional aspects. The two needed to be brought together, as did the work of different research disciplines, both with one another and with clinical practice. By way of example, as he indicated, it would be interesting to know if Page Faulk's reported findings could be replicated throughout the course of pregnancy, and also whether his transferrin receptor work would prove to be applicable to fresh tumour material as well as to cultured cell lines. Clinical application clearly depends on further information of this kind.

Future improvements in the understanding and management of habitual abortion and pre-eclamptic toxaemia may also depend on immunological work - for identifying those at risk and possibly for preventing or treating abortion and/or toxaemia by immunological means. But, here too, interdisciplinary collaboration would be required to correlate immunological findings with the endocrinology of these conditions and quite probably with placental biochemistry, cell replication and ageing as well. Equally, progress in preventing or controlling graft rejection and enhancing tumour rejection seems more likely to grow from continuing cross-fertilisation between disciplines than from an isolated breakthrough in any one research field. Other pointers to the future, indicated by Maxwell Anderson, included Guy Voisin's observations of ontogeny tending to mimic philogeny - which might suggest starting points for further research - and the need to apply Arthur Wild's elegant techniques for studying selective immunoglobulin transport to man, or at least to preparations more directly concerned with human pregnancy. The role of the placenta as an active, selective filter transmitting information freely between mother and offspring should prove a rewarding field for further investigation, which might also shed light on the thymus involution which takes place during pregnancy but remains unexplained. All in all, much remains to be done before the immunology of pregnancy in general, and of the placenta in particular, comes to be well understood. However further research holds out prospects of progress in many fields - as noted above and amplified later in this discussion.

Tumour enhancement and immunosuppression

Studies of tumour enhancement, reported by Guy Voisin, have confirmed that

IgG_1 antibodies, directed against histocompatibility antigens of a tumour, were capable of enhancing growth under any circumstances, at any dose. This contrasts with IgG_2, which is inhibitory at high doses, but also becomes enhancing under two conditions. During progressive dilution, IgG_2 changes from being inhibitory to enhancing, as it does if mixed with the corresponding soluble antigen - a procedure which does not much increase the enhancing power of IgG_1. In practice, this means that IgG_2 can be rendered enhancing by dilution and, specifically, by adding the inhibitory antigen from the tumour graft in question, to form an enhancing immune complex.

There are of course other means of producing immune suppression - notably by means of suppressor T-cells, which appear quite early in pregnancy - and Guy Voisin stressed the need to consider all the possibilities and how they might interact _in vivo_. It would be surprising if enhancing antibody and suppressor cells acted independently, and recent studies have shown some synergism between them. In the ordinary way, immune sera containing enhancing antibody suppress mixed lymphocyte reactions (MLR). But if suppressor cells are eliminated from the mixed cell population (_in vivo_, by adult thymectomy, or _in vitro_ by removing cells with histamine receptors), then the power of enhancing immune sera to suppress the MLR is drastically reduced - suggesting that the suppressor cells are necessary for the enhancing antibodies to exert their action. The effect is not complete, however. The MLR suppression cannot be reduced beyond a certain point, perhaps due to a peripheral action of the antibodies on target cells. Nevertheless, this recent work indicates active collaboration between the two regulatory systems - and the need for more research into its mechanisms.

On the other hand, as Eva Klein pointed out, the interaction of certain antibody classes with certain lymphocyte subsets is not confined to graft survival. Antibodies and cells can also participate in lymphocyte-mediated antibody-dependent cytotoxicity, and it is hard to say which is the more important reaction _in vivo_. In her view, it is oversimplified to think that tumour cells survive in the face of immunity solely because of T-cells and enhancing antibodies. Similarly, although the fetus appears to be protected in this way, it must also be immunologically privileged by its location. Nature, Dr. Klein stressed, would regard this as much too important to rely on nothing more than the balance between antibodies and T-cells. In pregnancy, they may be slightly the more important mechanism, but with regard to tumours, she felt that the role of blocking antibodies had been greatly overestimated by other speakers.

Antigen receptors

This led to discussion of the role of Fc receptors, which have not been demonstrated on tumour cells - where, in Arthur Wild's view, they may function like those he described in the placenta. He postulated a shedding process, in which antigen/antibody might first bind and then be shed. The part of the antibody molecule that actually becomes bound was then queried by Guy Voisin, who contested the statement in Dr. Wild's paper that an antibody could only bind by its Fab or Fc components. There is evidence of double binding in mouse cells incubated with an anti-H_2 antibody directed against their antigens. Repeated studies have confirmed that the mechanism here is double binding of the Fc and the Fab segments. This not only shows that the two types of binding are not mutually exclusive; it may also provide a model for the triggering of cellular activity by antibody.

Expanding on his paper, Page Faulk then drew attention to a miscellaneous grouping of trophoblast receptors, particularly on the syncytium, which could act antigenically. If antibody were made to these receptors - and there are known to be antibodies to, for instance, insulin receptors in human disease - its possible effects on the fetus and/or placental metabolism would need to be considered. Three candidates for study are the Fc receptors, the insulin receptor, and the transferrin receptors known to be present on the syncytium. The transferrin receptor, whose role in iron transport is poorly understood, is found in very high density all round the chorionic villus in the human, the baboon and the macaque monkey. (It is not, however, found in the placentae of rabbits, rats, mice or guinea pigs.) Page Faulk and his co-workers have suggested that maternal transferrin is bound to the receptor from maternal blood in the intravillous space. This normal maternal protein may then serve to mask the syncytium.

Could a similar process protect tumour cells? Probably, because Page Faulk's group have demonstrated transferrin receptors on all 48 tumour cell lines examined, but not in a single type of normal cell. In his words, the tumour cells seem to have learned, from the trophoblast, the trick of developing a receptor for transferrin - which apparently does other things, apart from transporting iron. (The placenta's usefulness as an experimental model for studying tumour immunology is further discussed below - see subheading 'Value of placental studies'.)

'Porosity' of placenta

Discussion then turned to the question of placental porosity, Leslie Brent challenging David Billington's statement about the mother making a full-blown immunological response against fetal antigens, which conflicted with what he said about the placenta as a barrier. If the maternal immunological response is truly full-blown, there can be little effective placental barrier preventing the mother from recognising the presence of alien tissue, though some kind of one-way barrier and/or more specific mechanisms could prevent the maternal response from reaching the fetus.

There is in fact, as Leslie Brent pointed out, some doubt about the porosity of the placenta, and he asked to what extent there might be cellular traffic between mother and fetus during pregnancy (as opposed to parturition when fetal red cells are known to appear in maternal blood). In reply, David Billington reaffirmed that in speaking about the placenta as a barrier, he was referring only to cellular traffic. As Arthur Wild showed in his paper, it is not a barrier to immunoglobulins, nor indeed to many other things. The crucial question is whether maternal lymphoid cells can gain access to the fetus, and there is no convincing evidence of that. If small numbers do get across, they would not survive very long, because they could be dealt with by the developing fetus.

In the reverse direction, the position is not so clear. As regards fetal erythrocytes entering maternal blood, it is generally accepted that this usually takes place at parturition, when haemorrhage occurs at the placental site. Only on rare occasions does it appear to occur otherwise, perhaps in cases of disclosed or undisclosed early abortion, for example. It might be argued that lymphocytes could enter the maternal blood in large numbers under these or other conditions, but David Billington described the only evidence of this as very suspect indeed. And Albert Neuberger pointed out that the specific mechanisms for gammaglobulin transport - acting independently of molecule size - are hardly compatible with a large structure like a lymphocyte normally crossing from one circulation to the other. These arguments may not be conclusive, however. The lymphocyte is not passive, like the red cell; it is an active migratory cell able to push itself between the cells of vascular endothelium and even bore through endothelial cells. Leslie Brent felt that this could enable it to cross the placenta, though David Billington doubted it because there are no intercellular spaces in the syncytiotrophoblast. But, whatever the mechanism, there is an early maternal immune response to the conceptus. Stressing that cytotoxic antibodies, of the kind mentioned by Eva Klein, were found in 80% of mothers at a very early stage, Maxwell Anderson quoted this as proof that some immunological information passes across the placenta, whether via lymphocytes or by some other means.

The possibility of lymphocyte transfer across the placenta was the subject of further inconclusive discussion, including the unsubstantiated notion that the placenta might be less porous in first pregnancies than in later ones, and the rather better founded hypothesis that certain forms of stem-cell deficiencies underlying congenital agammaglobulinaemia might be due to the transfer of maternal lymphocytes into the fetus. Page Faulk proposed a relatively simple experiment to resolve this question. When certain maternal allotypes, for instance the genetic markers on IgG, are transported across the placenta into the fetus, they lead to antibodies which can be detected in the baby 10 to 12 months after birth. These antibodies are of course specific to the allotype of the mother's IgG and can be used as a marker of lack of tolerance in utero, since they represent a fetal immune response to maternal immunoglobulin received during pregnancy. If anti-HLA antibodies were looked for in the child at the same time, that should reveal whether the fetus had also reacted immunologically to maternal cells, such as lymphocytes.

Value of placental studies

Discussion of the placenta as an experimental model was opened by Leslie Brent who favoured studies of its unique properties for their own sake, but questioned their value as a means of studying other complex phenomena such as malignancy, graft rejection and senescence. This would be asking for trouble, in his view, and unlikely to help resolve these other problems. Yet as Peter Beaconsfield pointed out, the placenta is accepted by the mother and then rejected - in strictly clinical terms - and he sought the opinion of other immunologists on the relevance of these processes to immune tolerance and rejection generally. For Eva Klein, the placenta was more likely to serve as a model for organ transplantation, because both are concerned with recognition of major histocompatibility antigens, different from those of the host, and with suppression of immune responses to them - vital alike to the survival of fetus and transplanted tissue. By contrast, the extent to which the antigenicity of many malignant tumours in man differs from that of the host remains a largely open question. Tumour immunology tends to be regarded with suspicion by those not working in the field because it focuses on clearly antigenic systems, like virus-induced tumours, of which there are few examples. While the extent to which naturally occurring tumours may be antigenic remains uncertain, the immunological response against them is nowhere near as strong as that against histocompatibility antigens. A parallel can be made with autoimmune diseases, where there is no dramatic rejection of an organ, but only some relatively minor impairment. Yet similar processes, perhaps activated by similar (or lesser) degrees of antigenicity one expected to reject tumours.

Eva Klein felt that this was expecting too much. Even in strongly antigenic animal systems, there is only a very brief interval after a tumour has arisen when its growth can be curtailed by immunological means. The opportunity is soon lost even with experimental tumours that provoke a powerful immune response. While a few spontaneous, naturally occurring tumours are sufficiently antigenic for immunosurveillance to be effective, their growth will often outstrip the immunological resources available for rejection. Most manifest tumours have hardly any antigenic features to stimulate an immunological response. Indeed, an important feature of many malignant cells is that they are 'immunologically unattractive', in Albert Neuberger's phrase, though that may not be the only factor determining their acceptance.

However, David Billington doubted whether the usefulness of the placenta as an experimental model should be rejected on these grounds. The human trophoblast may not carry major histocompatibility antigens, but the placenta does appear to possess a whole range of other antigens - and little is yet known about the maternal responses to them. He thought there were two possible reasons for this: because the techniques for testing the response have not yet been refined, and/or because the placental antigens provoke little response. Further studies might well show close parallels with tumour antigenicity and host response. Guy Voisin took a rather different view, stressing the need to distinguish between the immune mechanisms that are generally available and the efficiency with which they are applied in particular circumstances, according to the type of target, the intensity of the antigenic stimulus, the accessibility of the antigen, and so on. In considering an experimental model, it is necessary to know whether similar mechanisms are at work. In autoimmune states, for example, it is quite usual to speak of a rejection reaction, even if the organ is not actually rejected. The immune agents concerned and the type of reaction are similar to those in graft rejection, though the antigens are different. It may be that there are no major histocompatibility antigens on the trophoblast, as noted by Page Faulk, though this needs to be confirmed in other species, and at other stages of pregnancy. But even if it proves to be generally true, there are still enough other trophoblast antigens to raise an immune reaction in the mother. The main point stressed by Dr. Voisin is to identify the type of immune response they provoke and see whether this explains the lack of rejection. That might be relevant to rejection or enhancement of tumours.

Also reluctant to discard the placenta as a model for immunological research was E. C. Amoroso, who suggested investigating the reactions of surrogate mothers to wholly unrelated fetuses. Now that fertilised ova are being transferred from cattle bred in America to cattle in England, for example, an ideal model for studying immunological reactivity already exists. On the other hand, as he went on to point out, pregnancy is an endocrinological syndrome that should not be viewed in purely immunological terms. In the absence of pregnancy hormones, progesterone for example, pregnancy does not endure. Might not the immunological protection mechanism, whatever its nature, be dependent on the appropriate hormone levels at each stage of pregnancy to prevent rejection of the conceptus? It has, after all, been demonstrated that progesterone promotes the survival of allogeneic skingrafts. Other such experiments are required to determine whether the hormone dependence of pregnancy affects immunological reactivity. There may be other parallels here - between pregnancy and tumours that are hormone dependent. Choriocarcinoma, hepatomas and intestinal tumours all produce and/or influence the levels of hormones concerned in pregnancy (of both steroid and polypeptide type). Might not those hormones be exerting an immunosuppressive function, preventing rejection of the tumour? In choriocarcinoma, a fall in hormone production has been shown to indicate a good prognosis for this most malignant of tumours, and Prof. Amoroso proposed further studies of the interrelationship between hormones, immunosuppression and tumour growth. Conceptuses in surrogate mothers might provide suitable experimental models, among other possibilities.

In the present state of knowledge, there was unanimous agreement with Claude Villee's conclusion that no simple explanation can be given for the mammalian fetus not being rejected. Indeed Albert Neuberger thought it likely that three or four parallel mechanisms might collaborate in so vital a matter, to give the necessary degree of security. That the placenta had been neglected as an experimental animal - as the symposium's title suggested - was emphasised by Arthur Wild, who believed that there was much interesting work to be done - which could yield information useful in other fields. Among these are the novel methods of drug delivery mentioned in his paper. There are now techniques for isolating coated vesicles in bulk, especially from the human placenta and study of these should improve understanding of endocytosis. It might also enable coated vesicles to be used for transporting drugs otherwise unable to cross the placenta to the fetus. Of more general application is the idea of targeting drugs onto specific tissues by means of IgG, to produce the maximum desired effect at the site of action, with minimum dosage and little danger of adverse or other effects elsewhere in the body. Here too, placental studies might be of value. Moreover, in pregnancy itself, it may sometimes be desirable to stop a fetus receiving any passive immunity in the form of maternal antibodies. Examples are rhesus incompatibility, and maternal autoimmune diseases such as thrombocytopenia. As Arthur Wild suggested, greater knowledge of the Fc receptor might make it possible to manufacture innocuous compounds which would bind specifically - and competitively - to the Fc receptor, and thus prevent antibodies from being transported to the fetus.

Conclusion

That the placenta is an important organ to study - whether for its own sake or as an experimental model - was recognised by everyone who spoke and emphasised by Albert Neuberger in his concluding remarks. Immunologically, the still unexplained reasons why the placenta and the fetus are not rejected continue to be of fundamental importance. They may also be relevant to understanding of infertility, some at least of which may have immunological causes, as may spontaneous abortion. Immunological studies of these questions should prove to be of considerable clinical interest and importance. Equally the transport of large molecules, even outside the placenta, is a field of study that promises direct clinical benefit, as noted above.

The relationships between hormonal and immunological influences on biological function should also repay detailed study. Whether placental studies will prove of value in understanding tumour immunology and graft rejection, only the future can show. Meanwhile, exchange of information and ideas - like those outlined above - should serve both to stimulate interdisciplinary interest in placental research and to refine the uses to which it is put.

REFERENCES TO PAPERS IN SECTION III

THE PLACENTA AND THE TUMOUR : VARIATIONS ON AN IMMUNOLOGICAL ENIGMA

W. D. Billington

1 Trotter, W. (1941). Collected Papers of Wilfred Trotter. Oxford University Press.

2 Beer, A. E. & Billingham, R. E. (1976). The Immunobiology of Mamalian Reproduction. Prentice-Hall, New Jersey.

3 Edidin, M. & Johnson, M. H. (1977). Immunobiology of Gametes. Cambridge University Press.

4 Beer, A. E. & Billingham, R. E. (1974). Host responses to intrauterine tissue, cellular and foetal allografts. J. Reprod. Fert. Suppl. 21, 59.

5 Beer, A. E. & Billingham, R. E. (1977). Histocompatibility gene polymorphisms and maternal-foetal interactions. Transplant. Proc., 9, 1393.

6 Marti, J. J. & Hermann, U, (1977). Immunogestosis : A new etiologic concept of essential EPH gestosis, with special reference to the primigravid patient. Am. J. Obstet. Gynec. 128, 489.

7 Hancock, R. J. T. (1978). Sperm antigens and sperm immunogenicity. In Sperms, Antibodies and Infertility. Blackwell, Oxford.

8 Jones, W. R. (1976). Immunological aspects of infertility. In Immunology of Human Reproduction, p.375. ed. J. S. Scott & W. R. Jones. Academic Press, London.

9 Johnson, M. H. (1976). Fertilisation and implantation. In Immunology of Human Reproduction,p.33. ed. J. S. Scott & W. R. Jones. Academic Press, London.

10 Folkman, J. (1978). Tumour angiogenesis. In Immunological Aspects Cancer p.267. ed. J. E. Castro. MTP Press, Lancaster.

11 Kovithavongs, T., McConnachie, P. R. & Dossetor, J. B. (1974). Immunity to tissue sensitization, HLA and non-HLA as detected by the Abcil system. Transplantation 17, 453.

12 Merwin, R. M. & Hill, E. L. (1954). Fate of vascularised and non-vascularised subcutaneous homografts in mice. J. nat. Cancer Inst. 14, 819.

13 Medawar, P. B. (1953). Some immunological and endocrinological problems raised by the evolution of viviparity in vertebrates. Symp. Soc. exp. Biol., 7, 230.

14 Tuffrey, M., Bishun, N. P. & Barnes, R. D. (1969). Porosity of the mouse placenta to maternal cells. Nature 221, 1029.

15 Billington, W. D., Kirby, D. R. S., Owen, J. J. T., Ritter, M. A., Burtonshaw, M. D., Evans, E. P., Ford, C. E., Gauld, I. K. & McLaren, A. (1969). Placental barrier to maternal cells. Nature 224, 704.

16 Adinolfi, M. C. (1975). The human placenta as a filter for cells and plasma proteins. In Immunobiology of the Trophoblast, p.193. ed. R. G. Edwards, C. W. S. Howe & M. H. Johnson. Cambridge University Press.

17 Billington, W. D. & Jenkinson, E. J. (1975). Antigen expression during early mouse development. In The Early Development of Mammals, p.219. ed. M. Balls & A. E. Wild. Cambridge University Press.

18 Little, C. C. (1924). Genetics of tissue transplantation in mammals. J. Cancer Res. 8, 75.

19 Palm, J., Heyner, S. & Brinster, R. L. (1971). Differential immunofluorescence of fertilized mouse eggs with H-2 and non-H-2 antibody. J. exp. Med. 133, 1282.

20 Muggleton-Harris, A. L. & Johnson, M. H. (1976). The nature and distribution of serologically detectable alloantigens on the preimplantation mouse embryo. J. Embryol. Exp. Morph. 35, 59.

21 Krco, C. J. & Goldberg, E. H. (1977). Major histocompatibility antigens in preimplantation mouse embryo. Transplant. Proc. 9, 1367.

22 Sellens, M. H. (1977). Antigen expression on early mouse trophoblast. Nature 269,60.

23 Sellens, M. H., Jenkinson, E. J. & Billington, W. D. (1978). Major histocompatibility complex and non-major histocompatibility complex antigens on mouse ectoplacental cone and placental trophoblastic cells. Transplantation 25, 173.

24 Adinolfi, M. C. & Billington, W. D. (1976). Ontogeny of acquired immunity and feto-maternal immunological interactions. In Fetal Physiology and Medicine, p. 17. ed. R. W. Beard & P. W. Nathanielsz. Saunders, London.

25 Gusdon, J. P. (1976). Maternal immune responses in pregnancy. In Immunology of Human Reproduction, p.103. ed. J. S. Scott & W. R. Jones. Academic Press, London.

26 Murgita, R. A. (1976). The immunosuppressive role of alpha-foetoprotein during pregnancy. Scand. J. Immunol. 5, 1003.

27 Beer, A. E. (1979). Immunological recognition mechanisms during pregnancy. In Maternal Recognition of Pregnancy. CIBA Found. Symp. (in press).

28. Adcock, E. W., Teasdale, F., August, C. S., Cox, C., Meschia, G., Battaglia, F. C., & Naughton, M. A. (1973). Human chorionic gonadotrophin : its possible role in maternal lymphocyte suppression. Science 181, 845.

29 Tamerius, J., Hellstrom, I. & Hellstrom, K. E. (1975). Evidence that blocking factors in the sera of multiparous mice are associated with immunoglobulins. Int. J. Cancer 16, 456.

30 Price, M. R. & Robins, R. A. (1978). Circulating factors modifying cell-mediated immunity in experimental neoplasia. In Immunological Aspects of Cancer, p.155. ed. J. E. Castro. MTP Press, Lancaster.

31 Gershon, R. K. (1974). T cell control of antibody responses. Contemp. Top. Immunol. 3, 1.

32 Skowron-Cendrzak, A. & Ptak, W. (1976). Suppression of local GVH reactions by mouse foetal and newborn spleen cells. Eur. J. Immunol. 6, 451.

33 Oldstone, M. B., Tishon, A. & Moretta, L. (1977). Active thymus derived suppressor lymphocytes in human cord blood. Nature 269, 333.

34 Chaouat, G. (personal communication).

35 Smith, G. (unpublished results).

36 Chaouat, G., Voisin, G. A., Daëron, M. & Kanellopoulos, J. (1977). Anticorps facilitants et cellules suppressives dans la réaction immunitaire maternelle antifoetale. Ann. Immunol, (Inst Pasteur) 128, 21.

37 Smith, R. N. & Powell, A. E. (1977). The adoptive transfer of pregnancy-induced unresponsiveness to male skin grafts with thymus dependent cells. J. exp. Med., 146, 899.

38 Hamilton, M. S. (1977). Suppressor cells in pregnant mice. Fed. Proc. 36, 1183.

39 Beverley, P. C. L. (1978). T effector cells. In Immunological Aspects of Cancer Cancer, p.101. ed. J. E. Castro, MTP Press, Lancaster.

40 Eccles, S. A. (1978). Macrophages and cancer. In Immunological Aspects of Cancer, p.124. ed. J. E. Castro, MTP Press, Lancaster.

41 Nicklin, S. & Billington, W. D. (1979). Macrophage activity in mouse pregnancy. J. Reprod. Immunol. (in press).

42 Billingham, R. E. & Silvers, W. (1971). The Immunobiology of Transplantation, Prentice-Hall, New Jersey.

43 Kirby, D. R. S., Billington, W. D. & James, D. A. (1966). Transplantation of eggs to the kidney and uterus of immunised mice. Transplantation 4, 713.

44 Simmons, R. L. & Russell, P. S. (1967). Immunologic interactions between mother and foetus. Adv. Obstet. Gynec. 1, 38.

45 James, D. A. (1965). Effects of antigenic dissimilarity between mother and foetus on placental size in mice. Nature 205, 613.

46 Iles, S. A. (1973). Immunological aspects of mammalian pregnancy. D. Phil. thesis. University of Oxford.

47 Beer, A. E., Scott, J. R. & Billingham, R. E. (1975). Histoincompatibility and maternal immunological status as determinants of foetoplacental weight and litter size in rodents. J. Exp. Med., 142, 180.

48 Clarke, A. G. (1971). The effects of maternal preimmunization on pregnancy in the mouse. J. Reprod. Fert. 24, 369.

49 Humber, D. P., Mahouy, G., Chinn, S. & Barnes, R. D. (1974). The influence of parity and maternal preimmunisation on foetal survival in mice. J. Reprod. Fert. 41, 193.

50 Hetherington, C. M. (1978). Absence of effect of maternal immunisation to paternal antigens on placental weight, foetal weight and litter size in the mouse. J. Reprod. Fert. 53, 81.

51 Scott, J. S. (1976). Immunological aspects of trophoblastic neoplasia. In Immunology of Human Reproduction, p.329. ed. J. S. Scott & W. R. Jones. Academic Press London.

52 Billington, W. D. (1976). The immunobiology of trophoblast. In Immunology of Human Reproduction, p.81. ed. J. S. Scott & W. R. Jones. Academic Press, London.

53 Håkansson, S., Heyner, S., Sundqvist, K. G. & Bergström S. (1975). The presence of paternal H-2 antigens on hybrid mouse blastocysts during experimental delay of implantation and the disappearance of these antigens after onset of implantation. Int. J. Fertil. 20, 137.

54 Searle, R. F., Sellens, M. H. Elson, J., Jenkinson, E. J. & Billington, W. D. (1976). Detection of alloantigens during preimplantation development and early trophoblast differentiation in the mouse by immunoperoxidase labelling. J. exp. Med., 143, 348.

55 Jenkinson, E. J. & Billington, W. D. (1977). Cell surface properties of early mammalian embryos. In Concepts in Mammalian Embryogenesis, p.235. ed. M. I. Sherman. The MIT Press.

56 Billington, W. D., Jenkinson, E. J., Searle, R. F. & Sellens, M. H. (1977). Alloantigen expression during early embryogenesis and placental ontogeny in the mouse : immunoperoxidase and mixed haemadsorption studies. Transplant. Proc. 9, 1371.

57 Swinburne, L. M. (1970). Leucocyte antigens and placental sponge. Lancet ii, 592.

58 Billington, W. D. & Jenkinson, E. J. (1975). Antigen expression during early mouse development. In The Early Development of Mammals, p.219 ed. M. Balls & A. E. Wild, Cambridge University Press.

59 Wegmann, T. G. & Carlson, G. A. (1977). Allogeneic pregnancy as immunoabsorbant. J. Immunol. 119, 1659.

60 Goodfellow, P. N., Barnstable, C. J., Bodmer, W. F., Snary, D. & Crumpton, M. J. (1976). Expression of HLA system antigens on placenta. Transplantation 22, 595.

61 Faulk, W. P., Sanderson, A. R. & Temple, A. (1977). Distribution of MHC antigens in human placental chorionic villi. Transplant. Proc., 9, 1379.

62 Jenkinson, E. J. & Owen, V. (in preparation).

63 Voisin, G. A. & Chaouat, G. (1974). Demonstration, nature and properties of maternal antibodies fixed on placenta and directed against paternal antigens. J. Reprod. Fert. Suppl. 21, 89.

64 Robertson, W. B., Brosens, I. Dixon, G. (1975). Uteroplacental vascular pathology. Europ. J. Obstet. Gynec. Reprod. Biol. 5. 47.

65 Liggins, G. C., Fairclough, R. J., Grieves, S. A., Kendall, J. Z. & Knox, B. S. (1973). The mechanism of initiation of parturition in the ewe. Rec. Prog. Horm. Res., 29, 111.

66 Simmons, R. L. & Russell, P. S. (1967). Xenogeneic antigens in mouse trophoblast. Transplantation 5, 85.

67 Currie, G. A. (1967). Immunological studies of trophoblast in vitro. J. Obstet. Gynaec. Brit. Cwlth., 74, 841.

68 Beer, A. E., Billingham, R. E. & Yang, S. L. (1972). Further evidence concerning the auto-antigenic status of the trophoblast. J. exp. Med., 135, 1177.

69 Searle, R. F. & Jenkinson, E. J. (1978). Localization of trophoblast-defined surface antigen during early mouse embryogenesis. J. Embryol. exp. Morph. 43, 147.

70 Currie, G. A. & Bagshawe, K. D. (1967). The masking of antigens on trophoblast and cancer cells. Lancet i, 708.

71 Abelev, G. I. (1974). α-foetoprotein as a marker of embryo-specific differentiation in normal and tumour tissues. Transplant. Rev. 20, 3.

72 Laurence, D. J. R. & Neville, A. M. (1972). Foetal antigens and their role in the diagnosis and clinical management of human neoplasms : a review. Brit. J. Cancer 26, 335.

73 Coggin, J. H. & Anderson, N. G. (1974). Cancer differentiation and embryonic antigens : some central problems. Adv. Cancer Res. 19, 105.

74 Moore, M. (1978`. Antigens of experimentally-indiced neoplasms : a conspectus. In Immunological Aspects of Cancer, p.15. ed. J. E. Hastro, MTP Press, Lancaster.

75 Currie, G. A. (1974). Cancer and the Immune Response. Edward Arnold, London.

76 Baldwin, R. W. & Vose, B. M. (1974). The expression of a phase-specific foetal antigen on rat embryo cells. Transplantation 18, 525.

77 Klein, G. (1966). Tumour antigens. Ann. Rev. Microbiol., 20, 233.

78 Steel, G. G. (1973). Cytokinetics of neoplasia. In Cancer Medicine, p.125. ed. J. F. Holland & E. Frei, Lea & Febiger, Philadelphia.

79 Tubiana, M. & Malaise, E. P. (1976). Growth rate and cell kinetics in human tumours : some prognostic and therapeutic implications. In Scientific Foundations of Oncology, p.126. ed. T. Symington & R. L. Carter. Heinemann, London.

80 Currie, G. A. (1973), The role of circulating antigen as an inhibitor of tumour immunity in man. Brit J. Cancer 28 Suppl.1, 153.

81 Currie, G. A. & Alexander, P. (1974). Spontaneous shedding of TSTA by viable sarcoma cells : its possible role in facilitating metastatic spread. Brit. J. Cancer 29, 72.

82 Beard, J. (1904). The problems of cancer. Lancet ii, 1200.

IMMUNE AGENTS OF THE FACILITATION REACTION THEIR POSSIBLE ROLE IN PROTECTION OF THE PLACENTAL ALLOGRAFT

G. A. Voisin

1 Voisin, G. A. (1966).Le phénomène de facilitation immunologique, concept élargi de "enhancement-phenomenon". in: IVth International symposium on Immunopathology Monte Carlo, 1965. (Schwabe & co.,) Bâle, Stuttgart 1, 165.

2 Voisin, G. A. (1971). Immunity and tolerance : a unified concept. Cell. Immunol. 2, 670.

3 Voisin, G. A. (1975). Rejet et facilitation : le double aspect de la réaction immunitaire. La Recherche 6, 1044.

4 Goldberg, E. H. & Tokuda,S. (1976). Immunological enhancement of Sarcoma 1 by antibodies to fetal antigens in syngeneic mice. Transplantation 21, 263.

5 Le Mevel, B. P. & Wells, S. A. Jr. (1973). Foetal antigens cross-reactive with tumour-specific transplantation antigens. Nature New Biol. 244, 183.

6 Sören L. (1967) Immunological reactivity of lymphocytes in multiparous females after strain-specific matings. Nature, 213, 621.

7 Hellström, K. E., Hellström, I. & Brawn, J. (1969) Abrogation of cellular immunity to antigenically foreign mouse embryonic cells by a serum factor. Nature, 224, 914.

8 Voisin, G. A. & Chaouat, G. (1974). Demonstration, nature and properties of antibodies fixed on maternal placenta and directed against paternal antigens. J. Reprod. & Fertil., Suppl., 21, 89.

9 Chaouat, G., Voisin, G. A., Escalier, D. & Robert, P. (1978) Facilitation reaction (enhancing antibodies and suppressor cells) and rejection reaction (sensitized cells) from the mother to the paternal antigens of the foetus. Clin. exp. Immunol. in press

10 Chaouat, G. & Voisin, G. A. In preparation.

11 Chaouat, G., Voisin, G. A., Daëron, M. & Kanellopoulos, J. (1977) Anticorps facilitants et cellules suppressives dans la réaction immunitaire maternelle anti-foetale. Ann. Immunol. 128, 21.

12 Badet, M. T., Chateaureynaud-Duprat P., Voisin, G. A. (1974). Etude des réactions immunitaires chez l'amphibien urodèle Salamandra salamandra. Modalités de la réaction de transplantation. C. R. Acad. Sci. 278,1297.

13 Badet M. T., Chateaureynaud-Duprat, P. & Voisin G. A. (1975).In vitro demonstration and study of a complex immune reaction (rejection and facilitation) of mothers towards embryos in urodel amphibian Salamandra salamandra, C. R. Acad. Sci. 281, 199.

14 Badet, M. T., Chateaureynaud-Duprat, P. & Voisin, G. A. (1977). Etude de la réaction de protection maternelle contre une réaction de rejet de la mère à l'égard de ses larves chez Salamandra salamandra. C. R. Acad. Sci. 284, 2443.

15 Chateaureynard-Duprat, P., Badet, M. T. & Voisin, G. A. In preparation.

16 Loblay, R. H., Pritchard-Briscoe, H. & Basten, A. (1978). Suppressor T cell memory, Nature 272, 620.

17 Beer, A. E. & Billingham R. E. (1973). Maternally acquired runt disease. Science, 179, 240.

18 Hamilton, M. S. & Hellström, I. (1977). Altered immune responses in pregnant mice. Transplantation 23, 423.

19 Kanellopoulos-Langevin, C., Kanellopoulos, J. & Voisin, G.A. (1976). Role of suppressor cells in antibody-induced inhibition of mixed lymphocyte reactions. Ann. Immunol. 127, 5.

20 Searle, R. F., Sellens, M. H., Elson, J., Jenkinson, E. J. & Billington W. D. (1976). Detection of alloantigens during implantation development and early trophoblast differentiation in the mouse by immunoperoxydase labelling. J. exp. Med. 143, 348.

21 Bernard, O., Ripoche, M-A. & Bennett,D. (1977). Distribution of maternal immunoglobulins in the mouse uterus and embryo in the days after implantation. J. exp. Med. 145, 58.

22 Dumble, L. J., Tait, B. D., Whittingham, S. & Ashton, P. W. (1977). The immunological privilege of the fetus : decreased expression of paternal HLA. Immunogenetics 5, 345.

23 David, G. & Volkringer, P. (1967). Tolérance à l'homogreffe cutanée dans le post partum chez la souris. Ann. Inst. Pasteur 113, 483.

24 Heron, J. (1972). Prolonged survival of heart allografts transplanted in rats and rabbits following pregnancy. Transplantation 14, 551.

25 Jenkinson, E. J., Billington, W. B., & Elson, J., (1976). Detection of receptors for immunoglobulin on human placenta by EA rosette formation. Clin. exp. Immunol. 23, 456.

26 Brambell, F. W. R, (1970). The transmission of immunity from mother to gonodotropin : effects of crude and purified preparations on lymphocyte responses to phytohemagglutinius and allogeneic stimulation. J. Immunol. 115, 1249.

27 Vuagnat Ph., Neveu, T. & Voisin, G. A. (1973). Immuno-deviation by passive antibody, an expression of selective immuno-depression. I-Action of guinea-pig IgG1 and IgG2 anti-hapten antibodies. Eur. J. Immunol. 3, 90.

28 Vuagnat Ph., Neveu, T. & Voisin, G. A. (1973). Immuno-deviation by passive antibody, an expression of selective immuno-depression. II-Action of guinea-pig IgG1 and IgG2 anti-carrier antibodies. J. exp. Med. 137, 265.

29 Caldwell, J. L., Stites, D. P. & Fudenberg, H. H. (1975). Human chorionic gonodotropin : effects of crude and purified preparations on lymphocyte responses to phytohemagglutinins and allogeneic stimulation. J. Immunol. 115, 1249.

30 Maillard, J. & Favreau, C. (1977). Rôle immunitaire de la plasmine. II-La plasmine modifie la résponse-anticorps primaire des cultures de cellules spléniques. Ann. Immunol. 128, 999.

31 Fauve, R., Hevin, B., Jakob, H., & Jacob, F. (1974). Anti-inflamatory effect of murine malignant cells. Proc. Nat. Acad. Sci. USA 71, 4052.

32 Murgita, R. A., Goidl, E. A., Kontiainen, S. & Wigzell, H. (1977). α-fetoprotein induces suppressor T cells in vitro. Nature 267, 257.

33 Voisin, G. A. (1974). The impact of mother-foetus immunological relationships on fundamental immunological concepts. Excerpta Medica, Amsterdam, 109.

ROLE OF THE MAJOR HISTOCOMPATIBILITY COMPLEX IN THE IMMUNOBIOLOGY OF TROPHOBLAST ANTIGENS

J. A. McIntyre and W. Page Faulk

1 McIntyre, J. A., Turner, R. E., & LeRoy, E. C. (1978). Human leukocyte antigens (HLA) I. Biology of the HLA system; II. Clinical applications of HLA typing. South. Med. J., In Press.

2 Fudenberg, H. H. & Fudenberg, B. R. (1964). Antibody to hereditary gamma globulin (Gm) factor resulting from maternal/fetal incompatibility. Science, 145, 170.

3 Faulk, W. P., van Loghem, E., & Stickler, G. B., (1964). Maternal antibody to fetal light chain (InV) antigens. Am. J. Med. 56, 393.

4 Boyd, J. D., & Hamilton, W. J., (1970). The Human Placenta, p.282. W. Heffer & Sons, Ltd., Cambridge.

5 Ikle, F. A., & Gallen, S. T. (1964). Dissemination von Syncytiotrophoblast-zellen inn mutterlichen Blut wahrend der Graviditat. Bull Schweiz. Akad. Med. Wiss., 20, 62.

6 Thomas, L., Douglas, G. W. & Carr, M. C. (1959). The continual migration of syncytial trophoblasts from the fetal placenta into the maternal circulation. Trans. Assoc. Am. Physicians. 72, 140.

7 Park, W. W., (1959). Aspects of choriocarcinoma in the female. Ann. N.Y. Acad. Sci., 80, 152.

8 Park, W. W. (1958). Experimental trophoblastic embolism of the lungs. J. Pathol. Bacteriol., 75, 257.

9 Basdawil, W. A., & Toy, B. L. (1959). The natural history of choriocarcinoma: Problems of immunity and spontaneous regression. Ann. N.Y. Acad. Sci., 80, 197.

10 Seegal, B. C. & Loeb, E. N. (1940). Effect of anti-placental serum on development of foetus in the pregnant rat. Proc. Soc. Exp. Biol. Med., 45, 248.

11 Pressman, D. & Korngold, L. (1956). Localizing properties of anti-placenta serum. J. Immunol., 78, 75.

12 Boss, J. H. & Craig, J. M. (1963). The distribution patterns in the rat placenta of antigens common to the rat glomerulus as revealed by immunofluorescent techniques. Am. J. Obstet. Gynecol., 42, 443.

13 Boss, J. H., (1965). Antigenic relationships between placenta and kidney in humans. Am. J. Obstet. Gynecol., 94, 574.

14 Gaugas, J. M., Wright, C. & Curzen, P. (1974). Human placental heteroantigens demonstrable by immunodiffusion. Brit.J. Exp. Pathol., 55, 478.

15 Smith, N. C., Brush, M. G. & Luckett, S. (1974). Preparation of human placental villous surface membrane. Nature, 252, 302.

16 Faulk, W. P., Lovins, R. E., Yeager, C. & Temple, A. (1977). Antigens of human trophoblasts: Immunological and biochemical characterization. In Immunological Influence on Human Fertility. ed. B. Boettcher p.153. Academic Press, Sydney New York, London.

17 Galbraith, G. M. P., Galbraith, R. M. Faulk, W. P. & Wachtel, S. S. (1978). Detection of H-Y antigen by fluorescence microscopy. Transplantation. 26, 25.

18 Faulk, W. P., Temple, A., Lovins, R. E. & Smith, N. C. (1978). Antigens of human trophoblast: A working hypothesis for their role in normal and abnormal pregnancies. Proc. Nat. Acad. Sci. USA 75, 1947.

19 Dobrowatski, M. (1903). Bull. Int. d l'Acad. de Sci. de Cracovie 5, p.256.

20 Cohen, H. R. & Nadzel, A. J., (1940). Specific action of an antiserum for placental proteins on placenta and normal progress of pregnancy. Proc. Soc. Exp. Biol. & Med., 48, 249.

21 Seegal, B. C. & Loeb, E. N. (1964). The production of chronic glomerulonephritis in rats by the injection of rabbit anti-rat placenta serum. J. Exp. Med. 84, 211.

22 Beer, A. E., Billingham, R. E. & Yang, S. L. (1972). Further evidence concerning the auto antigenic status of the trophoblast. J. Exp. Med., 135, 1177.

23 Fawcett, D. (1950). The development of mouse ova under the capsule of the kidney. Anat. Rec., 108, 71.
Fawcett, D. W., Wislocki, G. B. & Waldo, C. M. (1947). The development of mouse ova in the anterior chamber of the eye and in the abdominal cavity. Am. J. Anat., 81, 431.

24 Kirby, D. R. S. (1960). Development of mouse eggs beneath the kidney capsule. Nature, 187, 707.

25 Simmons, R. L. & Russell, P. S. (1962). The antigenicity of mouse trophoblast. Ann. N.Y. Acad. Sci., 99, 717.

26 Simmons, R. L. & Russell, P. S. (1965). Histocompatibility antigens in transplanted mouse eggs. Nature 208, 698.

27 Simmons, R. L. & Russell, P. S. (1966). The histocompatibility antigens of fertilized mouse eggs and trophoblast. Ann. N.Y. Acad. Sci. 129, 35.

28 Simmons, R. L. & Russell, P. S. (1967). Xenographic antigens in mouse trophoblast. Transplantation, 5, 85.

29 Currie, G. A., van Doorninck, W. & Bagshawe, K. D., (1968). Effect of neuraminidase on the immunogenicity of early mouse trophoblast. Nature, 219, 191.

30 Currie, G. A. & Bagshawe, K. D. (1968). The role of sialic acid in antigenic expression: Further studies of the Landschultz Ascites Tumor. Brit J. Cancer. 22, 843.

31 Bagshawe, K. D. & Currie, G. A. (1968). Immunogenicity of L1210 murine leukemia cells after treatment with neuraminidase. Surgery, 218, 1254.

32 Currie, G. A. (1970). The conceptus as an allograft: Immunological reactivity of the mother. Proc. R. Soc. Med., 63, 61.

33 Simmons, R. L., Lipschultz. M. L., Rios, A. & Ray, P. (1971). Failure of neuraminidase to unmask histocompatibility antigens on trophoblast. Nature, New Biol., 231,111.

34 Kaneko, Y. & Nishimura, T. (1978). Factors affecting trophoblast growth in extrauterine sites. Transplantation, 25,309.

35 Furuya, N. & Hirao, T. (1976). A substrain mouse serologically classified in ddN strain and its behavioral characteristics. Tohoku. J. Exp. Med., 118, 355.

36 Kirby, D. R. S. (1968). The immunological consequences of extrauterine development of allogeneic mouse blastocytes. Transplantation, 6, 1005.

37 Hulka, J. F. & Mohr, K., (1968). Trophoblast antigenicity demonstrated by altered challange graft survival. Science, 161, 696.

38 Kirby, D. R. S. (1969). Is the trophoblast antigenic? Transplant. Proc. 1,53.

39 Vandeputte, M. & Sobis, H. (1972). Histocompatibility antigens on mouse blastocysts and ectoplacental cones. Transplantation, 14, 331.

40 Jenkinson, E. J. & Billington, W. D. (1974). Differential susceptibility of mouse trophoblast and embyronic tissue to immune cell lysis. Transplantation, 18,286.

41 Sellens, M. H., Jenkinson, E. J. & Billington, W. D. (1978). Major histocompatibility complex and non-major histocompatibility complex antigens on mouse ectoplacental cone and placental trophoblastic cells. Transplantation, 25, 173.

42 Johnson, M. H. (1975). Antigens of peri-implantation trophoblast. In Immunobiology of Trophoblast ed. R. G. Edwards, C. W. S. Howe, & M. H. Johnson, p.87. Cambridge University Press, Cambridge, England.

43 Muggulton-Harris, A. L. & Johnson, M. H. (1976). The nature and distribution of serologically detectable alloantigens on the preimplantation mouse embryo. J. Embryol. Exp. Morphol., 35, 59.

44 Palm, J., Heyner, S. & Brinster, R. L. (1971). Differential immunofluorescence of fertilized mouse eggs with H-2 and non H-2 antibody. J. Exp. Med. 133, 1282.

45 Searle, R. F., Johnson, M. H., Billington, W. D., Elson, J. & Clutterbuck-Jackson, S. (1974). Investigation of H-2 and non H-2 antigens on the mouse blastocyst. Transplantation, 18, 136.

46 Searle, R. F. Sellens, M. H., Elson, J., Jenkinson, E. J. & Billington, W. D. (1976). Detection of alloantigens during periimplantation development and early trophoblast differentiation in the mouse by immunoperoxidase labeling, J. Exp. Med., 143, 348.

47 Heyner, S. (1973). Detection of H-2 antigens on the cells of the early mouse embryo. Transplantation, 16, 675.

48 Carter, J. (1976). Expression of maternal and paternal antigens on trophoblast. Nature, 262, 292.

49 Sellens, M. H., (1977). Antigen expression on early mouse trophoblast. Nature, 269, 60.

50 Webb, C. G., Gall, W. E. & Edelman, G. M. (1977). Synthesis and distribution of H-2 antigens in preimplantation mouse embryos. J. Exp. Med., 146, 923.

51 Nilsson, K., Evrin, P. E. & Welsh, K. (1974). Production of 2-microglobulin by normal and malignant human cell lines and peripheral lymphocytes. Transplant. Rev., 21, 53.

52 Faulk, W. P., Temple, A.(1976). Distribution of 2-microglobulin and HLA in chonionic villi of human placentae. Nature, 262, 799.

53 Faulk, W. P. & Johnson, P. M. (1977). Immunological studies of human placenta: Identification and distribution of proteins in mature chorionic villi. Clin. Exp. Immunol., 27, 365.

54 Johnson, P. M. & Faulk, W. P. (1978). Immunological studies of human placentae: Identification and distribution of proteins in immature chorionic villi. Immunology, 34, 1027.

55 Faulk, W. P., Sanderson, A. & Temple, A. (1977). Distribution of MHC antigens in human placentae, Transplant. Proc., 9, 1379.

56 Goodfellow, P. M., Barnstable, C. J., Bodmer, W. F., Snary, D. E. & Crumpton, M. J. (1976). Expression of HLA system antigens on placenta. Transplantation, 22, 59.

57 Lawler, S. D. (1976). Immunogenetics of trophoblast tumours. J. Clin. Pathol., 29; Suppl. (Roy. Coll. Path.), 10, 132.

58 Zinkernagel, R. M. & Doherty, P. C. (1977). Major transplantation antigens, viruses, and specificity of surveillance T-cells. Contemp. Top. Immunobiol., 7, 179.

59 Zinkernagel, R. M. & Doherty, P. C. (1977a). The concept that surveillance of self is mediated via the same set of genes that determines recognition of allogeneic cells. Cold Spring Harbor Symp. Quant. Biol., 41,(2), 505.

60 Faulk, W. P. & Galbraith, G. M. P. (1978). Trophoblastic transferrin and transferrin receptors. Proc. R. Soc. Med. (B). In Press.

61 Loke, Y. W., Joysey, V. C. & Borland, R. (1971). HLA antigens in human trophoblast cells. Nature, 232, 403.

62 Hare, D. B., Harris, C. E., Kayhoe, D. E., Ray, J. G. & Scott, R. C. (1972-1973) Catalog of tissue typing antisera. DHEW Publication No. (NIH) 73-97., p.748.

63 van Rood, J. J. (1972). Joint Report: w4 and w6. In Histocompatibility Testing. eds. J. Dausset and J. Colombani , p.645. Munksgaard, Copenhagen.

64 Iwaki, Y., Park, M. S., Terasaki, P. I. & Billing, R. (1978). Enhancement of human kidney allografts by cold B-lymphocyte cytotoxins. Lancet, i, 1228.

65 Bresnihan, B., Grigor, R. R., Oliver, M., Lewkonia, R. M., Lovins, R. E., Faulk, W. P. & Hughes, G. R. V. (1977). Spontaneous abortion in systemic lupus erythematosis: An association with trophoblast-reactive lymphocytotoxic antibodies. Lancet, ii, 1205.

66 Szulman, A. E. (1973). The A, B and H blood group antigens in human placenta. New Engl. J.Med.,286, 1028.

67 McCormick, J. N., Faulk, W. P., Fox, H. & Fudenberg, H. H. (1971). Immunohistological and elution studies of the human placenta. J. Exp. Med., 133, 1.

68 Middleton, J., Crookston, C., Faulk, J. A., Robson, E. B., Cook, P. J. C. Batchelor, J. R., Bodmer, J., Fersara, G. V., Festenstein, H., Harris, R., Kissmeyer-Nielsen, F., Lawler, S. D., Sachs, J. A. & Wolf, I. (1974). Linkage of Chido and HLA. Tissue Antigens, 4, 366.

69 Snell, G. D., Dausset, J. & Nathenson, S. (1976). In Histocompatibility. p.216. Academic Press, New York.

70 Race, R. R. & Sanger, R. (1975). Blood groups in man (6th ed.) p. 164. London, Blackwell.

71 Levine, P. (1978). Blood group and tissue genetic markers in familial adenocarcinoma:potential specific immunotherapy. Seminars in Oncology, 5, 25.

72 Oliver, R. T. D. (1976). Histocompatibility matching and renal graft survival Proc. R. Soc. Med., 69, 531.

73 Grunnet, N., Kristensen, T. & Kissmeyer-Neilsen, F. (1976). Cell mediated lympholysis in man. The impact of HLA-C antigens. Tissue Antigens, 7, 301.

74 Kirby, D. R. S., McWhirter, K. G., Teitelbaum, M. S. & Darlington, C. D. (1967). A possible immunologic influence on sex ratio. Lancet. ii, 139.

75 Kirby, D. R. S. (1970). The egg and immunology. Proc. R. Soc. Med., 63, 59.

76 Artzt, K., Bennett, D. & Jacob, F. (1974). Primitive teratocarcinoma cells express a differentiation antigen specified by a gene at the T-locus in the mouse. Proc. Nat . Acad. Sci., 71, 811.

77 Edidin, M., Patthey, H. L., McGuire, E. J. & Sheffield, W. D. (1971). An antiserum to "Embryoid body" tumour cells that reacts with normal mouse embryos. In Embryonic and Fetal Antigens in Cancer ed. N. G. Anderson and Coggin, J.H., Jr. Oak Ridge National Laboratory, Oak Ridge, Tennessee.

78 Gooding, L., Hsu, Y. & Edidin, M. (1976). Expression of teratoma-associated antigens on murine ova and early embryos. Dev. Biol., 33, 403.

79 Jacob, F. (1977). Mouse teratocarcinoma and embryonic antigens. Immunol. Rev., 33, 3.

80 Vitetta, E. S., Artzt, K., Bennett, D., Boyce, E. A. & Jacob, F. (1975). Structural similarities between a product of the T/t locus isolated from sperm and teratoma cells, and H-2 antigens isolated from splenocytes. Proc. Nat . Acad. Sci., 72, 3215.

81 Morello, D., Gachelin, G., Dubois, P. H., Yanigaki, N., Pressman, D. & Jacob, F., (1968). Absence of reaction of a xenogeneic anti-H-2 serum with mouse embryonal carcinoma cells. Transplantation, 26, 119.

82 McClay, D. R. & Gooding, L. R. (1978). Involvement of histocompatibility antigens in embryonic cell recognition events. Nature, 274, 367.

83 Kasakura, S. (1971). A factor in maternal plasma during pregnancy that suppresses the reactivity of mixed leukocyte cultures. J. Immunol., 107, 1296.

84 Buckley, R. H., Schiff, R. I. & Amos, D. B., (1972). Blocking of autologous and homologous leukocyte responses by human alloimmune plasmas: A possible in vitro correlate of enhancement. J. Immunol., 108, 34.

85 Ayoub, S. & Kasakura, S. (1971). In vitro response of foetal lymphocytes to PHA, and a plasma factor which suppresses the PHA response of adult lymphocytes. Clin. Exp. Immunol., 8, 427.

86 Riggio, R. R., Parrillo, J. E., Bull, F. G., Schwartz, G. H., Stenzel, K. H. & Rubin, A. L., (1971). Inhibition of lymphocyte transformation by a placental glycoprotein. Transplantation, 12, 400.

87 Youtananukorn, V. & Matangkasombut, P., (1972). Human maternal cell mediated immune reaction to placental antigens. Clin. Exp. Immunol., 11, 549.

88 Youtananukorn, V. & Matangkasombut, P., (1973). Specific plasma factors blocking human maternal cell-mediated immune reaction to placental antigens. Nature New Biol., 242, 110.

89 Rocklin, R. E., Zuckerman, J. E., Alpert, E. & David, J. R. (1973). Effect of multi-parity on human maternal hypersensitivity to foetal antigen. Nature, 241, 130.

90 Pence, H., Petty, W. M. & Rocklin, R. E. (1975). Suppression of maternal responsiveness to paternal antigens by maternal plasma. J. Immunol. 114, 525.

91 Rocklin, R. E., Kitzmiller, J. C. Carpenter, C. B., Garovoy, M. R. & David, J. R. (1976). Maternal-fetal relation: absence of an immunologic blocking factor from the serum of women with chronic abortions. New Engl. J. Med., 295, 1209.

92 Taylor, P. V. & Hancock, K. W., (1975). Antigenicity of trophoblast and possible antigen-masking effects during pregnancy. Immunology, 28, 973.

93 Faulk, W. P., Jeannet, M., Creighton, W. D. & Carbonara, A. (1974). Immunological studies of human placentae: Characterization of immunoglobulins on trophoblastic basement membranes. J. Clin. Invest., 54, 1011.

94 Faulk, W. P., Jeannet, M., Crieghton, W. D., Carbonara, A. & Hay, F. (1974a) Studies of the human placenta. II. Characterization of immunoglobulins on the trophoblastic basement membrane. J. Reprod. Fertil., Suppl. 21, 43.

95 Voisin, G. A. & Chaouat, G. (1974). Demonstration, nature and properties of maternal antibodies fixed on placenta and directed against paternal antigens. J. Reprod. Fertil., Suppl., 21,89.

96 Jeannet, M., Wearner, C., Ramirez, E., Vassalli, P. & Faulk, W. P. (1977). Anti-HLA, anti-human "Ia-like" and MLC blocking activity of human placental IgG. Transplant. Proc., 9, 1417.

97 McIntyre, J. A. & Faulk, W. P. (1978). Suppression of mixed lymphocyte cultures (MLC) by antibodies against human trophoblast membrane antigens. Transplant. Proc. In press.

98 Kaku, M. (1953). Placental polysacchride and the etiology of the toxemia of pregnancy. Am. J. Obstet. Gynecol., 60, 148.

99 Levanon, Y. & Rossetini, S. M. O. (1968). Presence of circulating placental antigens and antibodies in toxemic and normal pregnancy patients. Immunoforsch., 136, 178.

100 Hulka, J. F., Hsu, K. C. & Beiser, S. M., (1961). Antibodies to trophoblast during the post-partum period. Nature, 191, 510.

101 Hulka, J. F., Brinton, V., Schaaf, J. & Baney, C. (1963). Appearance of antibodies to trophoblast during the post-partum period in normal human pregnancies. Nature, 198, 501.

102 Hulka, J. F. & Brinton, W. (1963). Antibody to trophoblast during early postpartum period in toxemic pregnancies. Am. J. Obstet. Gynecol., 86, 130.

103 Gaugas, J. M. & Curzen, P. (1974). Complement fixing antibody against solubilized placental microsomal fraction in pre-eclampsia sera. Brit.J. Exp. Pathol., 55, 570.

104 Tal, C. (1965). The nature of the cell membrane receptor for the agglutination factor present in the sera of tumour patients and pregnant women. Proc. Nat . Acad. Sci. 54, 1318.

105 Hersey, P., Honeyman, M., Edwards, A., Adams, E. & McCarthy, W. H. (1976). Antigens on melanoma cells detected by leukocyte dependent antibody assays of human melanoma antisera. Int. J. Cancer, 18, 564.

106 Hirsch, M. S., Kelly, A. D., Chapin, D. S., Fuller, T. C., Black, P. H. & Kurth, P. (1978). Immunity to antigens associated with primate C-type oncoviruses in pregnant women. Science, 199, 1337.

107 Tamerius, J., Hellstrom. I. & Hellstrom, K. E. (1975). Evidence that blocking factors in the sera of multi-parous mice are associated with immunoglobulins. Int. J. Cancer, 16, 456.

108 Brambell, F. W. R. (1970). The transmission of passive immunity from mother to young. North Holland Publishing Co., Amsterdam. p.234.

109 Johnson, P. M., Natvig, J. A., Ystehede, U. A. & Faulk, W. P. (1977). Immunobiology of human placentae: An immunofluorescence study of the distribution and character of immunoglobulins in chorionic villi. Clin. Exp. Immunol., 30, 145.

110 Faulk, W. P., Lovins, R. E., Goust, J. M. & Ainsworth, S. K. (1977). Immunological and biochemical studies of human trophoblasts. Fed. Proc., 36, 1064.

111 Masson, P. L., Delire, M. & Cambiaso, C. L., (1977). Circulating immune complexes in normal human pregnancy. Nature, 266, 542.

112 Medawar, P. B.. & Hunt, R. (1978). Vulnerability of methylcholanthrene-induced tumours to immunity aroused by syngeneic foetal cells. Nature, 271, 164.

113 Doll, R. (1975). The epidemiology of cancers of the breast and reproductive system. Scott. Med. J., 20, 305.

114 Bramwell, M. E. & Harris, H. (1978). An abnormal membrane glycoprotein associated with malignancy in a wide range of different tumors. Proc. R. Soc. Med. Lond. B., 201, 87.

PLACENTAL ANTIBODY TRANSPORT AND IMMUNOLOGICAL PROTECTION - THEIR CELLULAR MECHANISMS

Arthur E. Wild

1 Freda, V. J., (1962). Placental transfer of antibodies in man. Am. J. Obstet. Gynec. 84, 1756.

2 Brambell, F. W. R. (1970). The transmission of passive immunity for mother to young. Frontiers of Biology, 18, Amsterdam: North Holland Press.

3 Solomon, J. E., (1971). Foetal and neonatal immunology. Frontiers of Biology, 20 Amsterdam: North Holland.

4 Billington, W. D. (1976). The immunobiology of trophoblast. In Immunology of Human Reproduction, ed. J. S. Scott & W. R. Jones, pp. 81-102. London Academic Press.

5 Needham, J. (1931). Biochemistry of the placental barrier. Chemical Embryology Vol. 3 pp. 1485-1533 Cambridge: University Press.

6 Brambell, F. W. R., Brierley, J., Halliday, R. & Hemmings, W. A., (1954). Transference of passive immunity from mother to young. Lancet, i, 964.

7 Dancis, J., Lind, J., Oratz, M., Smolens, J. & Vara, P. (1961). Placental transfer of proteins in human gestation. Am. J. Obstet. Gynec. 82,167.

8 Gitlin,D., Kumate, J., Urrusti, J. & Morales, C. (1964). The selectivity of the human placenta in the transfer of plasma proteins from mother to foetus. J. Clin. Invest. 43, 1938.

9 Bangham, D. R. (1960). The transmission of homologous serum proteins to the foetus and to the amniotic fluid in the rhesus monkey. J.Physiol. 153,265.

10 Quinlivan, W. L. G. (1967). Gamma globulin-^{131}I transfer between mother and offspring in the rhesus monkey. Am. J. Physiol. 212, 324.

11 Wasz-Hockert, O., Wager, T., Hautala, T. & Widholm, O. (1956). Transmission of antibodies from mother to foetus. A study of the diphtheria level in the new-born with oesophageal astresia. Ann. Med. Exp. Biol. Fenn. 34, 444.

12 Nöschel, Von H., Stelzner, A., Seewald, H-J. & Klinger, G. (1975). Untersuchungen zur plazentapassage von Virus-Antikörpern und Immunglobulinen an der in vitro perfundierten menschlichen plazenta. Zbl. Gynäk. 97, 180.

13 Wilk, A. E. (1973). Transport of immunoglobulins and other proteins from mother to young. In Lysosomes in Biology and Pathology ed. J. T. Dingle, Vol.3 pp. 425-64. Amsterdam: North-Holland.

14 Hemmings, W. A. (1974). The relative decay of Fc and Fab fragments of homologous IgG from the circulation of the foetal rabbit. IRCS 2, 1453.

15 Virella, G., Nunes, M. & Tamagnini, G. (1972). Placental transfer of human IgG subclasses. Clin. exp. Immunol. 10, 475.

16 Schar, P. H., Alpert, E. & Alpert, C. (1973). Gamma G subgroups in human foetal cord and maternal sera. Clin. Immunol. Path. 2,62.

17 Chandra, R. K. (1976). Levels of IgG subclasses, IgA, IgM and tetanus antitoxins in paired maternal and foetal sera: findings in healthy pregnancy and placental insufficiency. In Maternofoetal Transmission of Immunoglobulins, ed. W. A. Hemmings, Clinical and Experimental Immunoreproduction. Vol. 2, pp. 77-90. Cambridge, University Press.

18 Gitlin, D. (1971). Development and metabolism of the immune globulins. In Immunological incompetence, ed. B. M. Kagan & E. R. Steihm, pp. 3-13. Chicago: Year Book Medical Publishers.

19 Brambell, F. W. R. (1966). The transmission of passive immunity from mother to young and the catabolism of immunoglobulins. Lancet. ii, 1087.

20 Matre, R., Tønder, O., & Endresen, C. (1975). Fc receptors in human placenta. Scand. J. Immunol. 4, 741.

21 Thomas, J. M., MacArthur, R. I. & Humphrey, L. J., (1976). Fc receptors on the human placenta. Obstet. and Gynec. 48, 170.

22 Matre, R. & Johnson, P. M., (1977). Multiple Fc receptors in the human placenta. Acta path. microbiol. Scand. Section C. 85, 314.

23 Wood, G., Reynard, J., Krishnan, E. & Racela, L. (1978a). Immunobiology of the human placenta. 1. IgGFc receptors in trophoblastic villi. Cell. Immunol. 35, 191.

24 Jenkinson, E. J., Billington, W. D. & Elson, J. (1976). Detection of receptors for immunoglobulin on human placenta by EA rosette formation. Clin. exp. Immunol. 23, 456.

25 McNabb, T., Koh, T. Y. Dorrington, K. J. & Painter, R. H., (1976). Structure and function of immunoglobulin domains. V. Binding of immunoglobulin G and fragments of placental membrane preparations. J. Immunol. 117, 880.

26 Elaon, J., Jenkinson, E. J., & Billington, W. D. (1975). Fc receptors on mouse placenta and yolk sac cells. Nature, 255, 412.

27 Wild, A. E., & Dawson, P. (1977). Evidence for Fc receptors on rabbit yolk sac endoderm. Nature, 262, 443.

28 Jones, E. A. & Waldman, T. A. (1972). The mechanism of intestinal uptake and transcellular transport of IgG in the neonatal rat. J. Clin. Invest 51, 2916.

29 Borthistle, B. K., Kubo, R. T., Brown, W. R. & Grey, H. M. (1977). Studies on receptors for IgG on epithelial cells of the rat intestine. J. Immunol. 119, 471.

30 Morris, B. & Morris R. (1976). Globulin transmission by the gut in young rats, and the effects of cortisone acetate. In Maternofoetal Transmission of Immunoglobulins, Ed W. A. Hemmings, Clinical and Experimental Immunoreproduction Vol. 2, pp. 359-70. Cambridge: University Press.

31 Martin, B. J. & Spicer, S. S., (1973). Multivesicular bodies and related structures of the syncytiotrophoblast of human term placenta. Anat. Rec. 175,115.

32 Wild, A. E. (1974). Protein transport across the placenta. In Transport at the cellular level, ed. M. A. Sleigh, & D. H. Jennings, Society for Experimental Biology Symposium XXVIII pp. 521-46. Cambridge: University Press.

33 Wild, A. E. (1975). Role of the cell surface in selection during transport of proteins from mother to foetus and newly born. Phil.Trans. R. Soc. Lond. B. 271, 395.

34 Moxon, L. A., Wild, A. E. & Slade, B. S. (1976). Localisation of proteins in coated micropinocytotic vesicles during transport across rabbit yolk sac endoderm. Cell Tiss. Res. 171, 175.

35 Rodewald, R. B. (1973). Intestinal transport of antibodies in the newborn rat. J. Cell, Biol. 58, 189.

36 Rodewald, R. B., (1976). Intestinal transport of peroxidase-conjugated IgG fragments in the neonatal rat. In Maternofoetal Transmission of Immunoglobulins, ed. W. A. Hemmings, Clinical and Experimental Immunoreproduction, Vol. 2, pp. 137-53. Cambridge: University Press.

37 Wild, A. E. (1979). Coated vesicle - a morphologically distinct subclass of endocytic vesicles. In Coated Vesicles, ed. C. D. Ockleford & A. Whyte, Cambridge: University Press, (in press).

38 King, B. F., & Enders, A. C. (1971). Protein absorption by the guinea pig chorioallantoic placenta. Am. J. Anat., 130, 409.

40 Ockleford, C. D. & Whyte, A. (1977). Differentiated regions of human placental surface associated with exchange of materials between maternal and foetal blood coated vesicles. J. Cell, Sci. 25, 293.

41 King, B. F. (1977). An electronmicroscopic study of absorption of peroxidase-conjugated immunoglobulin G by guinea pig visceral yolk sac in vitro. Am. J. Anat. 148, 447.

42 Bardawil, W. A., Toy, B. L. & Hertig, A. T. (1958). Localisation of homologous plasma proteins in the human placenta by fluorescent antibody. Am. J. Obstet. Gynecol. 75, 708.

43 McCormick, J. N., Gaulk, W. P., Fox, H. & Fudenberg, H. H. (1971). Immunohistological and elution studies of the human placenta. J. Exp. Med. 133, 1.

44 Thoumsin, H., Salmon, J. & Lambotte, R. (1972). Etude en immunofluoresence de placentas humains du dernier trimestre de la grossesse. Revue Europ. Etudes Clin. et Biol. 17, 976.

45 Johnson, P. M., Natvig, J. B., Yestehede, U. A. & Faulk, W. P. (1977). Immunological studies of human placentae: the distribution and character of immunoglobulins in chorionic villi. Clin. exp. Immunol, 30, 145.

46 Johnson, P. M. & Faulk, W. P. (1978). Immunological studies of human placentae: identification and distribution of proteins in immature chorionic villi. Immunology 34, 1027.

47 Wild, A. E. (1970). Protein transmission across the rabbit foetal membranes. J. Embryol. exp. Morph. 24. 313.

48 Slade, B. S. & Wild, A. E.(1971). Transmission of human Y-globulin to rabbit foetus and its inhibition by conjugation with ferritin. Immunology 20, 217.

49 Contractor, S. F. & Krakauer, K. (1976). Pinocytosis and intracellular digestion of 1251-labelled haemoglobin by trophoblastic cells in tissue culture in the presence and absence of serum. J. Cell. Sci. 21, 595.

50 Pearse, B. M. F. (1976). Clathrin: A unique protein associated with intracellular transfer of membrane by coated vesicles. Proc. Nat. Acad. Sci. USA. 73, 1255.

51 Billington, W. D. (1969). Immunological processes in mammalial reproduction. In Immunology and Development, ed. M. Adinolfi, Clinics in Developmental Medicine, No. 34, pp. 89-113, London: Spastics International Medical Publications.

52 Beer, A. E. & Billingham. R. E. (1976). The Immunobiology of Mammalian Reproduction, New Jersey: Prentice-Hall.

53 Rocklin, R. E., Kitzmiller, J. L., Carpenter, C. B., Garovoy, M. R. & David, J. R. (1976). Absence of an immunologic blocking factor from the serum of women with chronic abortions. New Engl. J. Med. 295, 1209.

54 Hellström, K. E., Hellström, I. & Brawn, J. (1969). Abrogation of cellular immunity to antigenetically foreign mouse embryonic cells by a serum factor. Nature, 224, 914.

55 Voisin, G. A. & Chaouat, G. (1974). Demonstration nature and properties of maternal antibodies fixed on placenta and directed against paternal antigens. J. Reprod Fert. Suppl. 21, 89.

56 Faulk, W. P., Jeannet, M., Creighton, W. D. & Carbonara, A. (1974). Immunological studies of human placentae: Characterisation of immunoglobulins on trophoblastic basement membranes. J. Clin. Invest. 54, 1011.

57 Faulk, W. P. & Jeannet, M. (1976). Immunological studies of immunoglobulins from human placentae. In Maternofoetal Transmission of Immunoglobulins, ed. W. A. Hemmings, Clinical and Experimental Immunoreproduction, Vol. 2 pp.47-60.

58 Ockleford, C. D. (1977). Antibody clearance by micropinocytosis: a possible role in foetal immunoprotection. Lancet, i, 310.

59 Jenkinson, E. J. & Billington, W. D. (1974). Studies on the immunobiology of mouse foetal membranes: the effect of cell-mediated immunity on yolk sac cells in vitro. J. Reprod. Fert. 41 403.

60 Tønder, O. & Thunold, S. (1973). Receptors for immuno-globulin Fc in human malignant tissues. Scand. J. Immuno. 2, 207.

61 Tønder, O., Morse, P. A. Jr. & Humphrey, L. J. (1974). Similarities of Fc receptors in human malignant tissue and normal lymphoid tissue. J. Immunol. 113, 1162.

62 Hellström, K. E. & Hellström, I. (1974). Lymphocyte-mediated cytotoxicity and blocking serum activity to tumour antigens. Adv. Immunol. 117, 587.

63 Faulk, W. P. & Temple, A (1976). Distribution of β_2 microglobin and HLA in chorionic villi of human placentae. Nature, 262, 799.

64 Faulk, W. P., van Loghen, E. & Stickler, B. B. (1974). Maternal antibody to fetal light chain (Inv) antigens. Am. J. Med. 56, 393.

65 Johnson, P. M., Faulk, W. P. & Wang, A-C. (1976). Immunological studies of human placentae: subclass and fragment specificity of binding of aggregated IgG by placental endothelial cells. Immunology 31, 659.

66 Wood, G., Reynard, J., Krishnan, E. & Racels, L. (1978b). Immunobiology of the human placenta. 11. Localisation of macrophages, in vivo bound IgG and C3. Cell. Immunol. 35, 205.

67 Dancis, J., Braverman, N. & Lind, J. (1957). Plasma protein synthesis in the human foetus and placenta. J. Clin. Invest. 36, 398.

68 Furth, van R. & Adinolfi, M. (1969). In vitro synthesis of α1-fetoprotein in man. Nature, 222, 1296.

69 Adinolfi, M., & Wood, C. B. S. (1969). Ontogenesis of immunoglobulins and components of complement in man. In Immunology and Development, M. Adinolfi, Clinics in Developmental Medicine, No. 34, pp. 27-61.

70 Dancis, J., Douglas, G. W. & Fierer, J. (1966). Immunologic competence of mouse placental cells in irradiated hosts. Am. J. Obstet. Gynec. 94, 50.

71 Anderson, R. G. W., Goldstein, J. L. & Brown, M. S. (1977). A mutation that impairs the ability of lipoprotein receptors to localise in coated pits on the cell surface of human fibroblasts. Nature, 270, 695.

72 Gregoriadis, G. (1977). Targeting of drugs. Nature, 265, 407.

SECTION IV

AGEING

MATURATION OR AGEING?

Editors' note: Nobody doubts that the normal placenta grows, differentiates, matures - in keeping with the changing needs of the developing fetus. Few if any obstetricians doubt that the placenta also ages in the latter part of pregnancy, and especially after full term, sometimes to an extent that seriously impairs its capacity to support further fetal development or even survival. But does the placenta really age? Or can the changes obstetricians regard as ageing be explained in other ways? That was the crucial question underlying much of the discussion in this session - and highlighted by an exchange between Alan Browne, putting the obstetric viewpoint, and Harold Fox who agreed fully with his observations but had alternative explanations for every one of them.

So should we conclude that the placenta does not age? Well, hardly. In a remarkably comprehensive review of age changes in other organs and tissues, Harold Fox was unable to point to much conclusive, or indeed exclusive, evidence of ageing in man or other animals. Lack of such evidence for the placenta should probably be seen against that surprisingly negative background.

We might almost draw a parallel with cancer. Clinically, its features are only too familiar, as with ageing. Yet, on closer inspection, it becomes much harder to define precisely what we mean by a neoplastic or ageing cell. Could this be because we are looking in the wrong places? Does the clue in both cases lie in the DNA? Is it possible that the age changes the eye perceives - and the microscope so easily misses - really represent the subtle consequences of minor DNA faults? Would more major faults produce overt disease? Could that be where the fundamental distinction lies between ageing and pathology?

We do not, as yet, know any of the answers, but it would perhaps be premature - on the evidence presented here - to conclude that the placenta does not undergo ageing of a kind, in some if not all its tissues.

In other fields, Jan Pontén reviewed the relationship between the ageing cell and malignant change, and Willi Hijmans described recent developments in the paradoxically youthful discipline of immunogerontology. It was reassuring to learn from the latter that ageing is not just an illusion - it can be objectively observed in the body's immune responses. What the observed changes mean remains a largely unanswered question, however. And it is still not really possible to say why older cells should be more susceptible to malignant change. If the answer really does lie in the DNA, the line of research proposed earlier for malignant disease might also enable the riddle of ageing to be solved. But that would only pose another if prevention and treatment were to become practical possibilities ...

SECTION IV

AGEING

Chairman: Hamish Munro

Ageing is a process in which control of body functions becomes gradually impaired. How it can be broken down into convenient areas for study and to what extent the ageing placenta can serve as a model are the main questions to which we shall be seeking answers. In recent years, so much attention has been paid to the molecular biology of ageing that its features have been relatively neglected. These may be summarised as progressive impairment of tissue function and increasing frequency of chronic disease, together with a rising incidence of certain acute conditions. The nutritional and other needs of the elderly must also be considered. Then we have to ask when the ageing process begins and at what rate its various aspects proceed. Perhaps its most consistent feature is loss of active tissue, from an early age, with gradual replacement by body fat. Metabolically, although overall activity declines, it does so in parallel with the loss of active protoplasmic mass. The remaining cells must therefore be functioning at normal levels of metabolic activity, but they will not necessarily be carrying out their functions as efficiently as youthful cells.

Within the overall pattern of impaired function and cell loss, there are considerable differences between tissues and in the ways they are affected by ageing. Voluntary muscle is, for instance, lost at a higher rate than other metabolically active tissues, from nearly 50% of body weight in fit young adults to about 27% at the age of 80. Why should muscle become selectively diminished? Probably because the anterior motor neurones in the spinal cord are quietly dying off - with consequent trophic damage to muscle cells. This is just one of the complexities of ageing. Bones break more easily as we get older because they lose calcium progressively through most of adult life, and especially after the menopause in women. This normal feature of ageing is less apparent in black populations,where the bones tend to be heavier - and consequently less likely to fracture with ageing - presumably because more bone was laid down during adolescence, among other factors. The rate of bone loss may be controllable by adding calcium to the diet or by so-called hormone replacement in menopausal women, or by administration of 1,25-dihydroxycholecalciferol, which may be less efficiently produced by ageing kidneys. On the other hand, high protein intakes slowly deplete bone calcium by inducing negative calcium balance - a long-term consequence of western-style diets rather than ageing as such. These examples should serve to highlight a fundamental point: that ageing is a highly complex process, difficult to study in all its aspects.

In discussing the causes of ageing, it is necessary to try and distinguish changes that can properly be attributed to age itself from those due to extraneous influences. To what extent true ageing processes may be genetically preprogrammed or simply the result of accumulating faults remains uncertain. Either way, cause and effect would not necessarily reside in the same tissue, as with motor neurone loss and muscle wasting. And the rate at which faults accummulate in a tissue could well be influenced by a variety of external influences during the whole course of its existance. Clearly, neither ageing processes nor their control can be studied as a whole. But we may usefully consider such features as error accummulations in cells of certain systems - as exemplified by cell replication in particular immunological processes, for instance. Many such aspects of ageing and their control can be studied in the placenta, though caution is required in applying the results to ageing in man or other animals.

THE PLACENTA AS A MODEL FOR ORGAN AGEING

Harold Fox

The ageing process is presumed to be universal, progressive, decremental, intrinsic - and manifested in irreversible loss of functional capacity, impaired ability to maintain homoeostasis, and decreased ability to repair damage. It is quite clear that in humans this process can be influenced by a wide range of social and environmental factors for, to quote a trite example, a wealthy American woman of 60 wintering in Palm Beach often both looks and feels younger than a 30-year-old Indian woman living in the slums of Calcutta. Even if these extrinsic influences are ignored, man - with his long lifespan, high incidence of age-related disease, and unavailability for experimental manipulation - presents the gerontologist with a series of problems that have not yet been overcome. Much ageing research has therefore been carried out on animals which have a relatively short lifespan and can be studied under experimental conditions; most animal species are however, just as subject as humans to age-related diseases, the effects of which are extremely difficult to disentangle from those due solely to ageing. Some gerontologists have concentrated their attention on nematodes or insects, but while these make excellent subjects for both observational and experimental ageing studies they are biologically so remote from man that the findings are of doubtful relevance. Tissue culture studies have been widely utilised in recent years to study ageing, but their validity must await proof that senescence of an organism is due simply to a summation of ageing in its constituent cells and that the changes observed in vitro are an accurate reflection of those occurring in vivo.

An ideal vehicle for the study of ageing would be a tissue or organ which is readily available, has a short and well-defined lifespan and is not subject to age-related disease processes. The placenta, whether human or animal, meets all these requirements - and has the further advantages that it is readily grown in culture and can be manipulated experimentally in animals. At first sight, it appears to be an excellent model for the study of ageing. Implicit in this statement are, however, two presumptions which require critical examination: first, that we are able to define, recognise and describe the ageing process and, second, that the placenta actually does age during its short span of functional activity. It is a matter for debate which of these two assumptions rests on the more insecure foundations.

NATURE OF THE AGEING PROCESS

To a pathologist who has unwittingly strayed into the field of gerontology there is a dismaying array of theories of ageing and an equally disconcerting number of apparently unanswered basic problems. Amongst the latter are such fundamental questions as the distinction between maturation, differentiation and ageing, the difficulty of separating the effects of ageing from those of age-related diseases, the nature of the interrelationships between cellular, organ and body ageing, the problem of whether ageing is a single universal process in all creatures or a complex myriad of ageing mechanisms and - the ultimate challenge - whether death is a component or consequence of the ageing process.

Current gerontological interest is focused on cellular ageing, based on a widespread belief that body or organ senescence represents the summation of changes occurring at the cellular or molecular level. This dates back to the demonstration by Hayflick and Moorhead[1] that human embryonic fibroblasts cultured in vitro have a finite replicative capacity, being able to undergo only about 50 ($\pm$10) population doublings. This now classical experiment destroyed the previously held belief in the immortality of cultured, non-transformed cell lines.[2] It was subsequently shown that embryonic cells have a much greater lifespan in culture than cells obtained from adults, and that the population-doubling capacity of adult cells is inversely related to the age of the donor.[3] These experiments have led to the belief that ageing of organisms, expressed in vivo as a continuous decrease in viability, is reflected in the limited lifespan of somatic cells in vitro. Attempts to explain this phenomenon of cellular senescence have fallen into two broad groups: those suggesting that ageing is genetically programmed, and those arguing that loss of viability is due to a random accumulation of errors or damage in macromolecules.

Genetic programming

The fact that a fully differentiated cell loses the ability to replicate suggests that terminal differentiation is coupled to loss of proliferative potential and, therefore, that differentiation and ageing are parts of a single programmed process. Programmed clonal ageing is assumed to be under the control of some form of clock mechanism which measures either the number of cell divisions or some other sequential or recurrent process. Several possible models of such a clock have been proposed:

1. Gene depreciation. Two theories base their clock model on gene loss. One suggests that somatic cells lose a terminal segment of DNA at each replication, so that as vital genetic information incidentally contained in the terminal segment is deleted, the cell eventually loses viability. The other postulates a sequential modification of bases in repeated sequences of DNA by specific enzymes. According

to this theory, the number of cell divisions is directly related to the number of repeats in the sequence, so that, when all the sequences have been modified, promoter or operator regions originally adjacent to structural genes are widely separated and the apposition of DNA-dependent RNA polymerase becomes impossible; if the affected gene is a vital one the cell will lose viability.[4]

2. Codon-restriction. This hypothesis of Strehler et al[5] postulates a sequential activation of synthetase genes during development and ageing - which could lead to an accumulation of synthetase suppressors and so to failure of RNA translation, with eventual loss of cellular viability.

3. Transcription failure. Von Hahn[6,7] proposed that the control of cellular ageing functions at the level of transcription of genetic information into RNA resulted from a control mechanism operating in the nuclear chromatin. An age-related increase takes place in the stability of the DNA double helix; this is dependent upon the degree of binding of certain proteins, and the process of strand separation (which is essential for transcription) becomes progressively blocked as the cell ages.

4. Isozymic shift. Krooth[8] suggested that isozymes of various structural genes become activated during ageing, and that these operate with decreased accuracy, resulting in progressive cell damage.

5. DNA repair fault. In senescent cells DNA repair occurs at a reduced rate,[9-11] and this could be due to a programmed change in the genes controlling synthesis of repair enzymes.

Accumulated errors

Arrayed against, and in contrast to, these theories of genetic programming are those arguing that ageing is a random 'wear and tear' type of process which results from accumulation of errors. Two broad types of error theory have been proposed, one favouring random somatic mutation and the other an accumulation of defects in protein synthesis. The random point mutation theory, once very popular,[12] is now generally thought to lack plausibility for it not only implies that there must be an extremely high mutation rate but that these mutations must occur initially in non-essential genes.

Medvedev's[13] 'redundant message' theory could, however, overcome these difficulties; he argues that essential genes are present in multiple copies, that the mutation rate in suppressed genes must be far higher than in active genes, and that as mutation errors occur in active genes reserve sequences containing the same information take over. This process continues, according to the theory, until the redundancy in the system is exhausted - at which stage cell ageing will occur.

Medvedev's theory combines some features of the accumulated errors and clock hypothese. It also has the merit of offering an explanation for the diverse lifespans of different species, these being dependent upon the degree of gene repetition and the amount of redundant message.

Decreased fidelity of protein synthesis was postulated by Orgel[14] to be the cause of ageing. According to this theory, mis-specifications in the structural genes coding for the protein synthesising machinery would lead to errors accumulating - until a stage of 'error catastrophe' was reached, and cell function became fatally impaired. He later modified this proposal, suggesting that a steady-state of error could be attained within a cell but that mis-specified proteins could operate by a feedback mechanism to produce new gene mutations and further errors in protein synthesis.[15] The error hypothesis has been taken as the basis of:

The 'commitment theory' of Holliday and his colleagues[16,17] who suggest that normal cells have a steady-stage of protein errors, but that there is a given probability that a critical error will move a cell into a 'committed' state in which, though the cell is still outwardly healthy, the level of errors gradually increases until the stage of lethal error catastrophe is reached. If, in a culture, both committed and uncommitted cells grow at the same rate until the lethal catastrophe occurs, then there will be a progressive increase in the number of committed cells. This is because uncommitted cells can give rise to committed cells, but not vice versa. The population density of uncommitted cells will therefore eventually reach a very low level and may be lost from the culture by a dilution process.

Kirkwood[18] has looked at the error hypothesis in evolutionary terms. He has suggested that while there must be a high level of translation stability in germ-cell lines, such regulation is less stringent in somatic cells. Accuracy requires energy expenditure, and there may be an energy-saving switching off of the mechanisms responsible for high translation accuracy at or around the time somatic cells are differentiated from the germ lines; this would leave the somatic cells in a relatively unstable state in which a small random increase in errors commits them to eventual error catastrophe. Kirkwood's theory thus envisages ageing as the price we must pay for conserving energy.

Rival concepts

These two main concepts - of programming and error accumulation - dominate ageing theory, but a number of older hypotheses still retain their adherents and fresh theories continue to proliferate. The view that attributed ageing largely to changes in extracellular connective tissue was at one time very widely held,[19] senescence being thought to be accompanied by progressive cross-linking of collagen molecules. However, Jackson[20] has pointed out that most, probably all, of the temporal changes in collagen occur during development and maturation, and that there is little evidence of any significant physicochemical change in collagen during ageing. Immunological mechanisms are thought by some to play a primary role in ageing, possible mechanisms including the running down of a thymic clock, programmed failure in the homoeostatic control of tolerance, without development of autoimmune or graft-versus-host reactions, and derepression of genes controlling the mutation rates of histocompatibility antigens.[21] Yet others have postulated that ageing is due to such things as accumulation of free radicals causing widespread lipid peroxidation,[22,23] a build-up of noxious substances,[24] or the secretion of 'ageing' hormones by the hypothalamic-pituitary axis.[25]

Despite this plethora of theories, some of which smack more of the armchair than of the laboratory, the central role of the cell in ageing dominates much current gerontological thought, and the proponents of the two major conflicting schools of programmed senescence and error theory remain locked in controversy. I am in no position to choose, and have no particular preference, between these two basic concepts, whose merits and demerits have been debated in a number of reviews.[4,26-36] It is in any case clear that in vitro models of replicating cells play a central role in contemporary ageing theory.

The original studies of cell replication have been repeated and extended by a number of other workers who have confirmed Hayflick's findings,[37-39] but Schneider and Chase[40] have questioned whether there is really an inverse relationship between donor age and the doubling capacity of cultured fibroblasts. This challenge has been sustained in the recent report of Goldstein et al[41] who have shown that while the inverse relationship holds true for fibroblasts derived either from diabetics or from individuals with a genetic predisposition to diabetes mellitus, it does not apply to fibroblasts from carefully chosen normal donors. If these findings are confirmed they must cast some doubt on the validity of the in vitro replicative cell system as a model for in vivo human ageing. It remains apparently true that fetal fibroblasts have a greater replicative capacity than those from adult donors, but they also contain growth promoting factors that are absent from adult cells.[42] It is also noteworthy that the replicating cell model offers little insight into the reasons why cells that have ceased replication should undergo senescent change or into the mechanism of ageing in such post-mitotic differentiated cells. Many discussions of the in vitro model imply that ageing is due to a loss of replicative capacity or, alternatively, that it is manifested in loss of doubling potential. However, there is no evidence, in humans or other mammals, that the actual limit of replicative cell life is reached in a normal lifespan; the ageing mammal retains its capacity for self-renewal of skin, intestine and blood, though at reduced rates.[43-44] Furthermore, as Martin[35] has pointed out, many of the pathological processes thought to be age-related are characterised by excessive proliferation of cells rather than loss of replicative activity.

Finally, we must ask whether cellular ageing really is the fundamental basis of senescence. Kohn[19] and Franks[45] reviewed the evidence for cell loss or malfunction limiting the lifespan of an individual and concluded that the functional reserve in most organs is so large that cell loss or functional impairment could be of little importance; a man can survive quite normally after removal of one kidney, over half his liver and large areas of brain and intestine. To cause ageing in these organs cell loss would have to be of enormous degree and accompanied by gross interference with regenerative cell proliferation - events that have not been shown to occur.

The present position may be summarised by saying that: the relevance of in vitro models to in vivo ageing remains unproven, the mechanism of cellular ageing obscure, the role of cell loss or malfunction in organ ageing doubtful and the process of which the whole body ages unknown.

STRUCTURAL AND FUNCTIONAL CHANGES DURING AGEING

We can recognise an aged body, but can we identify a senescent organ or cell? This section is concerned with the functional, biochemical and morphological changes thought to characterise the ageing cell or organ.

Structural changes

The conventional techniques employed by the anatomist or pathologist to study the body, namely naked-eye examination and light microscopy, shed little light on the morphology of human senescence. Changes attributed to ageing have been described in many organs, but the almost insuperable difficulty in distinguishing between those attributable solely to senescence and those due either to specific disease processes (such as atherosclerosis) or to altered physiological states (such as inactivity or malnutrition) has not been overcome. Consider the aged heart, a popular subject for morphologically orientated gerontologists. It may be unduly small or abnormally heavy in old people and embody changes presumed to be senescent, including patchy thickening of the endocardium, increased rigidity, thickening and calcification of the valves, increased interstitial fibrous and adipose tissue in the myocardium, shrinkage of some myocardial fibres and hypertrophy of others, fibrosis of the sino-atrial node, increased collagen in the valves together with disruption of valvular architecture, excess elastic fibre content in the pericardium and an accumulation of lipofuscin pigment in muscle cells.[46-50] It has however, been demonstrated that heart weight does not alter with age in completely healthy, atheroma-free subjects.[51] Moreover, it is possible that the other changes noted, with the exception of lipofuscin accumulation, may be due to such factors as atherosclerosis of the coronary vessels, disease of the fine cardiac vasculature, old rheumatic heart disease, cigarette smoking or respiratory inadequacy, rather than to ageing per se.

Studies of the ageing brain and liver have yielded similarly conclusive results. It has long been held that there is a progressive loss of neurones from the brain with increasing age, but - as Brody[52] has pointed out - cell loss in most areas of the brain occurs principally between birth and maturity, an observation supported by the remarkable constancy of total DNA in the rat or mouse brain throughout adult life.[53,54] In humans, there is some neuronal loss during adult life but this shows a very variable and inexplicable distribution, being quite marked in the locus coeruleus, for instance, but not in the trochlear or inferior olivary nuclei.[55-57] Several non-specific and inconstant nuclear changes have been described in ageing cerebral neurones, but the only abnormality consistently noted in such cells has been an accumulation of lipofuscin, a change discussed in more detail later in this section.

The non-diseased liver of the aged individual is usually normal to the naked eye, but histological examination often reveals variation in the size of hepatocytes and their nuclei, nuclear inclusions, multiple nucleoli and an abundance of lipofuscin.[58-60] These changes are by no means consistent however, many aged livers being histologically normal in all respects. Although considerable emphasis has been laid upon the presence of hyperdiploid cells in senescent livers, Hollander[61] found the incidence of such cells to increase with age in rat liver until maturity (i.e. 12 months), after which they remain constant.

Histological studies of other organs, such as the intestine, testis or lung, have yielded a rich variety of apparently age-related changes, all of which are inconsistent and none of which can be confidently attributed to ageing rather than to age-associated disease.

Electron microscope studies

The introduction of the electron microscope raised hopes that the study of cellular fine structure would reveal a characteristic morphological picture of cellular decline with senescence. These hopes have not been fulfilled, though ultrastructural studies have yielded information less meagre than that obtained by light microscopy. The plasma membrane of senescent cells does not show any structural abnormality, though it does increase in surface area in old rat hepatocytes.[62,63]

The most consistently noted nucelar change in aged cells has been deep invagination or indentation of the nuclear membrane - observed in rodent myocardial cells, hepatocytes and neurones[64-67] and in cultured human or chick fibroblasts.[68,69] The actual volume and surface area of the nucleus does not, however, appear to change with increasing age.[62] Clumping of nuclear chromatin has been described as an ageing change in periosteal osteocytes,[70] but the chromatin pattern appears to remain unaltered in senescent hamster myocardial cells[67] and in long-cultured human fibroblasts.[69] Fibrillary rod-like or lattice-type nuclear inclusions have been observed in neurones of senescent mice or rats[66,71] but have not been noted in any other type of aged cell.

Age-related nucleolar changes have not been widely commented upon, but ring-shaped nucleoli have been described in senescent rat hepatocytes,[64] while Mann et al[72] have noted a progressive decline in nucleolar volume in human cerebral neurones with advancing age. Adamstone and Taylor[73] have demonstrated that in the epithelial cells of the rat jejunum there is a progressive change in nucleolar morphology as the cells move up from the basal crypts to the tips of the villi, the nucleoli originally being large and polymorphous and later becoming smaller and showing re-organisation into two clearly defined components (amphinucleoli), which eventually break up to form a separate plasmosome and karyosome. This change has been attributed to ageing, but it should perhaps be considered a feature of differentiation.

The appearance of the Golgi apparatus does not alter with advancing age in mouse intestinal cells or in the cerebral neurones and hepatocytes of the rat,[65,66,74,75] though it has been observed to become unduly prominent in the myocardial cells of aged rats[76] and in cultured human fibroblasts after multiple passages.[69,77] Dilation and vacuolation of the Golgi cisternae has been described in spinal neurones of senescent mice,[78] but this is an isolated observation.

Comments on the endoplasmic reticulum in senescent cells have been rather conflicting. The amount of smooth endoplasmic reticulum in aged rat hepatocytes has been variously reported as increased,[62,79] decreased, and unchanged,[80] while the quantity of rough endoplasmic reticulum in these cells has been described as decreased by some observers[62,79,80] and as unchanged by others.[74] The amount of endoplasmic reticulum appears to decline with age in hamster myocardial cells[67] whilst, in senescent neurones, there is a tendency for the cisternae of endoplasmic reticulum to become disorganised and disrupted,[65] a change not noted in other aged cells.

A number of observers have commented on a decline with age in the number of mitochondria neurones, and in human liver cells,[81-85] but an age-dependent increase in mitochondrial density has been noted in rat hepatocytes[62] and in both rat and hamster myocardial cells.[67,76,86] To confuse the issue still further, the number of mitochondria appears to be unchanged in senescent rat neurones[66] and mouse small intestine,[75] and it remains constant in cultured human fibroblasts even after many sub-passages.[69] Age-related changes in mitochondrial size have been the subject of equally conflicting findings. Increased mitochondrial volume has been noted in senescent rat and human hepatocytes,[62,81,83] but mitochondrial size appears to remain unchanged with age in mouse hepatocytes, mouse small intestine,[66,67,75,84,85] hamster myocardial cells and rat neurones, and tends to decrease in aged rat myocardial cells and human liver cells.[76,87]

There has been a measure of agreement that the mitochondrial cristae usually shorten with age and that the volume of the organelle they occupy decreases.[67,83,85] A similar change has been noted in human fibroblasts retained for a lengthy period in culture,[69] whilst in elderly cultures of chick fibroblasts the cristae tend to realign themselves along the long axis of the mitochondria.[68] In ageing mouse hepatocytes, decreased density and vacuolation of the mitochondrial matrix has been described, together with loss of matrical granules,[83] but similar changes have not been observed in senescent rat hepatocytes or neurones.[66,76] The formation of giant mitochondria has been frequently noted as a feature of aged insect flight muscle, but there has been only one report of such a phenomenon in senescent mammalian tissues, megamitochondria having been described in aged human hepatocytes.[87]

The literature on age-related changes in cell lysosomes is somewhat confusing, largely because of differing morphological definitions. Some have considered the term lysosome to include primary lysosomes, dense bodies, residual bodies and autophagic vacuoles. Others have restricted their definition to one or other of these structures. Within the limitations of this nosological farrago, the number of lysosomal structures has been reported to increase with age in rat neurones, myocardial cells and hepatocytes[63,74,88] and in hamster myocardial cells;[67] and their number also increases in cultured human fibroblasts after multiple passages.[69] By contrast, Pieri et al[62] observed no change with ageing in the number of lysosomes in rat hepatocytes, though an increase in their volume and permeability was noted - a change also detected in senescent rat neurones.[88]

The most consistent change seen at the ultrastructural level in ageing cells is an accumulation of lipofuscin, confirming the earlier observations of light microscopists. This pigment has been observed in senescent neurones and myocardial cells both in humans and in a wide range of animal species[65,66,76,89-99] and has also been noted in aged: rodent adrenocortical cells,[100] mouse osteocytes,[101] cat thyroid,[102] and mouse testes.[103] Only in human and rodent neurones, however, have quantitative studies shown that the amount of lipofuscin increases in a uniform manner throughout life,[84,99] but even in cells of the same age in the same organ there is a very variable degree of pigment accumulation. In the brains of aged individuals, the cells of the inferior olivary nucleus invariably contain large amounts of pigment, while the Purkinje cells of the cerebellum are virtually pigment-free.[99,104,105] The origin of lipofuscin pigment has been much disputed, it being variously thought to be derived from mitochondria, endoplasmic reticulum, lysosomes or Golgi-derived bodies which act as traps for damaging substances.[106-109] Currently it is widely believed that lipofuscin granules represent the modified indigestible remains of lysosomes and that the lipoproteins which constitute the pigment are formed by the interaction of the products of fatty acid peroxidation with biologically useful molecules.

Whether the lipofuscin pigment can be regarded simply as 'inert slag'[110] or whether it interferes with cell metabolism and contributes to the process of cellular senescence is a moot point. Mann and Yates[99] found that cytoplasmic RNA content remained steady in neurones during the initial accumulation of lipofuscin but declined progressively after a certain critical level of intracellular pigment was attained. The same workers have, however, subsequently shown that cytoplasmic RNA levels in neurones in different areas of the brain decrease by much the same amount despite widely differing degrees of pigment accumulation; the relationship between declining cellular function and lipofuscin increase therefore remains uncertain.[72]

It will be clear from this brief review of the structural aspects of senescence that cellular ageing cannot at present be defined in morphological terms. To a limited extent, an increase in lysosomes, a loss of rough endoplasmic reticulum and increasing nuclear identation appear to be characteristics of the aged cell, but these changes are by no means consistent. The composition and turnover of cell membranes does not appear to alter with age[111] and it would therefore probably be unrealistic to expect clear-cut and permanent changes in renewable cell structures such as mitochondria. These organelles are, however, in what is probably an altered microenvironment and it is possible that a more dynamic attitude to their morphological characteristics should be adopted. Mitochondria in liver cells from young rats appear to withstand hypoxia with apparent ease, while those in hepatocytes from senescent rats become swollen and fragmented.[112] This altered response to stress is probably more significant than minor variations in volume and density detected by a static morphometric approach. The abnormality seen with greatest consistency in ageing cells is the presence of lipofuscin, but this can also occur in unrelated pathological states, such as starvation; it is by no means a constant feature of aged cells and it can occur in young and clearly non-aged cells.[113] Furthermore, lipofuscin accumulation is a reversible change.[114] Neuronal pigment accumulation is greatest in those areas which show least age-related cell loss and less in those regions in which there is appreciable cell loss.[57]

FUNCTIONAL CHANGES

It is usually thought that nearly all body functions decline in efficiency with advancing age, and texts on clinical geriatrics generally state that physiological activities as diverse as muscle strength, tactile sensitivity, dark adaptation, cardiac output, gastric acid secretion, colonic peristaltic activity, pulmonary vital capacity, maximum breathing capacity, renal glomerular filtration rate, conduction velocity in peripheral nerves, and thyroid hormone secretion all decrease in old age.[114,115] Three points need to be made about these assumptions. First, there have been few, if any, longitudinal studies in individuals over their lifespan, to show whether there is a true age-related decline in these activities after maturity has been reached. Second, there is no agreed consensus about either the existence or the degree of many of these decreases in functional efficiency. Third, it is extremely difficult to prove that the decreased efficiency of a particular physiological activity in old age is not due either to an age-related disease process or to factors such as nutritional deficiency or inactivity.

Conflicting results

It is even harder to demonstrate that ageing is associated with impairment of functional efficiency at the cellular level. Three specific cellular functions which have been particularly examined are respiration, protein synthesis and mitotic activity, but these studies have not allowed any consistent pattern of physiological decline to emerge. It has long been thought that reduced oxygen uptake and a decreased rate of oxidative phosphorylation characterise aged tissues, and there is indeed evidence that liver and brain homogenates from aged rats take up less oxygen than do those from young animals,[116] the oxidative metabolism of glucose is diminished in brain slices from senescent rats,[117] and metabolic rate, glucose consumption and oxygen utilisation decline in cerebral tissue from aged humans, mice and dogs.[118-120] By contrast, however, other studies have shown that there is no age-related decline in oxygen consumption, glucose utilisation or oxidative phosphorylation in hamster brain slices,[121] rat liver slices of homogenates,[122-5] or isolated rat hepatocytes[126] or in isolated mitochondria from the heart, liver and muscle of senescent hamsters and rats.[127-30] Furthermore, although unselected elderly humans exhibit a reduced cerebral oxygen consumption, elderly men free from atherosclerosis have rates which do not differ from those of healthy young males.[131]

Equally conflicting views have been expressed about the protein synthetic ability of aged cells. A number of workers have shown that the ability of isolated microsomes from mouse liver or heart to synthesise protein is reduced in aged tissues,[131-3] but others have been unable to demonstrate any age-related decline in the protein synthetic capacity of hepatic microsomes,[134,135] rat liver slices[136] or mouse heart tissue.[137] Yet others have maintained that the ability of mouse liver microsomes and isolated rat hepatocytes to synthesise protein increases with advancing age,[138] and the capacity of rat liver for albumin synthesis appears to be augmented in old age.[136,139]

Studies of the effects of age on RNA synthesis have yielded particularly confusing results. They can be summarised as showing that, while RNA levels tend to be generally high in aged tissues, the rate of RNA synthesis with advancing age shows a decrease in some organs, an increase in others and no alteration in yet others.[140-2]

The results of studies of cell proliferative capacity in animal tissues give a more consistent picture. The mitotic index appears to decline with age in both rapidly and slowly renewing tissues,[143-5] and there is a similar age-related decrease in the number of cells entering DNA synthesis.[144,146-8] The cell-cycle time increases in aged tissues,[147-50] this being apparently due to a progressive lengthening of the time spend by cells in the G1 phase;[145] and the renewal time of epithelia, such as those lining the mouse gastrointestinal tract, is increased.[145,149,151] However these studies of cellular proliferative capacity have been carried out largely in animals. In the only two human tissues which seem to have been investigated, namely abdominal wall epidermis and gingival epithelium, the mitotic index appears to increase with advancing age.[152,153]

Of interest in connection with placental studies is the effect of ageing on the synthesis of steroid hormones. The circulating levels of many hormones decrease during old age, but this does not necessarily mean that the ability of aged cells to synthesise such hormones is diminished. An example of this is the testicular secretion of testosterone, the levels of which fall in senescent males of most species. Nevertheless, although the aged mouse testis secretes a reduced amount ot testosterone, the ability of senescent mouse testicular tissue to metabolise C21 steroids by the delta-4 pathway is in no way diminished; indeed it actually appears to be increased.[154] Similarly, the biosynthesis of testosterone in vitro by the delta-5 pathway is increased rather than decreased.[155] Such findings indicate that a decrease in the function of a tissue may be due more to the effects of extrinsic influence than to an intrinsic failure of functional capacity in the tissue concerned. In the human, however, the situation may be more complex. In vivo studies show that the testicular production of testosterone in the aged is reduced,but that of androstenodione remains unaltered,[156] suggesting an age-related defect in the delta-4 pathway.

ENZYME CONTENT

A good deal of effort has been expended on attempts to define, by biochemical or histochemical techniques, a pattern of enzymatic change characteristic of senescent cells. The results of these labours have been the subject of a number of reviews,[157-60] which make discouraging reading for anyone attempting to draw an enzymatic map of the aged cell. This can be illustrated by considering the results obtained for a number of key enzymes, and as it is impractical to review changes in every enzyme we will concentrate on those which have also been extensively studied in placental tissue.

Amongst the enzymes concerned with surface transport mechanisms the one receiving the most attention has been alkaline phosphatase. Its levels have been variously reported to decrease, increase and remain unchanged in the liver of aged rats and mice.[161-3] They appear to decrease with age in rat and female mouse kidney[164-165] and in mouse adrenal gland and salivary gland,[166,167] while remaining unaltered in the lungs of aged female mice.[163] Alkaline phosphatase levels in the small intestine of the mouse have been reported to decrease, [168] to increase,[169] and to remain unchanged[75,77] with advancing age. The levels of another transport enzyme, 5-nucleotidase, have been noted to decrease in the liver and lungs of senescent male mice while remaining unchanged in those of aged female mice and increasing in senescent mouse kidney.[163,165]

Hydrolytic lysosomal enzymes show an equally variable pattern of change. Acid phosphatase activity has been reported both as increased[163,170] and decreased[171,172] in senescent mouse liver, and as increased[173] and unchanged[171,174] in aged rat liver. The activity of this enzyme appeared to decrease with age in some studies of rat and mouse kidneys[172,175] and to remain unchanged in others.[165] In the lungs, acid phosphatase activity declines with age in male mice but does not alter in females,[165] and although the levels of this enzyme increase in aged rat salivary glands[166] they remain unchanged in senescent mouse and rat prostatic tissue[176,177] and in rat small intestine.[178] Beta-glucuronidase activity has been reported to decline with age in rat liver[179] and increase in mouse liver[163] but to increase markedly in the lungs of old mice.[180]

Respiratory enzymes tend to show a more consistent pattern of age-related change. Succinic acid dehydrogenase activity has been reported to decrease in the liver, lungs and prostate of aged mice,[163,165,176,181] and in the liver, kidney, salivary glands, striated muscle, myocardium and periosteal cells of senescent rats,[166,182-5] the only ageing tissue in which levels of this enzyme appear to increase being the human brain.[186] Cytochrome oxidase activity declines with advancing age in many mouse and rat tissues but does not alter in rat liver and mouse kidney.[163,176,183-5] Again, the only senescent tissue in which the activity of this enzyme appears to increase is the human brain.[186]

The glycolytic enzyme lactate dehydrogenase shows a strikingly non-consistent pattern of change in ageing cells. Thus, its activity increases with age in human myocardium and brain,[186,187] male mouse liver, lung and prostate[163,176] and rat liver, but decreases in the stomach, heart, muscle and brain of the senescent rat[188-90] and in aged mouse kidney and muscle,[191,192] while remaining unchanged with age in horse heart[193] and in female mouse liver and lung.[163] Almost equally variable are the findings for the glycogenolytic enzyme glucose-6-phosphatase. Its activity diminishes with age in mouse liver and male mouse lung[163,194] but has been variously reported to increase [165] and decrease in aged mouse kidney, and to decrease and remain unchanged in senescent rat liver.[163,194,195]

The Krebs'cycle enzymes have received relatively little attention, but the activity of malate dehydrogenase has been reported to increase with age in rat liver, human brain[174,186] and human heart;[187] it does not,however, show any age-related change in rat liver mitochondria,[165] but has been reported to decrease in aged rat brain and heart.[196]

It is easy to dismiss this wide variability of results as being due to faulty technique, and it is true that in some studies the definition of 'old' has not been fully satisfactory. Moreover, histochemical studies which indicate (albeit in a rough manner) the amount of enzyme per cell may give results differing widely from those of biochemical studies, which may be considerably influenced by changes in cell number. It is nevertheless clear that there is a considerable variation in age-associated enzyme changes in different organs of the same animal, in different sexes, in different species and even in differing strains of the same species.[163,167] This variability defies any attempt to give a systematic and cohesive account of enzymatic changes in ageing cells. Possibly a more dynamic approach is required; changes such as an altered isozyme pattern, a changed inductive capacity or the synthesis of inactive or heat-labile enzyme in the course of ageing may be of more importance than a simple determination of enzyme content. It must be admitted, however, that recent reviews of such changes in old age have given little support to these concepts.[198,199]

AGEING OF THE PLACENTA

It is widely accepted that the placenta ages as pregnancy progresses and that at term the organ is in, or on the verge of, a decline into morphological and functional senescence. This belief is due to the apparent convergence of a number of clinical, morphological, functional and biochemical studies, but their results have rarely been subjected to critical evaluation. We shall therefore consider what is known about such changes in the human placenta and discuss placental ageing against the backcloth of general ageing studies outlined above.

Clinical findings

The clinical concept of placental senility is based almost entirely on observations of the effects of prolongation of pregnancy. Between 10 and 12% of all gestations extend to 42 weeks, while 5% persist for 43 weeks or more.[200,201] In most series of such prolonged pregnancies, the mean birthweight has tended to flatten out at the 42nd week of gestation and then to decline slightly,[202,203] while both the perinatal mortality rate and the incidence of clinically detectable intrauterine hypoxia have been moderately or markedly elevated.[204-15] In addition between 20 and 40% of infants born after an unduly long pregnancy show clinical evidence of intrauterine malnutrition, manifested by the 'postmaturity syndrome' at birth.[203-216]

These ill-effects of prolonged pregnancy have traditionally been attributed to placental senescence, but not all observers have agreed that extended gestation is of any detriment to the continuing growth and wellbeing of the fetus.[217-22] Even if the highest figures for fetal hypoxia and death in prolonged pregnancy are accepted as accurate, it becomes clear that the majority of infants born after a protracted gestation are healthy and well oxygenated. It could be argued that many such babies were probably born to mothers who had miscalculated their date of conception, but this suggestion is not in accord with the fact that, although mean birthweight tends to decrease in prolonged pregnancy, the proportion of unusually heavy babies actually increases. Indeed, the majority of non-diabetic women who give birth to a baby weighing more than 4kg do so after a pregnancy extending beyond term[200,211,212,218] - fetal growth having presumably continued during the extra weeks of intrauterine life.

Such clinical observations permit the conclusion that a decrease in the efficiency of materno-fetal transfer occurs in only a minority of prolonged pregnancies and that any presumed decline in the functional capacity of the ageing placenta is not a universal phenomenon. Clinically, a decline in placental capacity can only be presumed, because reduced materno-fetal transfer might equally well be decreased maternal utero-placental bloodflow or deficient fetal uptake of oxygen and nutrients.

Placental growth

Placental weight increases progressively throughout a normal gestation, not only to term but also throughout the extra weeks of a protracted gestation.[203,223] The rate of increase does, however, tend to flatten out quite markedly during the later weeks of pregnancy, and it has been claimed that true placental growth ceases well before term. This concept of a pre-term cessation of growth, which is often adduced as evidence of placental senescence,[224] is based largely on the work of Winick and his colleagues. They have shown that the total DNA content of the human placenta rises steadily until the 36th week of gestation, and thereafter remains static while total placental RNA and protein levels continue to rise[225] - indicating that growth of the placenta after 36 weeks is due solely to hypertrophy of cells already present. Similar results were obtained for the rat placenta, in which total DNA levels rise to reach a steady plateau by the 17th day of a 21-day gestation.[226] This latter finding has been supported by an autoradiographic study demonstrating an absence of DNA synthetic activity after 17 days,[227] and an ultrasonic study of the in situ human placenta has indicated that its volume tends to remain static after the 36th week of gestation.[228]

These apparently conclusive findings have, however, not remained unchallenged. A recent study in Manchester has shown that total DNA levels in the human placenta rise in a linear fashion until, and beyond, term.[229] Although this conflicts with the findings of Winick et al[225] it is in accord with histological observations showing that nearly all term placentae from uncomplicated pregnancies contain small groups of highly immature villi of first trimester pattern. These are scattered throughout an otherwise fully mature villous population.[230-2] The suggestion that they are freshly-formed villous offshoots from the villous stems[233] has received support from the demonstration that they are invariably situated in the centre of a lobule and can be shown, by autoradiography, to be actively synthesising DNA.[234,235] Quite apart from these observations, quantitative morphometry of human placentae has shown a linear increase in placental volume and villous surface-area to term[236,237] and a continuing growth of the trophoblast beyond the 40th gestational week.[238]

It is now almost certain, in my view, that a degree of placental growth continues until term; indeed, there is some evidence of trophoblastic mitotic activity and DNA synthesis still being detectable at 40 weeks.[239,240] There is clearly a marked decrease in placental growth rate in the later stages of pregnancy, but this cannot be argued as evidence of placental senescence unless it is also shown that the decrease in growth rate is irreversible - and a mild degree would not be of concern unless it endangered the continued growth and oxygenation of the fetus. Quite obviously the placenta does not usually show evidence of functional failure during the last weeks of pregnancy, since the vast majority of term infants are well oxygenated and adequately nourished. Moreover, even at term the placenta has a very considerable functional reserve capacity enabling it to withstand the loss of between 30 and 40% of its functioning villi without any obvious detrimental effects on the fetus.[241,242] The decrease in growth activity is by no means invariable or irreversible, but there seems no valid reason why the placenta should continue to grow once it has attained a sufficient size to fulfill its transfer function. If required to perform a greater workload, the placenta can continue to increase its size very considerably, as shown by the unusually large placentae that are often encountered in cases of severe maternal anaemia[243-4] or decompensated heart disease[245] and in pregnancy at high altitude.[246] The potential for a recrudescence of placental growth is clearly seen whenever the villous syncytiotrophoblast is damaged. The best example is pre-eclampsia in which syncytiotrophoblast suffers ischaemic damage that is invariably accompanied by marked proliferation of the villous cytotrophoblastic cells.[248-9] These are the only trophoblast component capable of DNA synthesis, and they can be considered as stem cells constituting a germinative zone which is, in normal pregnancy, largely quiescent at term. The proliferation of these cells in response to syncytial damage is clearly an attempt to repair and replace the damaged tissue. That the cytotrophoblast cells undergo true hyperplasia is shown by the presence of mitotic figures and by their active synthesis of DNA under experimental <u>in vitro</u> conditions that mimic those obtaining <u>in vivo</u> in the pre-eclamptic patient.[250]

Those arguing that a decrease in the rate of placental growth during the late stages of pregnancy is evidence of senescence often appear to be comparing the placenta, perhaps unconsciously, with an organ such as the small intestine, in which continuing viability is dependent upon a constantly replicating stem cell layer producing short-lived post-mitotic cells. A more apt comparison would be with the liver, which is composed largely of relatively long-lived post-mitotic cells and which, once optimal size has been reached to meet the demands of the body, shows very little evidence of DNA synthesis or cell replication, while retaining a demonstrable capacity for considerable regenerative growth. The available evidence therefore suggests that the decreased growth rate of the placenta during the later weeks of gestation may be better considered as an indication of morphological and functional maturity than as evidence of senility.

<u>Macroscopic morphology of placenta</u>

The first trimester placenta is almost invariably free from gross lesions of any type, but at term the organ often contains infarcts or plaques of perivillous fibrin and is not infrequently overtly calcified. These changes are thought by many to be accentuated in placentae from prolonged pregnancies and to be evidence of placental senescence.[251-3] In reality in uncomplicated pregnancies both the infarcts due to thrombosis of maternal arterioles and the fibrin plaques which result from haemodynamic turbulence witbin the intervillous space are invariably too small to dissipate the physiological reserve of the placenta. They do not therefore impair its functional capacity. Neither is the incidence of either lesion increased in placentae from prolonged gestations.[254] Despite their lack of functional significance both these lesions are, in the strict sense of the word, pathological. Their presence is no more indicative of placental senescence than is a myocardial infarct of cardiac senescence.

Macroscopic calcification of the placenta is certainly an age-related change, because it only develops during the later months of gestation; there is,however, no excess of calcification in placentae from pregnancies extending beyond 40 weeks.[255,256] The pathogenesis of placental calcification remains obscure, but it is difficult to regard as a senescent change, since it is found most commonly in placentae from young primigravid women, and even extensive calcium deposition does not impair the functional efficiency of the placenta.[255-8]

Light microscopy of placenta

During the nine months of gestation, the placental villi undergo progressive histological metamorphosis manifest by: a decrease in their diameter, gradual disappearance of the cytotrophoblastic cells, thinning and focal attenuation of the syncytiotrophoblast, clumping of the syncytial nuclei, thickening of the trophoblastic basement membrane, condensation and fibrosis of the stroma, loss of Hofbauer cells and lateral movement together with sinusoidal dilatation of the fetal vessels. Many early students of placental histology interpreted these changes as being the morphological expression of an ageing process and regarded the villi of the term placenta as degenerate and senescent.[259-260] This view has been, and still is, uncritically repeated in many accounts of placental morphology. For example, an otherwise excellent paper [261] published as recently as 1976 says, in part: 'the placenta exhibits histologic signs of deterioration and tissue degeneration as term approaches, similar to senescence in the individual at old age'.

A more rational approach to time-related structural changes in the placental villi is to regard them as an indication, not of ageing, but of maturation and differentiation - processes designed, in teleological terms, to increase the area of trophoblast in contact with the maternal blood, and so approximate the maternal and fetal circulations as closely as possible to promote optimal trophoblastic transfer. The decreased size of the villi is due to a process of continuous branching, which results in a progressive increase in the ratio between placental area and volume, while the dilatation of the fetal vessels and their move from a central to a peripheral position steepens the materno-fetal gradients and crowds the flow lines. The overall result of these changes is a six-fold increase in the transfer efficiency of the placenta as pregnancy progresses to term. [237]

The focal attenuation of the syncytiotrophoblast, often regarded as degenerative in origin, is actually evidence of topographic differentiation of the trophoblast. The markedly thinned, anuclear areas of the syncytium usually overlie, and appear almost to fuse with the wall of, a dilated fetal vessel and are now generally known as 'vasculosyncytial membranes'.[262] These differ histochemically and ultrastructurally from the non-membranous areas of the trophoblast[263,264] and have come to be widely regarded as specialised zones specifically adapted for facilitating gas transfer across the placenta. Failure to develop these membranes during the later stages of pregnancy is associated with a high incidence of intrauterine fetal hypoxia.[265]

Changes increasing the functional efficiency of the placenta can hardly be regarded as evidence of senescence, and it is equally difficult to attribute most of the other morphological changes in the term placenta to senility. The villous cytotrophoblast cells do not, as was once thought, disappear, but persist as a germinative zone which, though largely inactive, retains its proliferative potentiality.[248-9,266, 267] Similarly, the stromal Hofbauer cells are not truly lost; the apparent decrease in their number is largely due to their compression and distortion by collagen fibres during the process of stromal fibrosis.[230,268-70] This latter change is often cited as evidence of villous ageing but, although accurate estimates of placental collagen content are not available, I have the impression, shared by others, that the stromal content of fibrous tissue begins to increase at the end of the first trimester and reaches a plateau by the end of the second trimester, with little or no subsequent change.[271-3] The early onset and lack of progression argue against this being a senescent change.

The only age-related change in the placental villi which merits serious consideration as a possible ageing phenomenon is the presence of syncytial 'knots'. These are focal aggregations of syncytial nuclei at one or more points on the villous circumference to form multinucleated protrusions into the intervillous space. They do not appear until quite late in pregnancy and then increase steadily in number until term.[274] The nuclei which form these knots are, unlike those elsewhere in the same villus, small and markedly basophilic with markedly clumped chromatin. It has been suggested that they may result from a sequestrational process which arranges for effete, aged nuclei to be segregated away from the metabolically active areas of the trophoblast.[275] This concept is based upon several observations: the continuing formation of syncytial nuclei from the cytotrophoblast throughout pregnancy, the fact that the nuclei in a term villus are therefore heterogeneous with respect to age, the lack of basophilia and nuclear chromatin clumping in the non-aggregated nuclei of a villus bearing a knot, and the fact that the number of syncytial nuclei is greater in villi with knots than in those of comparable size which are devoid of knots.[274,276]

Accordingly, the cytotrophoblast is thought to produce syncytial nuclei throughout pregnancy, and these terminally differentiated, post-mitotic structures have a lifespan of possibly between six and ten months. At term, the proportion of them formed during the earliest stages of pregnancy become senile, but they cannot readily be shed as happens in the skin or gut (though a few do break off to enter the maternal circulation). The placenta, again arguing teleologically, therefore sequestrates this aged and unwanted nuclear material away from the functionally active areas of the trophoblast. Subsequently, it is often utilised by the placenta to form the intervillous bridges which may possibly play a mechanical role in buttressing the villi against the effects of sudden pressure changes during labour.[277] The presence of aged nuclei within the trophoblast does not, however, necessarily imply that this tissue is itself senescent, as the senile nuclei are not only adequately replaced, but also sequestrated and utilised. This dynamic situation shows that the trophoblast continues to be viable; if it were really senescent, there would probably be true deletion of nuclear material.

Nearly all term placentae contain occasional scattered villi which have undergone complete fibrinoid necrosis. This villous lesion has not, until quite recently, been regarded as a possible ageing change, but Burstein et al[278] have suggested that the fibrinoid material is actually amyloid, formed as a consequence of immunological attack on senescent trophoblastic cells that are synthesising mis-specified proteins. This not unattractive hypothesis gains support from the demonstration that the initial site at which the villous fibrinoid material appears is in a cytotrophoblastic cell.[279] But neither I nor others have been able to confirm that the villous fibrinoid material has the staining or electron microscopic characteristics of amyloid.[279] However, the most potent objection to the concept of fibrinoid necrosis as senile amyloidosis is that it does not appear to be truly age-related: villi showing this lesion are quite often found in first-trimester placentae, including those from pregnancies terminated for social reasons.

One final point about the light microscopy of the term placenta is that the presence of lipofuscin seems not to have been reported. Admittedly a specific search for this pigment does not appear to have been undertaken, but it is difficult to believe that its presence would have passed unnoticed by the many microscopists who have studied placental histology during the past century. Light microscopy therefore appears to yield no morphological evidence of senescence in the term placenta, so it appears logical to extend the search for ageing changes to placentae from prolonged pregnancies. The many studies of such placentae have reported findings which, although very variable, tend to polarise into two distinct concepts. On the one hand, placental morphology in prolonged pregnancies is not considered to differ materially from that normally found at term.[280-281] On the other, features have been described or interpreted as indicative of senility or even 'hypersenescence'.[251-3,282-8] Neither of these extreme views is correct, in my view, their findings being based upon too few specimens or histological misinterpretation.

In my own experience, a considerable proportion of placentae from prolonged pregnancies, about 30%, are fully normal and indistinguishable from term placentae. And about 10% show only those changes, i.e. cytotrophoblastic hyperplasia and trophoblastic basement thickening, which are characteristic of some degree of placental ischaemia - in consequence of reduced maternal utero-placental bloodflow (the cause of which is obscure, but discussed more fully in the next section on ultrastructural changes). A further 20% of placentae from extended gestations appear to be underperfused from the fetal side. Again, the reasons for this are not understood, but there appears to be either collapse or constriction of the villous fetal vessels which, instead of being sinusoidally dilated, are small and inconspicuous. The poorly vascularised villi are richly endowed with syncytial knots and have an increased amount of stromal fibrous tissue - which is not indicative of senescence but an invariable consequence of reduced villous fetal bloodflow, whether in early or late pregnancy.[254] In a further 40% of placentae from prolonged pregnancies the villi show a combination of both ischaemic change and fetal underperfusion and it is only the infants whose placentae show these combined changes that suffer the complications usually ascribed to prolonged pregnancy.

Although the pathogenesis of the two vascular changes that influence villous morphology in prolonged pregnancy are not fully understood, it is difficult to think of either as an ageing change in the true sense of the word, while the placenta itself appears to be almost a passive bystander, showing no changes which cannot be directly attributed to these circulatory alterations. In other words, the failure to define morphological features of senescence in the term placenta is equally apparent in placentae from prolonged pregnancies.

Ultrastructure of placenta

The fine structure of the placenta is now extremely well documented, but most reports comment only upon the ultrastructure of the first trimester or the term placenta; longitudinal studies throughout pregnancy have been few. Many comparisons between the fine structure of the placenta in early and late gestation have been principally concerned with delineating and confirming, at the ultrastructural level, the maturational changes already noted by light microscopists.

Comments upon age-related changes in trophoblastic organelles have been both few and conflicting. Although the height of the trophoblastic surface microvilli is generally agreed to decrease as pregnancy progresses,[289-291] the number of microvilli per unit area of the trophoblast has been variously noted to decline,[292] remain unchanged[293] or increase[294] as term is approached. While the profiles of smooth endoplasmic reticulum in the trophoblast become larger and more infrequent as the placenta matures,[289,292,295-6] this change does not occur in the placenta of the rhesus monkey.[297] Claims that the number of free syncytial ribosomes decline towards term[291,298] could not be substantiated by Jones.[293] Some workers have noted an age-related decrease in the number of syncytial mitochondria,[296] and others have commented on a progressive change in the appearances of the mitochondrial cristae,[290] but Jones[293] could not detect any age-related alterations in the number, size or configuration of these organelles. There has been rather more agreement that the large lipid droplets in the syncytiotrophoblast become progressively fewer after the first trimester,[292,296,299,300] but as these structures have been variously considered as nutritional fat in transit from mother to fetus, steroid hormones or steroid hormone precursors, the significance of the observation is debatable. There has, however, been no agreement whether the small osmiophilic granules in the syncytium, which are more acceptable to many as synthetic products, decrease[293,298] or increase[291] through pregnancy.

Changes in the number of lysosomes in the trophoblast during gestation have been little studied, but my impression, based largely upon ultracytochemical studies, is that these organelles are most numerous during the first trimester and then decrease in density. Certainly, a striking feature of the term placenta is the sparsity of dense residual bodies.

Martin and Spicer[301] made a specific search for ultrastructural evidence of ageing in the placenta. They described senescent syncytial nuclei with chromatin clumping and irregular notching in the term placenta but noted that these changes were seen only in aggregated nuclei; they were absent from dispersed nuclei, which confirms the aged nature of the nuclei forming syncytial knots. These workers did, however, also observe an age-related decrease in the size of the syncytial nucleoli, together with loss of the nucleolonemal channels, a decrease in nucleolar dense component and an accumulation of nucleolar heterochromatin. These changes closely resemble those observed by Adamstone and Taylor[73] in the nucleoli of rat intestinal cells as they pass from the crypts of the villous tips. Martin and Spicer consider these nucleolar changes to be indicative of true senescence and suggest that they may reflect impaired protein biosynthesis. It is however, possible that the change in nucleolar morphology is a muturational rather than an ageing phenomenon, as already noted, and especially so as Martin and Specer found that it could be observed as early as the third month of gestation.

Virtually all the comparative comments made so far in this section have been based upon subjective assessments of electronmicrographs, and there has been, to the best of my knowledge, only one morphometric study of the fine structure of the placenta in early and late pregnancy.[302] This demonstrated that the volume fraction of the syncytial trophoblast occupied by the mitochondria and endoplasmic reticulum decreased sharply at term, while that of the nucleus increased; there was no change in the volume fraction of lipid droplets or lysosomes.

All in all, the currently available electronmicroscope data offer no conclusive evidence of senescence in the term placenta. True, there are a few promising hints that further study at this level may provide more definitive proof of ageing but any optimism in this respect must be tempered by the extremely wide diversity of opinions on the ultrastructural characteristics of cellular senescence. The logical extension of electronmicroscopy to placentae from prolonged pregnancies has been undertaken by few workers and the results available are both inconclusive and contradictory.[303,304] In our own study of such placentae[305] it was observed that the villous syncytiotrophoblast showed small focal areas of necrosis together with changes suggesting decreased functional activity (i.e. a patchy decrease in the density of surface microvilli, dilatation of the rough endoplasmic reticulum, a reduction in the number and size of the mitochondria, a diminished number of lipid droplets and osmiophilic granules, a sparsity of Golgi bodies and a decreased number of pinocytotic vesicles). Other abnormalities noted were hyperplasia of the villous cytotrophoblastic cells, thickening of the trophoblastic basement membrane and contraction, vacuolation and blebbing of the endothelial cells in the fetal villous vessels.

It is clearly tempting to attribute these trophoblastic changes to senescence, but they could be ascribed rather more convincingly to uteroplacental ischaemia and were indeed qualitatively identical to those found in placentae from women with pre-eclampsia.[293] Utero-placental ischaemia is not usually thought an important factor in prolonged pregnancy, but it has been demonstrated that the utero-placental bloodflow usually decreases significantly in prolonged gestations.[306-8] This phenomenon is not confined to humans; a similar fall in maternal blood flow to the placenta has been shown to occur in post-term gravid rats.[309] The reduction in placental bloodflow in humans is of unknown pathogenesis and rarely as marked as that found in pre-eclampsia. It would nevertheless be capable of inflicting on the trophoblast the degree of morphological damage, and probable functional impairment, noted. Most of the other abnormalities encountered in these placentae could be similarly explained, though the lesions of the fetal endothelial cells are more probably due to either fetal hypoxia or acidosis. The possibility of the ultrastructural changes in placentae from prolonged pregnancies being due to an ageing change cannot be dogmatically refuted, but their appearances are more suggestive of ischaemic damage, and this would accord with the known reduction in maternal bloodflow.

Enzyme histochemistry

Although there have been numerous studies of the enzyme histochemistry of the placenta, again very few workers have made sequential studies of the changes in enzyme activity over the course of pregnancy. Despite this omission, the activity of both alkaline phosphatase and glucose-6-phosphatase in the trophoblast appear to be considerably greater at term than in the first trimester, and the activity of acid phosphatase decreases markedly as gestation progresses.[310-5] These changes are of some significance because alkaline phosphatase is thought to play an important, but as yet ill-defined, role in membrane transfer mechanisms and, as discussed earlier, the activity of lysosomal enzymes tends to increase in many senescent tissues.

Light microscope studies have suggested that the activities of the various respiratory dehydrogenases remain unchanged in the trophoblast throughout pregnancy,[314,316-9] but our own ultracytochemical findings indicate a distinct decline in both malate and lactate dehydrogenase activity towards term.[320] This evidence of decreased respiratory activity in placental tissue is not necessarily an ageing change; it may be an adaptive mechanism increasing the amount of oxygen available for transport to the fetus. Very little information is available about age-related changes in other placental enzymes, though Lobel et al[318] noted a significant decrease in demonstrable 3beta-hydroxy-delta^5-steroid dehydrogenase activity during the last few weeks of pregnancy (an observation of doubtful significance because the placenta contains both endogenous activator and inhibitor substances for this enzyme).[321]

In placentae from prolonged pregnancies there is continuing increase in trophoblastic alkaline phosphatase activity,and the decline in acid phosphatase levels also continues.[311,312,315] Malate dehydrogenase activity decreases sharply after the 42nd week of gestation, but that of lactate dehydrogenase begins to increase at this late stage.[320] These changes suggest a partial switch from aerobic oxidative phosphorylation to anaerobic glycolysis - a not inexpected finding, a view of the moderate degree of utero-placental ischaemia known to occur in prolonged pregnancy.

Functional and metabolic changes

It is difficult to draw a clear picture of the age-related changes in placental function from the scattered, fragmentary and often inconclusive information available. Although the most important placental function is to transfer oxygen and nutrients from mother to fetus, remarkably little is known about changes in this capacity as pregnancy advances. It has, however, been demonstrated that the rates of both sodium and water transfer across the human placenta increase steadily until the 36th week of gestation, but thereafter begin to decline.[322,323] In rats, the rate of transplacental passage of glucose and amino-acids increases dramatically between the 14th and 20th days of gestation, to reach a plateau; further artificial prolongation of pregnancy (by administration of progesterone) produces a marked decrease in the transfer rate of these substances by the 22nd day.[224] This apparent decline in the transfer capacity of the placenta in late pregnancy is often attributed to placental senescence, but a decline in maternal blood flow may serve as an equally valid explanation. Unfortunately very little is known about factors that limit transfer across the placenta, though the passage of some substances may be 'membrane limited' and others 'flow limited'. The ability of the placenta to transfer a substance whose passage is known to be largely membrane-limited has not yet been shown to decrease during late pregnancy when adequate maternal utero-placental bloodflow is maintained.

Alongside transfer hormone synthesis is the other principal function of the placenta - and the only trophoblastic activity that can be reasonably accurately assayed during pregnancy. While placenta plays a part in oestrogen synthesis, oestrogen assay is now regarded more as a test of fetal than of placental function; nevertheless it is worth noting that maternal urinary and plasma oestriol levels increase fairly steadily until the 32nd week of gestation and thereafter rise sharply until term.[324] This does at least indicate that the placenta is not failing in its role in oestrogen synthesis during the last weeks of gestation. Maternal urinary oestriol levels during prolonged pregnancy are extremely variable, showing no obvious or definite trend.[325]

Progesterone secretion during late pregnancy is almost entirely attributable to placental activity, and maternal <u>urinary pregnanetriol</u> levels rise steadily to reach a plateau at 34 weeks, which is sustained until term. Maternal <u>plasma progesterone</u> levels present a confusing picture however. A steady increase until about the 34th gestational week may be followed by no further rise,[326] a slight fall,[327,328] or a continuous rise until term.[329]

Placental secretion of human chorionic gonadotrophin (HCG) is highest during the first trimester, after which levels decline. This is clearly a change in physiological role rather than an ageing phenomenon since the fall in HCG levels is accompanied by a rise in human chorionic somatotrophin (HCS). The syncytiotrophoblast is solely responsible for HCS secretion, and plasma levels of this hormone rise steadily until the 36th week of pregnancy, after which they decline slightly. HCS levels during prolonged pregnancy show no consistent pattern of change.[331]

Taken together, studies of placental hormonal synthesis offer scant evidence for placental ageing. True, there is some evidence suggesting a decline in placental synthetic activity during the last few weeks of gestation, but it must be borne in mind that the control mechanisms for placental hormone production are unknown. Output may well be influenced by the rate of maternal bloodflow through the intervillous space.[332]

A third functional aspect of the placenta which is open to, but has received little, study is its replicative capacity. The only well-documented investigation of the proliferative potential of placental cells has been reported by Vincent et al.[261] who compared the in vitro doubling capacity of cells from a 13-week-old human placenta with that of skin from its own fetus. The cultured fetal skin cells underwent over 70 passages, but those derived from the placenta were capable of only just over 40 population doublings. This impressive evidence was however impaired by failure to identify with any degree of accuracy the type of placental cells grown in culture; the work needs to be both repeated and extended. Despite these in vitro findings, there is no doubt that the full-term placenta has not exhausted its replicative capacity, because it responds to hypoxia, under in vivo or in vitro conditions, with marked proliferation of villous cytotrophoblastic cells.[247-50,266,267] Whether the intensity of this response varies with the age of the placenta is a problem requiring further investigation.

The metabolic activity of the placenta that has been most widely studied is its in vitro oxygen consumption. There has been fairly good agreement that this is lower in the second half of pregnancy than during the first half - subject to some dispute whether this decline is progressive or not.[333-9] The oxygen consumption of placentae from prolonged pregnancies appears to be even lower than that at term.[340] This reduced respiratory activity is not necessarily indicative of placental senescence, however, since the metabolic demands of the placenta itself are less at term than during the first trimester, when it is growing rapidly. A subsequent reduction of oxygen consumption in the placenta, when its needs are lower, could be considered teleologically as an adaptive mechanism for increasing the proportion of maternal-placental oxygen supplies actually available to the fetus. It is no longer fashionable to consider the placenta as competing with the fetus for maternal oxygen, but as much as 20% of the oxygen supplied may be utilised by the placenta early in pregnancy and a reduction will clearly leave more for the fetus.

Further evidence suggesting an overall decrease in the metabolic activity of the placenta in late pregnancy comes from the demonstration of a decline in glucose production and utilisation[335] and of a decrease in the synthesis of nucleic acids and protein.[341] However, there does not appear to be any alteration in the protein synthetic capacity of isolated placental ribosomes as gestation progresses.[342,343] Finally, this rather impoverished account of age-related changes in placental functonal capacity may be concluded with an observation of special interest from the standpoint of ageing theory: the DNA-repairing capacity of the placenta does not alter throughout the course of pregnancy.[344]

CONCLUSIONS AND SUGGESTIONS FOR FUTURE STUDIES

As a model for the study of human ageing, the placenta has advantages not shared by any other organ, yet a critical review of the available data reveals little conclusive evidence of true placental ageing. Virtually all the morphological and functional changes observed in the placenta during normal gestation can be attributed to maturation and/or differentiation, while those found in prolonged pregnancy appear to be principally due to alterations in maternal utero-placental bloodflow. There is therefore little need to invoke a decline into senescence. This does not exclude placental ageing, however, there being no agreed or defined criteria for the recognition of ageing at either organ or cell level. Until such criteria are established - and the prospects are not bright at present - the question of placental ageing, and hence of the organ's value for gerontological research, must remain sub judice. Meanwhile, there seems no reason why the current techniques of gerontological study, unsatisfactory though they may be, should not be applied to the placenta with as much intensity as is currently going into ageing studies of the heart, liver and other organs. Indeed, the placenta probably merits greater attention because the theoretical and practical aspects of placental ageing could well prove to be of greater importance than those of hepatic, cardiac or cerebral senescence.

Possible future lines of investigation include:

1. Accurate studies of quantitative ultrastructural morphometry, extended to placentae from prolonged pregnancies. Organellar morphometry in placentae from pre-eclamptic women should also be undertaken in order to define those changes which are due solely to ischaemia, so enabling those, if any, due solely to ageing to be identified.

2. Studies of possible age-related changes in the proliferative capacity of the placenta. In vitro studies of the replicative lifespan of the various cell types from placentae of differing gestational age. The ability of the cytotrophoblast to replicate when maintained in vitro under conditions of low oxygen tension should be studied in placentae of differing gestational age.

3. Investigation of age-related changes in organellar stability, e.g. the effects of hypoxia on mitochondria from placentae of differing gestational age.

4. A study of age-related changes in placental function and metabolism,

e.g. protein synthesis in tissue slices and isolated microsomes from placentae of varying age.

5. Studies of placental transfer efficiency at differing stages of gestation, using the isolated cotyledon technique.

DISCUSSION

Looking at our fellow men and women, we can all recognise ageing - usually with some precision, since it is possible to guess most people's ages within five years or so. Yet this cannot be done on closer, histological inspection. Much the same applies to function, which clearly declines with age in most organs and tissues, yet functional changes often prove elusive at cellular levels. In short, ageing is difficult to study - and perhaps especially so in the placenta, where its very existence is in question.

Another instance, quoted by Dorothy Villee, is progeria - the rare disorder of children which has many of the manifestations we recognise as 'ageing'. These unfortunate children lose their hair, they have extensive atherosclerosis and highly crossed-linked collagen, and develop functional deformities of their joints. They often die of coronaries at around the age of eight, with the classic appearance of a diminutive 90-year-old. Yet, on closer inspection, only one of the many biochemical parameters of their cell functions studied by Dr. Villee has proved to be abnormal: both in vivo and in vitro, there is resistance to insulin. Administration of insulin in normal dosage to children with progeria does not produce a fall in blood sugar, two or three times the normal dose being required to elicit a response. Similarly, their fibroblasts are very resistant to insulin in vitro. This is in contrast to fibroblasts both from children of the same age and from elderly individuals at what appears to be a comparable stage of ageing. There is also a difference between early passage and late passage cells in this respect; even fibroblasts from progerics are more responsive to insulin in early passage than later on. These observations led Dorothy Villee to suggest that other membrane phenomena, involving the ability of receptors to respond to an exogenous stimulus, might provide opportunities for study of ageing processes.

While agreeing that progeria constitutes a potential model for the study of ageing, Harold Fox pointed out that here too the picture is complicated by age-related diseases. The link between ageing and altered carbohydrate metabolism he found particularly interesting, because it provides further confirmation that diabetic cells have a reduced lifespan - which is true not only in diabetics but also in some non-diabetics with a family history of the disease. As regards surface membrane changes, Hamish Munro noted that HLA surface antigens are defective in progeria cells studied *in vitro* (though not when fresh). Similarly, the number of corticosteroid receptors diminishes quite considerably in ageing rats. If an organ like the liver is challenged with hormone-inducing enzyme, the time taken to induce enzyme production gets progressively longer with the age of the animal - which may mean that the number of receptors for that hormone diminishes with age. Evidence of this kind suggests that the synthetic capacity of cells to make, or to conserve, receptors is altered by ageing. Another possibility, indicated by Page Faulk, is that there may be not so much a loss of receptors as a decline in receptor affinity. Studying such questions in progeria has to overcome both the rarity of the disorder and the difficulty of propagating these cells *in vitro*; they undergo mitosis reluctantly, at a very slow rate if at all. An alternative, proposed by Eluned Woodford-Williams, might be available in children with Down's disease, who also age prematurely though not at such an accelerated rate. In particular, their placentas might repay study - both at term and from earlier therapeutic abortions.

Turning to the two contrasting theories of ageing, Robin Holliday drew attention to a widespread misapprehension. While the 'programmed' theory postulates genetically determined ageing, which may well be correct, the 'error' theory is often assumed to be based purely on non-genetic mechanism. Yet the accuracy of Macronolecule synthesis and the efficiency of repair are known to be genetically controlled. Both theories are in fact compatible with genetic control. To what extent studies of cell ageing *in vitro* can shed light on these theories of ageing or on mechanisms of ageing *in vivo* remains a matter of controversy. When fibroblasts lose the capacity to divide *in vivo*, this could be related to mycoplasmic contaminants or a defective culture medium, or to the cells being derived from diabetics or their relatives - rather than to the age of their donor. All these questions remain open. However, fibroblast studies have revealed a novel mechanism to which cell errors might accumulate, as Hamish Munro pointed out, through failure to eliminate them. The capacity to remove error molecules has been shown by Hayflick and others to diminish with ageing. If an analogue of arginine is substituted for the real thing, proteins made in the fibroblast do not fold properly, and in young cells the faulty molecules are recognised by the lysosomal system and quickly removed. But in elderly cells, this mechanism becomes impaired, with reduction of the capacity for removing errors. That change may or may not be accompanied by increased production of errors in ageing cells, though the potential is there because the senescent fibroblasts studied have an increased rate of protein turnover.

Discussion next turned to the features of placental growth and development, or maturation, that could be regarded as evidence of an ageing process. Some possibilities, put forward by Hamish Munro, included: a reduced number of receptors, or impaired receptor function, a reduced capacity for biochemical transport, and lowered concentrations of normal cell constituents or accumulation of abnormal ones. Subsequent contributions showed that firm evidence of placental ageing is lacking, both in itself and because - as Robin Holliday put it - there is at present no well-defined single or multiple theory of ageing to set such evidence against. Dynamic studies are likely to prove most rewarding in Harold Fox's view. For instance, does cytotrophoblastic proliferation respond differently in young and ageing placentae, and, if so, in what ways? How do placental mitochondria react to hypoxic conditions in young and old placentae? Is there a real difference in response to various kinds of stress?

Such questions cannot yet be answered with any confidence, but Eric Newsholme voiced reservations about this method of enquiry, from a biochemical viewpoint. Suppose the mitochondria in a tissue showed no difference in oxygen uptake between young and old cells; unless one could be sure of studying maximum capacity the results might simply be misleading. Much the same applies to studies of enzyme activity - with added doubts about the exact functions of enzymes in vivo. Studying biochemical processes in vitro in such a way that the results are fully applicable to the living animal presents major problems. For this reason, Eric Newsholme and his group have long been seeking biochemical indices that are physiologically meaningful. Simple mitochondrial oxygen uptake, stimulated by EDP, was one possibility that did not appear to qualify. However, in the enzyme field, criteria of greater promise include both the maximum anaerobic glycolytic capacity and the maximum aerobic capacity of muscle. While lactic dehydrogenase studies have proved of little if any value, work on the kinetic and regulatory properties of phosphofructokinase at maximum capacity promises to be more rewarding. Even so, Eric Newsholme was cautious about its value to research on ageing.

As regards insulin resistance, he went on to report recent work which has revealed differences between young and old rats in the insulin sensitivity of adipose sites. But ageing and, of course, diabetes are not the only factors influencing insulin response. Environmental factors can also play a part. Swedish studies in middle-aged men have shown that those who trained every day had greater insulin sensitivity than their unfit contemporaries. If declining insulin sensitivity proves to be a feature of ageing in any tissues in vivo, there is a hint here that at least one aspect of ageing might be combated by physical fitness - though the present evidence would by no means confirm such a hypothesis.

Discussion of environmental influences led Harold Fox to ask whether ageing is completely intrinsic or partly extrinsic - and how independent is it of age-related disease processes. To these fundamental questions, he added others. Does ageing represent a summation of cellular or organ changes? Why do the various tissuse apparently age in different ways and at different rates? What accounts for the wide individual variation in ageing? And why do different species have different lifespans? Parrots and turtles, of all creatures, live for as much as 200 years, while most others have much shorter lives. This looks to be clear evidence of programming, but that does not necessarily exclude either the accumulation of errors or the influence of environmental factors in the broadest sense - embracing both those extrinsic to the body as a whole and internal influences that are extrinsic to particular organs or tissues.

From a clinical standpoint, Eluned Woodford-Williams expressed the view that we should go back to Claude Bernard's concepts of the external and internal milieu. In the latter sphere, she suggested that decline in the autonomic nervous system underlies most of the clinical signs of human ageing, those in other parts of the body resulting from autonomic deficiencies. Mid-brain changes may play an important part in bringing about such deficiencies. Not only in Parkinson's disease but also in mood disorders and the autonomic control of many basic functions, including glucose metabolism and fluid and electrolyte balance, the mid-brain centres are major determinants of the internal milieu to which other tissues and organs are exposed. But the internal milieu is also determined by the genes an individual is endowed with, and by his way of life. All such influences should be considered. For example, in osteoporosis the blood pH and some of the levels of blood components may be abnormal and these changes presumably influence the rate of bone loss. But respiratory and renal function affect the pH and composition of the blood and must influence the severity of osteoporotic changes. In Eluned Woodford-Williams' view, such interrelationships have not been sufficiently investigated.

A diminished capacity for repair she does not regard as a feature of old age, however. Following surgery, the speed at which elderly patients recover generally equals that in younger patients, despite evidence of impaired repair at cellular level and despite changes in the internal milieu with ageing. One of the most consistent of the latter, noted by Eluned Woodford-Williams, is an increase in extracellular water at the expense of intracellular water. Since it would presumably alter some cell functions, though apparently without impairing healing, that may be a more significant change than loss of lean body weight - which does not necessarily imply any deficiency in the remaining cells. Overall, her clinical view of ageing patterns suggests that they are pathological and largely secondary to other changes. That leaves little room, in the intact human animal, for the supposed distinction between ageing itself and age-related disease.

The importance of whole animal studies was stressed by Willi Hijmans. In his view, subcellular, cellular and organ findings should always be seen in this context, and studies of the lifespan of various species by Dr. Hollander at his own institute in Leiden has revealed many misconceptions - about the influence of sex and hybridity on longevity, for example. While sharing an interest in this important aspect of ageing research, Harold Fox voiced reservations about intact animal work, on the grounds that it rested on observational phenomenology. For Willi Hijmans, however, there was no clear distinction between observing changes in the whole animal and in its constituent biochemistry, say, or its DNA. What we recognise as ageing in toto must, after all, represent the combined effect of ageing processes in the body's organs and tissues. Clinically there is another complicating factor, though, as Harold Fox pointed out. Many elderly patients are taking drugs to combat age-related or other conditions, and their effects are hard to disentangle from a clinical picture that is already highly complex. Hence, in large part, the interest in experimental models of ageing.

But is the placenta such a model? Does it actually age? What, asked Harold Fox, is its natural lifespan? 'As long as the pregnancy continues' was his own answer - which suggests that it may not so much age as simply become expendable when no longer needed. Since an increase in variability is one of the more consistend features of ageing in Willi Hijmans' view, he suggested longitudinal studies of such criteria as the weight, number of cells, water content, and collagen content of the placenta, as an additional means of determining whether it does age or not. There is little data on this question at present. What of lipofuscin deposition, quoted in Harold Fox's paper as quite a consistent sign of senescence? Marcellino Dianzani enquired whether any longitudinal studies of the related lipid perodixation had been done on the placenta, since changes here might provide evidence of ageing. But no such work has been done, and Harold Fox expressed doubts about its value; no one knows whether lipid peroxidation changes as a cause or result of ageing, nor whether lipofuscin accumulation represents 'inert slag', as it were, or is itself capable of decreasing cellular function. In other words, basic studies of this kind seem to offer little early prospect of resolving the question of placental ageing.

Clinically, Maureen Young was firmly of the opinion that the placenta is not an aged organ at term, and perfectly capable of performing its main function of nourishing the fetus. Striking examples of this are to be seen in post-mature animals. For instance, rabbits which are usually born weighing 30-40 grams increase to 70-80 grams in three days if labour is artificially deferred. In cattle there is a rare gene which produces malformation of the head and prolongs gestation indefinitely, presumably because the hypothalamic /pituitary signal for parturition cannot be given. Gestation in the cow is normally around 250 days, but these animals will go on for 1½ or 2 years - during which the placenta keeps pumping away, and the animal continues to grow. Claude Villee cited this as evidence that the placenta does not age. Yet human placentas certainly show much variability at term, some looking 'really dreadful' with so many infarcts and calcium deposits that it seems astonishing they can manage to nourish the fetus, whereas others look superb. Biochemists tend to be selective, taking specimens of the better looking tissue - even from very tattered, aged-looking placentas - for analytical and other studies. This selectivity mighy be one reason for failure to identify age changes, if they were present only in the 'older' looking parts of the placenta. But that seems unlikely in the light of subsequent discussion.

The arterial lesions sometimes described do not, for example, appear to be evidence of ageing. They are confined, according to Harold Fox, to the maternal utero-placental vessels, which do not form part of the placenta, and are seen only in pre-eclampsia. The changes are pathological and he believes they should be described as atherosis, to distinguish them from true atherosclerosis. The actual lesion consists of accumulated fat-laden cells in the intima, whereas atheroma is a disease of the medial musculature. Whether changes also occur in the cytotrophoblast that replaces the endothelium around maternal utero-placental vessels is not clear. But, as Harold Fox pointed out, the nature of the atherotic changes is hardly relevant to ageing of the placenta, since the lesions are pathological and the affected vessels outside the placenta itself.

From an obstetrical viewpoint, calcification is the feature that marks an 'old' placenta from a genuinely post-mature labour. The difference, said Alan Browne, can be seen and felt. Moreover, many of the placentas associated with intrauterine disasters and deaths are not only calcified but very small. Recognition of associations between raised perinatal mortality, postmaturity, reabsorption of the liquor amnii and placental inadequancy though 'ageing' has been a major influence on obstetric practice during recent decades. Yet, as Alan Browne pointed out, the ageing placenta can only be seen 'through a glass darkly'. Intrauterine diagnosis depends on tests of placental function, the composition of the liquor, and the actual growth and behaviour of the fetus. Evidence of 'ageing' of the placenta is certainly taken seriously in obstetric practice. At the same time, Professor Browne agreed that the placenta can go on and on functioning over long periods, as in his case of anencephaly without extreme postmaturity, where 'the placenta was like a rock but went on supporting an enormous baby'.

These apparently conflicting observations were clarified by Harold Fox, who agreed with the facts outlined by Alan Browne but questioned his interpretation of them. While calcification is an age-related change, there is no evidence that it in any way interferes with placental function. Furthermore, it is reversible; total loss of calcium from the placenta can take place during a prolonged pregnancy. Placental calcification does not therefore fulfil the criteria for senescent change. Rather the opposite, for its presence is related to a good outcome of the pregnancy, being most frequently seen in primigravidae of social class I and more commonly in the spring. Curiously, monozygotic, dichorionic twins are sometimes born with one placenta calcified and the other not. All in all, Harold Fox concluded that placental calcification is an ill-understood age-related change, non-senescent in nature.

As regards small-for-dates babies, it is often assumed that the baby is small because the placenta is small, but he suggested the opposite - that the placenta is small because the baby is small, due almost invariably to extra-placental factors. In Harold Fox's view, the small placenta is normally quite adequate to meet its nutritional and oxygen demands. In prolonged pregnancy, where there is sometimes a decline in placental function, this appears to be entirely due to a critical decrease in maternal bloodflow - and not to any intrinsic change in the placenta itself. If this critical reduction in bloodflow does not occur, then the post-mature baby continues to grow. The majority of women who have a baby weighing more than 4 000 grams, and who are not diabetic, have had prolonged pregnancies. However, as Leslie Brent pointed out, even if the maternal utero-placental bloodflow is the crucial factor determining fetal growth and viability in these circumstances, it cannot be wholly dissociated from what is happening in the placenta or its vessels.

Confirmatory evidence that placental size may be determined by the embryo and/or fetus, rather than vice versa, came from Richard Gardner. In the mouse, the rate of initial proliferation and growth of the trophectoderm derivatives, which form a very important part of the placenta, is precisely determined by interaction with the inner cell mass. In other words, the size of the cell population initially deployed is dependent upon the growth of the early embryo. How long this interaction goes on in the mouse is uncertain, but the last stage at which the trophectoderm can be isolated and this interaction demonstrated is at 8½ to 9 days of a 20-day gestation.

Discussion of placental ageing concluded with two further proposals for objective assessment, both based on comparative studies in early and late placentae. Hamish Munro suggested looking for differences in cell replication, while Jean Ginsburg proposed investigation of enzyme changes known to be associated with senescence in fibroblasts or other tissues. But all such research will have to discriminate carefully between the placenta's unquestioned evolution to maturity and any real evidence of ageing. Willi Hijmans took the view that the placenta does not age but matures - which makes it an ideal subject of study by gerontologists. After all, the ideal we are looking for is not the usual decline of ageing, but continuation of good health right up to death. What better model could there be than something that matures and then remains in optimal condition until it stops functioning and disappears?

THE AGEING CELL AND MALIGNANCY*

Jan Pontén

The relationship between cellular ageing - or ageing in general - and malignancy is a complex one. The basic question, as with other age-related diseases, is whether tumours form part of the ageing syndrome or simply accompany it at times. A true component of ageing should eventually affect the whole population, without too much individual variation. Loss of accommodation of the eye provides a good example. In the twenties, there is slow decline in the elasticity of the lens, followed by rapid decline, so that by about 55 years there is practically no lens mobility left. This familiar change shows little variation. At first sight, the increase of malignancy, with age, in animals as well as man, follows a somewhat similar pattern, but when the figures are inspected more closely and broken down for different types of tumour, a rather different picture emerges. With prostatic carcinoma, for example, the incidence starts to increase at the age of 50, and then increases steeply, until at the age of 80 or so, it becomes difficult to follow the incidence further. Clinically, prostatic cancer affects about 15% of men, but the total incidence is higher as judged by post-mortem studies, regardless of whether the patients had any symptoms of carcinoma. The curve of incidence based on these figures rises more sharply, assuming a slightly different shape to reach much higher levels, before it flattens out at about the age of 80.

Studies of other types of human malignancy have usually revealed an upper shoulder of this kind at lower levels - and at different ages for different tumours. This levelling off is of some importance because it occurs at well below 100% for all tumours, except prostatic carcinoma diagnosed on pathological criteria. Composite curves for a range of tumours follow the same type of pattern, showing a late decrease in the risk of contracting malignancy. This speaks against malignancy being considered part of the ageing syndrome, in the strict sense.

* See also Handbook of the Biology of Ageing, Ed. Hayflick, L. & Finch, C.B. Van Nostrand, 1977.

Another argument telling against malignancy as part of the ageing syndrome is that the incidence of different tumour types varies widely between different animal species. Certain species, such as the dog, have a high incidence of malignant mastocytomas, which are virtually unknown in man. Taken together, leukaemias and lymphomas are fairly common in most animals, but when the tumour spectrum is broken down into different types of leukaemias, it turns out to differ substantially between species. For example, erythroleukaemia is common in the chicken, whereas it too is virtually unknown in man. It can occur in the mouse, but appears to be uncommon under natural conditions. Without going into much more detail, I should like to state that available statistics and for higher mammals provide no definite evidence that malignancy forms part of the ageing syndrome. Its features are much more like those of an acquired disorder.

This is a very important conclusion, because it means that cancer prevention is within our reach. If malignancy were really part of the ageing syndrome, prophylactic measures would be as futile as trying to prevent reading difficulties in the aged. But if malignancy does not form part of the ageing syndrome, is this also true for all types of proliferative disorder? For instance, are benign tumours also distinct from the ageing syndrome? Unfortunately, since researchers tend to work on dangerous conditions, there is an almost complete lack of factual data on this important question. However, there is one disease - the senile wart, or benign basal cell papilloma - which seems to occur in 100% of all old people and is commonly multiple. This might be a benign proliferative disorder that constitutes part of the ageing syndrome (but there is no known connection between those benign basal cell papillomas and carcinomas).

Another interesting neoplastic disorder which might be considered part of the ageing syndrome is so-called benign gammopathy - a condition in which the serum contains a monoclonal myeloma-like protein (the M-component). This disease has a surprisingly consistent age-dependent curve, from a linear increase starting at about 50 years, and reaching about 3% in persons over 70. This may sound low, but detection of M-component in the serum means that a considerable number of plasma cells, or B-lymphocytes, are producing this monoclonal immunoglobulin. The real incidence of benign gammopathy might be much higher, perhaps even reaching 100% in old age. One or two clones of benignly proliferating plasma cells producing monoclonal immunoglobulin would not necessarily be detected by serum testing - and not all such clones produce immunoglobulins. Non-producing lymphoctyes might also proliferate clonally.

In summary, while there is no conclusive evidence that malignant tumours in humans form part of the ageing syndrome, some benign proliferative disorders may do so. But these do not appear to undergo malignant transformation.

AGE RELATED SUSCEPTIBILITY TO CARCINOGENESIS?

If malignancy is not part of the ageing syndrome, why should cancer be more common in the old than in the young? This question has been debated under many headings - immunosurveillance or other immunological mechanisms, hormonal imbalances and so forth. Here I shall concentrate on one aspect: Is the aged cell more susceptible to carcinogenesis? This could plainly be tested by studying young and old animals, mice for example, to see if they respond differently to the same carcinogens. Unfortunately, most studies of this question have suffered from inadequacies, but the small series of experiments by Ebbesen at least suggests an answer. She took skin from old and young mice for transplantion into young syngeneic recipients, which were then subjected to chemical carcinogenesis by dimethyl-butyric acid. The result was that the old skin, even though it was in the same host as the young skin, responded with about three times the incidence of carcinoma. This is the only, rather insubstantial evidence to show that the aged cell, in the skin of a mouse, is really more susceptible to chemical carcinogens. Since the young host animals were the same, they presumably responded similarly to young and old transplants and to the carcinogen. Other possible causes of greater susceptibility to chemical carcinogens in old animals - such as more prolonged exposure, hormonal imbalance, or decreased general immune resistance - all seem to have been excluded by the methodology adopted.

Another way of studying age-related susceptibility to carcinogenesis is to culture cell lines of different ages in vitro and see whether they undergo malignant transformation on exposure to a carcinogen. In one such study SV40 virus was used as the transforming agent on aged and young human lung fibroblasts. The old fibroblasts showed evidence of greater susceptibility at two different stages. First, virus-specific T-antigen, revealed by intranuclear fluorescence, was found in about 30% of aged cells in late passages, compared with only about 1% of young cells. Secondly, the appearance of T-antigen was also followed by characteristic disturbances of growth and loss of contact inhibition. On the other hand, the chances of obtaining infinite growth transformation, i.e. establishing lines from these T-antigen carrying clones, were very much higher from the young cells.

The conclusion here is that aged cells appear to be more susceptible to infection by SV40, and to undergo disturbance of growth control, but that the final, and most important, step in carcinogenesis - the acquisition of infinite growth potential - still remains to be shown. A somewhat similar picture has been obtained by applying RNA tumour viruses to cells of differing age. In general, young cells are far more easily transformed into loss of contact inhibition than old cells, but there are wide species differences. With human cells, which are not prone to spontaneous transformation it is not possible to produce infinite growth transformation. That positive evidence of malignant changes can only be obtained in cells with an unstable background from particular species, such as the mouse or other rodents.

The whole question of the relationship between cell ageing and susceptibility to malignant transformation is still very much open to experimentation. What role placental studies can play remains to be seen, but it is possible that cultured fibroblasts from that organ could help provide answers to some of these questions. It would surprise me if hormonal imbalance or lack of immunosurveillance explain, to any substantial degree, why old people are more prone to carcinoma than young ones.

DISCUSSION

In studying malignant transformation it is obviously necessary to establish firm criteria that distinguish malignant call lines, but Robin Holliday queried how much reliance could be put on infinite growth potential in vitro - on the grounds that tumour cells do not always divide vigorously in vivo. Much depends on the type of tumour, in Jan Pontén's view. For human tumours there is overwhelming evidence of infinite growth potential - clinically, on transplantation into nude mice, and in cell lines in vitro. On transfer to mice or culture there is never slow growth; the cells either show infinite potential or die immediately. With human tumours that are transferable (see below), the likelihood that they will form infinite cell lines is so high that this can be regarded as an obligate component of malignancy in man. By contrast, attempts to transplant cells from normal human tissues and benign tumours into nude mice have failed, and even cultures of human fibroblasts have a finite life. The dividing line between malignant cell populations and normal or benign cells may not always be clear cut, but infinite growth potential provides an invaluable criterion of malignancy.

This conclusion is not seriously undermined by wide differences in the ease of establishing cell lines. In Burkitt's lymphoma, Jan Pontén reported a success rate of about 80%; for malignant gliomas and melanomas, only about 20% and for some tumours less than 1% The difficulty appears to be a technical one, in providing the cells with the right environment. If a proliferative cell line is once established from any of these human tumours, it shows infinite growth potential. However, Eva Klein pointed out that 'immortalization' of this kind is not synonymous with malignancy in vivo. Lymphoblastic cell lines which are 'immortal' in culture do not produce tumours when implanted in nude mice, for example. As regards the relative ease of establishing cell lines from Burkitt's lymphomas, she suggested that this might be due to the presence of the lymphoma virus, whose genome might contain important information on the acquisition of 'immortality'. Certainly, other lymphosarcomas not containing the virus are much harder to establish as cell lines.

Turning to Ebbesen's work on the carcinogen susceptibility of skin grafts from old and young mice, Leslie Brent wondered whether the higher incidence of tumours demonstrated in aged skin really excluded the possibility that the malignant changes might be due in part to ageing itself. Ageing and age-related susceptibility are, after all, not necessarily mutually exclusive. Jan Pontén agreed, describing the Ebbesen findings as no more than a fair experimental demonstration that aged skin cells may be more susceptible to chemical carcinogenesis, irrespective of hormonal imbalance or immunosurveillance. But this, as yet, unconfirmed evidence of greater susceptibility in old cells has to be set against many observations that young tissues are highly susceptible to chemical and other forms of carcinogenesis. Maxwell Anderson quoted as examples the higher incidence of cancer after irradiation of the infant thymus or thyroid and the fact that young women having frequent chest X-rays for pulmonary tuberculosis had a much higher incidence of breast cancer than controls. Quite possibly, as he suggested, young and old cells may both be susceptible - in different ways and to different carcinogens. But studying such differences is by no means easy, and Jan Pontén noted two major problems. First comparing the effect of X-rays or other carcinogens in young and old animals allows insufficient time for malignant changes to become manifest in the latter - because death from other causes intervenes. Second, there are tremendous differences, as noted earlier, in the internal milieu of young and old animals. Ebbesen's technique of transplantating young and old cells into young hosts largely overcomes these difficulties, to reveal intrinsic cellular differences. However, Arthur Wild doubted whether immunological problems are excluded, because an old donor mouse might have produced autoantibodies to its own skin cells. Those cells might then have antibodies on the cell surface which could make them more susceptible to carcinogens - although Eva Klein took the view that such antibodies would be shed quite fast in the new host, and not replaced. Clearly this is a field needing considerably more work before firm conclusions can be reached about age-related susceptibility to carcinogenesis.

Moreover, Leslie Brent stressed that the possible protective effects of immunosurveillance, initiating rejection of tumour cells, should not be overlooked. Among the findings which led Macfarlane Burnet to develop this very useful concept was that autopsies in people who had died violently in road accidents showed a much greater incidence of incipient tumours than actually becomes manifest clinically in the population as a whole. In other words, there is a much greater reservoir of incipient tumours in youngish people than would be expected from the observed incidence of those tumours. Whatever makes such incipient tumours go away is clearly a matter for debate, pending further research. Leslie Brent took the view that the basic finding could not be ignored, through Jan Pontén felt that it had not been fully substantiated, while other evidence in support of immunosurveillance was cited by Page Faulk. In children with immunodeficiency diseases - which are common enough to be well-documented - there is a very high incidence of tumours, principally but not exclusively affecting the lymphoid system. The implication of defective immunosurveillance here led Hamish Munro to question whether the greater susceptibility of older mouse skin to carcinogenesis,in Ebbesen's studies, is due to increased sensitivity or to failure of a protective mechanism. It seems not unreasonable to postulate that age might have both effects - if aged cells do indeed prove to be more susceptible to carcinogens.

This uncertainty was taken a stage further by Harold Fox who questioned what is meant by the term malignant cell. Many of the common epithelial tumours evolve slowly over many years, through a process which is neoplastic but not overtly malignant, and imperceptibly pass into what may be classed as malignancy at some ill-defined stage that cannot be identified. In his view, this prolonged process, differing from simple malignant transformation, is not mirrored in most experimental situations. Jan Pontén concurred, saying that mouse work often put too much emphasis on tumour progression - whereas, in human cancers, the pathological diagnosis is based on a certain degree of differentiation. This normally appears in metastases and if there is a recurrence ten years later, the same degree of differentiation is seen. Unlike mouse tumours, human malignancy has a fixed aberration, or degree of differentiation, from its inception that is maintained for years over hundreds and hundreds of cell doublings. Myeloma is a case in point, human myeloma being noted for its stability over many decades, faithfully producing the same immunoglobulin. By contrast, so-called mouse myelomas - really plasma cell tumours, as Willi Hijmans pointed out - are noted for their instability, with a high rate of mutation and all manner of secondary changes. Moreover, hormone dependence seems to disappear more quickly from murine than from human tumours. Admitting that he might be overstressing these points, Jan Pontén said he wanted to set the balance right, since so much reliance is placed on murine tumours as models for human cancer.

Turning to changes in the internal milieu, Dorothy Villee drew attention to the age-related increase in the serum glucose concentration after a feed. This slight but definite increase is of the order that increases the biosynthesis of collagen by fibroblasts growing in culture - and she suggested that any tissue which can take in as much glucose as there is in its milieu may be altered in its function with age. Eric Newsholme took this argument further. The elevated concentration of glucose in cells could produce, over a long period, high concentrations of polyols - sorbitol and fructose. These might lead to ion and water disturbance, and thus produce changes in protein structure - which we recognise macroscopically as the effects of ageing. In diabetic patients, the long-term secondary changes might also be mediated in this way (and it is noteworthy that some of them, e.g. lens opacities, could be regarded as accelerated ageing). Though these ideas need to be confirmed, Eric Newsholme emphasised that precise regulation of the concentrations of metabolic intermediates is vitally important to the well-being of cells, and tissues, and that glucose is a good example of such a metabolic intermediate.

Age-related changes in the hormonal milieu were stressed by Olga Genbačev, with special reference to the menopause - with its striking reduction in female hormone levels, involution of the ovaries and consequent changes in the adrenals. In addition to the many body tissues and functions affected by the changed hormonal milieu that follows the menopause, she also reported evidence from radioimmune assays, showing hormonal changes in prostatic adenoma and carcinoma. Moreover, longitudinal studies of hormonal imbalance are beginning to show predisposition to certain types of carcinoma, including breast cancer. And once attention has been directed to the long-term effects of milieu changes, it is but a step to recognising that the intra-uterine milieu must play a part in determining many subsequent events.

In both man and other animals, there is a carry over from intrauterine conditions which can be detected for several generations. By way of example, Hamish Munro described work on animals malnourished in utero by feeding an inadequate diet to their mothers. For two or three generations, the females are less capable of reproduction, and both sexes show behavioural abnormalities (but the male reproductive apparatus is not affected). This indicates that there must be long-term intra-uterine 'programming', which is still reflected later in the life of the offspring and adversely influences both pregnancy and fetal development of the next generation. Seeking possible parallels, Hamish Munro asked if there is any evidence that intra-uterine laying down of such 'programmes' affects the course of human or animal ageing. Different groups of animals might show different ageing rates, which could be related to intrauterine experience. And small-for-dates babies might have different obstetrical histories,even going back a generation or two, and/or be more or less likely to suffer from certain developmental deficiencies or disorders - conceivably including effects on their own pregnancy or the next generation. At present, this is pure hypothesis, though small-for-dates babies can be separated into those that are premature and others that are malnourished in utero. Developmentally, they appear to form a heterogeneous group, with at least two growth patterns, according to Dorothy Villee. Some 'catch-up' growth if they are well nourished in infancy and childhood, getting back to the normal percentiles for their age. But others can never get back, irrespective of the nutrition they receive.

The importance of placental studies to understanding of the intra-uterine milieu can hardly be overemphasised in these latter fields. Whether the placenta can provide a useful model for studying the ageing process in general, or in selected tissues, remains an open question - coupled with uncertainties about ageing itself and doubts whether the placenta actually undergoes ageing towards the end of pregnancy. More work is clearly needed to clarify these fundamental questions. In one field, the ageing of the immune system, a good start has been made - as Willi Hijmans showed in the final paper.

NEW DEVELOPMENTS IN IMMUNOGERONTOLOGY

Willi Hijmans

This is not the place to discuss the definition of ageing, but it seems appropriate to give an operational description. 'Systematic changes occuring as a function of time' may serve our purpose. These changes are usually associated with a decline of function. Judged from this angle, all systems are subject to ageing. It would be surprising if the immune system were exempt from this general rule or if its decline had different characteristics from those seen in other systems. Its usually gradual loss of function is characterised by:

a. Remarkable differences in the rate of decline of the different functions, and

b. Increased variability of the indices of function, associated with

c. Increased vulnerability.

Immunogerontology made its start more than half a century ago[1] when several authors convincingly demonstrated that serum titres and skin tests were lower and less frequently positive in the elderly than in the young. It took another few decades[2] for the first reports to be published, covering the entire lifespan of experimental animals. Radiation biology provided the impetus to carry out these studies because of the need for information on the long-term effect of irradiation. But since gerontology has established itself as a scientific discipline, there has been a regular flow of publications on this subject, which has recently been the subject of several reviews.[3-5] A major feature which has emerged in recent years is the need to acknowledge that the normal immune system is extremely complex, and any age-related changes should be evaluated against this background. Only some of these changes can be interpreted as dysfunctions, which could be the result of minor defects and therefore difficult to detect. A separate question is whether these dysfunctions can lead to age-related pathology.[6]

CELLULAR CHANGES

Accessory factors

Information on this aspect of the immune reaction remains scarce. One can only repeat what was said in a recent review: the ability of macrophages to collaborate with T- and B-cells in antibody production is not impaired with age.[3] In view of the difficulties in quantifying phagocytosis and the absence of data on phagocytosis of well-defined antigens in ageing studies, the possibility that age-related changes do indeed occur cannot be excluded. Even so, they can hardly be the cause of the impressive decrease in antibody production in old animals.

Information concerning the complement system is even scarcer; a recent survey on amplification mechanisms[7] fails to mention the influence of ageing.

Stem cells

The overwhelming majority of stem cells are found in the bone marrow and their number seems to remain constant. According to Harrison et al,[8] the often observed functional loss is due to transplantation, at least in mice, and not to ageing. Vacek et al,[9] working with rats, also conclude that the decline in the immune response is not due to a decrease in the number of stem cells. They did find a decreased harvesting ability in the spleen microenvironment during the first few months of life, but this is a phenomenon of maturation, not ageing. Albright and Makinodan[10] made young stem cells grow in old recipients and vice versa, and they suggest that old stem cells remain old, whereas young stem cells can be aged in an accelerated manner. These observations point to an influence of hormones and other factors. The conclusion that the stem cell should not be regarded as the main culprit in immunological ageing is important in view of the fact that immuno-rejuvenation has been suggested - and attempted [11] - to restore the aged immune system. Further experiments along these lines should not be limited to the stem cells.

The B-Cell system

The branch of the immune system responsible for the humoral immune response is called the B-cell system, because in birds its origin lies in the Bursa of Fabricius. The equivalent in mammals is unknown and probably does not exist as such, but because of the central role of the bone marrow in the humoral immune response, the use of the terms B-cells and B-cell system have become accepted.

The decline of B-cell function towards T-independent antigens late in life is a consistent finding,[12] although this decline is far less marked that in the immune response towards thymus-dependent antigens. The decline in B-cell function seems to be due to a reduction in the number of responding cells and not due to an alteration in the capacity of those cells that do respond. Abraham et al[13] came to this conclusion from their studies in mice, where they used lipopolysaccharide as a B-cell mitogen, and Kruisbeek[14] confirmed these conclusions in rats. Kishimoto et al[15] also ascribe the lipopolysaccharide-induced enhancement of the anti-TNP response in the spleens of old mice to diminished numbers of TNP plaque-forming precursor cells in this organ. There is, however, a strain dependence in this phenomenon: the C3H/HeJ strain of mice are, for instance, known to be unresponsive to the lipoplysaccharide-induced mitogenesis. Mason Smith[16] also stresses strain differences: BALB/c and C3H mice maintain their response to type III pneumococcal polysaccharide, whereas SJL mice show an early decline. Zharhary et al[12] noted a delayed peak response to TNP-KLH in old mice, but the number of cells at the time of the peak response remained constant. However, Callard et al[17] state that the reduction with age in B-cell function is due to a qualitative defect in the lymphocytes themselves; the numbers remain constant, but their function is impaired.

In man, the reaction of peripheral blood lymphocytes to pokeweed mitogen, which activates human B- and well as T-cells, remained stable according to Halbrecht et al.[18] But Weiner et al[19] mentioned a better response in young than in old individuals. In contrast, elderly individuals responded better to anti-IgG than young. Divergent results in man can be expected to occur more frequently than in experimental animals; numbers of human subjects are often small and the selection of individuals can have a greater influence on results than in studies of inbred animals.

Two new developments deserve special attention. The first concerns well-controlled experiments by Singhal et al,[20] who suggest that the depressed immune function in senescence is accompanied by an age-dependent increase in suppressor B-cell activity. This is a non-specific activity of these cells, which are mainly present in the bone marrow. The decreased immune response seen in ageing does not result - or rather, as the authors carefully state, does not only result - from a deficiency of a subpopulation of lymphocytes, quantitative, but from an active block, caused by an increased number of B-suppressor cells. The appearance of suppressor cells is an early event in the autoimmune F_1 hybrid, NZB/W mouse, preceding the appearance of autoimmune phenomena, and a casual relationship is easy to imagine.[21] The second new development is the recognition that the major compartment of antibody secreting cells shifts with age from the spleen to the bone marrow. In CBA mice the total number of cells which contain immunoglobulins remains constant from 6 weeks to 2 years of age, but the spleen's relative contribution decreases from approximately 65% to about 20%. In 2-year-old mice the relative contribution in terms of cytoplasmatically positive cells was 80%, which may well reflect a shift from the primary response to a secondary response pattern.[22]

IMMUNOGLOBULINS

The immunoglobulin level can be used as an overall index to the number and activity of immunoglobulin-secreting cells, on the reasonable assumptions that the humoral immune response is to a large extent under T-cell control, and that the serum level is determined by synthesis, catabolism, excretion, and pool-size. Different authors mention minor differences as a function of age, but agree that there is no general decrease as it advances. There is consensus on the following pattern in man: the IgE level remains steady, while those of IgA and IgG increase steadily with age. The graphs can be extrapolated to the maximum age group, in which paraproteins occur commonly (see below) and an imbalance is often seen in the kappa to lambda ratio.[23,24] More information is needed on IgE, but the elevation of IgG is known to be caused by increased levels of the IgG_1 and IgG_3 subclasses, which are more effective in binding complement than subclasses IgG_2 and IgG_4. The only subclass which fails to cross the placenta is IgG_2.

In mice, data are available for the CBA strain, bred under conventional conditions.[25] This is a long-lived strain, not prone to age-related pathology of the immunological system. Only the levels of subclasses IgG_1 and IgG_{2b} increase with ageing, but all classes and subclasses show increased variation, with the exception of IgM (the latter observation being in contrast to man). In C57BL mice, a plateau is reached at the age of 12 months, again with the exception of IgM, which reaches a steady level at 18 months. Large variations are already present at an early age, which could be due to the high frequency of idiopathic paraproteinaemia in this strain. These data are mentioned here to illustrate the complexity of the situation and the need to go into detailed analysis. Each strain may have its characteristic variation profile.[26]

Idiopathic paraproteinaemia

This condition is characterised by the presence of a homogeneous immunoglobulin peak or M-component in the serum, and it can be considered the benign counterpart of multiple myeloma. Its essentially benign character was clearly demonstrated in an eleven-year follow-up of a large number of persons in a health survey.[27] Its increase in incidence with ageing, which reaches a peak of 19%[23,28] makes it of special interest to immunogerontologists. As autoantibodies are also known to increase with age, it has been suggested that these paraproteins are associated with autoantibody activity, but no support for this suggestion was found in a recent study.[29] New analytical possibilities are now available, since the description of an animal model by Radl and Hollander.[30] They observed these homogeneous immunoglobulins frequently in aged mice of the C57BL strain, but far less in other strains.

Specific antibodies

In contrast to the overall immunoglobulin levels, the specific antibody response shows a clear age-related decrease. This was first described in man in 1926[1] and in mice in 1962.[2] The latter study showed that the number of antibody secreting cells in the spleens of old mice was only one-tenth of the maximum found in young adult animals. Cell transfer experiments established that the major part of the age-related decline could be attributed to the cells of the immunological system, rather than to changes in the microenvironment. In later studies,[31] spleen cells from old mice were mixed with those from young animals - with variable results which underlined the complexity of the system and could be due to suppressor cells and stimulatory effects. These findings illustrate the new perspectives in immunogerontology. The question is no longer whether an age-related decrease takes place in the immune response, but how it can be defined in terms of the most recent immunological concepts. These include the dichotomy of the immune system into the B- and T-cell systems, the interaction between these two, either negative or positive, the interrelationships within each system and, finally, the regulatory effect of the genetic make-up of the individual - with interest currently focusing on the major histocompatibility complex.

Further questions then arise. Does the age-related decline in the immune response affect only the primary reaction, or also the secondary reaction? And what differences, if any, are there between the so-called T-dependent and T-independent antigens? In several strains it has been established that the age-related decline occurs with primary and secondary immunisation, although the effect on the secondary response is less marked.[32] Other details have been studied mainly at the cellular level, and will therefore be discussed below.

Autoantibodies

It has long been known that the frequency with which autoantibodies can be detected in man increases with age, and Walford[33] has emphasised the significance of this observation. More recent investigations[29,34] have revealed that the general statement of an increase as a function of time needs modification in two seemingly trivial aspects. First, the increase is not observed in the very old and, second, the increase is not general, but selective - affecting in particular the latex test for rheumatoid factor, the antinuclear antibodies and only those organ-specific autoantibodies which are directed against the thyroid gland. The reason for this selectivity is not clear, but the levelling off in old age may be interpreted as the absence of autoantibodies conferring a survival advantage,

The NZB strain of mice and the B/W hybrid are the prime examples of spontaneous autoimmunity in animals, but the early death of these animals is no proof of early ageing. The cause of the autoimmunity remains unclear. The thymus has been implicated for a number of reasons, but more recently a defect at the level of the polyclonal activation of B-cells has been postulated. An attractive experimental model for the study of the relationship of autoimmunity to ageing involves the age-related response for the long-lived (B10C3) F_1 mice to their own TNP modified red cells. The suppressor T-cells, which are held responsible for the regulation of the immune response, were found to be severely impaired in the aged animals.[36]

Avidity

The same authors[36] confirmed and extended earlier findings[15,37] that there is a substantial decrease in the avidity of antibodies on ageing, at least for thymus-dependent antigens; the avidity of antibodies against a thymus-independent antigen was not found to be reduced significantly. However, others have failed to find a difference in the affinity of antibodies between old and young mice.[12] The reason for this discrepancy is not clear, though the use of an adjuvant may play a role, and studies using an adjuvant reported a preferential loss in the primary and secondary response to DNP-BGG in aged animals.[37]

The network system

Theoretical considerations have lead Jerne[61] to suggest the existence of a network of the variable domains of the immunoglobulin molecules as a regulation system governing the immune reaction. The basis for this concept is the observation that antibody molecules possess antigenic specificity at their antibody combining sites. Against these so-called idiotypes (antibody 1), anti-idiotype antibodies (antibody 2) can be raised in other animals of the same or of another species, but they also occur within the animal itself. The anti-antibodies in their turn carry specific idiotypes, which can act as antigens. Two independently working groups of investigators[38,39] have provided experimental evidence on the existence of such a regulatory system. The bearing of this new concept on immunogerontology is obvious. Selective defects may occur with ageing, and these may be the underlying cause of age-related pathology due to immune dysfunctions - which may be exceedingly difficult to detect as a result of the complexity of the system.

THE THYMUS AND THE T-CELL SYSTEM

The thymus and/or the T-cell system are widely implicated as major sites for studying the cause of the age-related decline of the immune reactivity. Classical morphology has shown that the thymus involutes rapidly after attaining maximum size about the time of sexual maturity.[40] The evidence has been so persuasive that the opinion has long prevailed that the thymus has no functional significance during adult life, despite several observations of accelerated decline in function after thymectomy.[41] The activity of the T-cell system used to be ascribed entirely to the presence of long-lived circulating and thymus-processed lymphocytes. This opinion has now been revised.[42] Partly in the light of morphological findings indicating that the decrease of the thymic gland is mainly due to involution of the cortex rather than the medulla. Transplantation experiments with thymus tissue clearly show a decline in function in the host animal[43] and thymectomy, performed in adult animals, accelerates the natural decline in cellular immunity.[44] In mice there is a specific subset of T-cells, which disappears very rapidly after adult thymectomy,[41] and in man a sharp decrease has been noticed in the level of a serum factor after thymectomy in patients suffering from myasthenia gravis.[45]

Thymic humoral factor and the thymus epithellum

In very general terms the role of the thymus is to process lymphocytes and humoral factors are thought to be responsible. A number have been described, and they have been obtained from the thymus, from serum, and most frequently from the supernatant of thymic epithelium in culture. The epithelium has been the most likely candidate for secretory activity, according to various workers,[46] and it is clear that not one single factor, but a series of substances, must be responsible for promoting the differentiation of precursor T-cells. A decreased activity of the serum with ageing has been reported, a strikingly early drop being observed in the NZB and B/W mouse.[47]

T-cells

The complexity of the immune system is also apparent from studies of the T-cells. Although the total number of T-cells is comparable in young and old mice[48] an increase has been described in the subpopulation which contains the T-suppressor cells. Makinodan et al[31] studied the effect of mixing cells from young and old animals on the antibody response. This either reduced, added to or elevated the reaction. The occurrence of all three types of response suggest the existence of multiple causes for a decreased T-dependent humoral immune response in old mice. Co-cultivation studies[49] showed an increase of specific T-suppressor cell activity in the spleen of immunodeficient primed old mice. Such a suppressor effect was not detected in old mice towards the T-independent antigen pneumococcal polysaccharide SIII.[17] In man, the T-suppressor activation of blood lymphoctyes concanavalin-A declines with age and this may explain the increased frequency of autoantibodies in aged persons.[50] Studies by Goidl et al[37] indicate that ageing, at least in their mouse strains, is associated with changes in both helper and suppressor T-cell function. In addition to these effects of the interaction of subpopulations of T-cells and the new findings on B-suppressor cells, the influence of the age-related changes in the carrier-primed T-cell fraction on hapten-primed B-cells have been studied.[51] The T-cell population proved to be greatly deficient in old mice. An aberration in this interaction is compatible with normal figures for total numbers of T- and B-cells.[52]

Reaction to mitogens

A number of recent studies have been devoted to the reaction of human and animal T-cells from different age groups to mitogens. Phytohaemagglutinin causes blast formation and proliferation; the latter can be monitored by thymidine incorporation and the effect becomes less prominent in aged mice. Usually this decline is considered to be due to a decrease in the number of reactive cells, but Callard et al[48] believe it to be the result of qualitative changes in these cells. In man results vary. Weiner et al[19] reported a decreased response in the elderly, but this was not found by Halbrecht et al.[18] These differences may be due to unknown factors affecting the selection of subjects. Numbers of individuals studied in these investigation are usually small, and the definition of health in the elderly is arbitrary. Ben-Zwi et al[53] mention the effect of spontaneous proliferation in the aged, and decreased values for the stimulation index might be expected with these increased background values. Preumont et al[54] observed a decreased binding of actinomycin by lymphocytes from aged persons after PHA stimulation, and they explain this phenomenon by an age-induced structural alteration of chromatin.

The effects of concanavalin-A have been investigated in mice by Abraham et al[13] who confirmed that the decreased response was due to reduced numbers of reactive cells. A decreased reaction has now also been found in aged rats,[14] not only with spleen lymphocytes, but also with lymphoctyes from the peripheral blood. In man, no age-related effects have been published,[18,53] but Antel et al[55] found the suppressor effect exerted by concanavalin-A activated T-cells to be greater in the elderly than in young adults, whereas Hallgren and Yunis[50] mention a variable loss of suppressor activity following concanavolin-A administration. Recent figures for pokeweed, which is a mitogen in man for both B- and T-cells, fail to show significant differences between old and young persons[18] or give small differences which are statistically lower in old than in young people.[19] In mice, the T-dependent one-way mixed lymphocyte reaction does show an age-dependent decrease,[56] most probably due to a reduced number of responding cells and not to altered cell sensitivity or to any changes in the cell cycle. Hirano and Nordin[57] found an age-associated decline in the development of cytotoxic lymphocytes in the in vitro mixed lymphoctye culture not only in the short-lived autoimmune NZB mice, but also in control mice of the DBA strain. There was no relationship between the decrease in cytotoxicity and the frequency of autoantibodies against erythrocytes, which are the hallmark of the NZB animals.

Tolerance and autoimmunity

At first sight the age-related decrease of the immune response is difficult to reconcile with the concomitant increase in the appearance of autoantiobdies, but the paradox is more apparent than real in such a complex system. A decreased function in a subset of cells may lead to an imbalance in such a way than another subset may respond with increased activity. Weigle and Parks[58] have recently introduced a new model to study the results of age on tolerance by analysing the different effects of the administration of lipopolysaccharide, in its twin capacity as a mitogen and polyclonal activator. The latter activity was undisturbed in two-year-old A/J mice, but was markedly decreased in the autoimmune NZB animals. These results could indicate a defect on the B-cell level. Cantor et al[41] conclude that the development of autoimmunity in this strain is associated with an absence of feedback suppression due to the absence or malfunction of a T-cell subset. In man, Hallgren and Yunis[50] associate the increased frequency of autoantibodies on ageing with a decline in a suppressive effect of concanavalin-A activated lymphocytes. Again, generalisations should be avoided. MacIntosh and Segre[59] report that the minimum tolerizing dose is ten times higher in young than in old mice, but when the thymus-dependent system is involved this conclusion is only applicable to the IgM response.

GENERAL CONSIDERATIONS

There is increasing evidence that the thymus is the major organ controlling the age-associated decline of immune function. Recent evidence shows that the B-system is also involved. This should not be surprising, since ageing is associated with a functional decline of all organs and systems. Precise information on the location of the immunological defects is of more than academic interest, since - among other considerations - it would be an essential requirement for any attempt at immunoengineering.[60] This task may be more complicated than used to be thought because multiple causes for the age-related decline would need to be taken into account.[31] Immunosenescence cannot be regarded as a single process; indeed it probably results from a number of different processes, many of them interrelated, which may occur simultaneously or separately. This multiplicity may call for multiple solutions of great sophistication, and is in line with growing awareness of the complexity of the immune system. It has been the subject of a recent review by Jerne,[61] in which he distinguishes four interacting levels: the B-system, the network, the T-system and the histocompatibility complex. This scheme could be very helpful to the immunogerontologist in planning his experiments, because each level should yield useful data. On the first level, that of the B-cells, there is a need to investigate the position of IgD because of its role in the development of tolerance during ontogeny.[62] On the second level, it can be asked if the network still operates adequately in the aged individual. And on the third level, now that the thymus is recognised as holding a central position in immunosenescence, we need to know if this decreased activity is due to a local autonomous process. The pituitary-thyroid axis has been referred to in this respect[63,64] and Kay[40] mentions the neuroendocrine system as the most probable extrathymic site for the central control mechanism.

Finally, at the fourth level, there is the major histocompatibility complex, a cluster of genes, which influences a large number of immunological activities. From observations on survival patterns of congeneic mice, Smith and Walford[65] have derived direct evidence that this complex exerts an effect on ageing. Their conclusions should stimulate further studies on the genetic aspects of the immune response, as related to ageing. This is not an easy task to perform in man, and it calls for longitudinal studies of certain genetic types. However, the recent report by Greenberg and Yunis,[66] who showed that women with a specific haplotype have a survival disadvantage, illustrates that short-term studies may also be rewarding.

DISCUSSION

Several of the main features of ageing in the immunological system were emphasised in discussion - notably that while there is no decrease in total immunoglobulin, thymus-dependent antibody levels are very much reduced with age, and antibody variance markedly increased. As noted earlier, this increase in variance has been postulated as a characteristic feature of ageing in general - though it is hard, at first sight, to see how it might be applied to the lens, which Jan Pontén cited as a classic example of ageing, largely on the grounds that its loss of elastricity is so consistent. However, more detailed examination could well reveal greater variance between ageing inelastic lenses than among younger flexible ones. Indeed, variance of molecular structure - corresponding to that in immunoglobulins - might prove to underlie the consistent loss of lens elasticity with age. This would fit well with Willi Hijmans' point that as various measures of function decrease with age, there is a striking increase in the coefficient of variation - the pooled variants for different observations rising from a figure of 10 to about 4 000.

Another immunological aspect of ageing, in the so-called 'natural killer cell', was described by Eva Klein. These recently discovered cells can kill cetain cell-lines. For example, spleen cells from a non-immunised animal or any sample of human blood will kill a certain proportion of the tumour cells in culture. This apparently non-specific process is now thought to be an important contributor to immunosurveillance in vivo. That has yet to be confirmed in man, but the activity of 'natural killer cells' is known to be age-dependent and genetically determined in mice, with a peak at about four months of age followed by decline. These cells are believed to play a part in immunosurveillance because thymusless nude mice do not come down with tumours, apparently thanks to 'natural killer cells' acting against incipient tumours and thus compensating, at least in part, for the other immunological deficiencies of this strain. The killer cells appear to be immature T-cells but it is not yet clear how they recognise tumour cells or what constituents they are directed against. It may seem paradoxical, as Eva Klein said, that thymusless nude mice should have immature T-cells, but that has been confirmed. And the fact that they not only possess anti-tumour activity but also decline with age could be relevant to two main themes of the foregoing papers - increasing susceptibility to tumours and ageing of the immune system.

The discovery of 'natural killer cells' should be seen in the context that T-cells in general have fallen into disfavour as mediators of immunosurveillance, if indeed that concept proves valid. Their role is in question because, in addition to the observations in nude mice, patients receiving immunusuppressant therapy do not suffer the plethora of tumours that would be expected if T-cell mediated immunosurveillance were a major protective mechanism. Another question, raised by Leslie Brent, is how the 'natural killer cells' - assumed to be immature T-cells - come to be present in nude mice with virtually no thymus and scarcely any T-cells. Where do they come from? Is the term thymus derived (or T) cell, a misnomer here? In reply, Eva Klein pointed out that while normal maturation of T-cells is thymus-dependent, they are originally derived from stem-cells in the bone marrow. In thymusless mice they do not mature to become T-cells but do apparently acquire the capacity to kill tumour cells non-discriminantly. Further research into the mechanisms of this action should reveal - among other things - why 'natural killer cells' do not attack foreign feto-placental tissue equally non-discriminately, at least in thymusless mice. Whether immature T-cells are as active in man and what functions they normally perform (apart from being T-cell precursrs) are other unanswered questions.

Discussing the evolution of T-cells, Guy Voisin drew attention to age-related changes in another population: the suppressor T-cells. The level of thymic hormones decreases with age, earlier in NZB mice than with other strains, at about the time suppressor T-cells decrease in number and activity - and autoimmune reactions develop. These are attributed to the declining protective effect of suppressor T-cell which would otherwise prevent the appearance of autoantibody. Whether this interpretation is correct remains to be seen. But meanwhile Hamish Munro wanted to know if the ageing defects in the immune system could be attributed primarily to impairment of cell division or to diminished cell function, such as the capacity to synthesise thymusine. Willi Hijmans had no doubt that thymic function decreases as shown by diminished production of thymusine in older animals. Moreover, Leslie Brent reported that a three-to-fourfold increase in the number of B-cells had been described in old mice. So there is no shortage of such cells, nor does there appear to be any problem in their maturation. The lesion seems to arise at a later stage, either during the activation process, or during interaction between B and T lymphocytes - but not associated with a decline in the proliferative powers of the B lymphocytes. However, Guy Voisin described a strong correlation between the decrease of number of T-cells and the decrease in thymic hormone, which appears to be secreted not by lymphocytes but by epithelial cells in the thymus. Since this hormone seems to be necessary for the maturation of T-cells, that might be the site of the defect. As regards thymic involution, which is not well-documented in the mouse, this has recently been shown to be localised in the cortex of the thymus, and associated with an impressive decrease in the number of mature T-cells.

That involution of the thymus takes place during pregnancy was pointed out by Maxwell Anderson, who quoted observations in inbred mice, in outbred rats, and to an extent in man. Is this widespread phenomenon, he asked, evidence that pregnancy might be regarded as resembling and perhaps contributing to ageing? Certainly there is decreased activity of the immune system during pregnancy, but - as detailed in the previous section - there are also many immunosuppressive factors active in pregnancy which appear to distinguish it immunologically from ageing. Perhaps the most obvious distinguishing factor is that the pregnancy changes are reversible, though - as Page Faulk indicated - the thymus involution does continue for as long as the mother breast-feeds the baby. A major influence to which Dorothy Villee drew attention is the powerful immunosuppressive action of adrenal glucocorticoids, whose production is increased in pregnancy. This relationship was supported by Guy

Voisin on the grounds that the number of lymphocytes in pregnancy and the changes in the thymus resemble those obtained in animals treated with corticoids. Another immunological feature of pregnancy, mentioned by Maxwell Anderson, is hyperplasia in the lymph nodes draining the pregnant uterus and those in certain other areas, notably the renal nodes. The significance of these diverse observations and their relationship with feto-placental immunology are fields crying out for further research and clarification, irrespective of any possible link with ageing.

Noting the age-related immunological changes now recognised in mice and in man which appear to represent a downward drift in responsiveness, Leslie Brent wondered whether this makes old people more susceptible to infectious diseases such as pneumonia. But, while agreeing that the incidence of pneumonia is age-related, Willi Hijmans thought there was no clinical or experimental evidence that old people are immune deficient and more subject to infection for that reason. The overwhelming majority of infections in older subjects, animal or man, can be explained by stasis - examples being prostatic enlargement, emphysema and pulmonary congestion - and he stressed that there is no deficiency in the immune response towards pneumococci. Hamish Munro agreed that loss of power in the intercostal muscles, preventing proper ventilation, must be a major aetiological factor in the pneumonias of old age. However, malnutrition might also play a part, and that could impair the immune response. Many old people, especially those with intercurrent infections, respond poorly to surface antigens, but improve when given vigorous nutritional support. Similarly, cancer patients with cachexia often show poor responses to antigenic stimulation but can be brought into a more responsive state by nutritional measures, enabling them to withstand operation, radiation, or chemotherapy much more positively. It should not however be assumed, as Willi Hijmans pointed out, that there is any age-related decline in immune responsiveness to malignant tumours - though autoimmune conditions and those involving immune complexes may be affected by ageing. He concluded by generalising from these observations to stress the need for precise methods of studying immune responsiveness in a wide range of different clinical and experimental circumstances. A start has been made with immune complexes but much remains to be done - painstakingly, step by step, for the many complexes already recognised as well as those yet to be identified. For all the rapid expansion of immunological knowledge in recent years, we still lack basic information on many of its aspects and cannot yet put the whole picture of humoral and cellular immune responses together - except by way of hypothesis. Research into ageing has not even reached that point. To what extent placental research can help to fill in the details or clarify the overall picture in these important fields remains to be seen.

REFERENCES TO SECTION IV

THE PLACENTA AS A MODEL FOR ORGAN AGEING

Harold Fox

1 Hayflick, L. and Moorhead, P. S. (1961). The serial cultivation of human diploid cell strains. Exp. Cell. Res. 25, 585.

2 Carrel, A. (1912). On the permanent life of tissues outside of the organism. J. Exp. Med. 15, 516.

3 Hayflick, L. (1965). The limited in vitro lifetime of human diploid cell strains. Exp. Cell. Res. 37, 614.

4 Holliday, R. (1975). Growth and death of diploid and transformed human fibroblasts. Federation Proceedings 34, 51.

5 Strehler, B., Hirsch, G., Gusseck, D., Johnson, R., and Bick, M. (1971). Condon-restriction theory of aging and development. J. Theor. Biol. 33,429.

6 von Hahn, H. P., (1966). A model of regulatory aging of the cell at the gene level. J. Geront. 21. 129.

7 von Hahn, H. P., (1970). The regulation of protein synthesis in the aging cell. Exp. Geront. 5, 323.

8 Krooth, R. S., (1974). A deterministic mechanism for cellular and organismic ageing. J. Theor. Biol. 46, 501.

9 Epstein, J., Williams, J. R. and Little, J. B. (1974). Rate of DNA repair in progeric and normal human fibroblasts. Biochem. Biophys. Res. Comm. 59,850.

10 Mattern, M. R., and Cerutti, P. A. (1975). Age dependant excision repair of damaged thymine from X-irradiated DNA by isolated nuclei from human fibroblasts. Nature, 254, 450.

11 Little, J. B. (1976). Relationship between DNA repair capacity and cellular ageing. Gerontology, 22, 28.

12 Curtis, H. J., (1971). Genetic factors in aging. Adv. Genet. 16, 305.

13 Medvedev, Z. A. (1971). Repetition of molecular-genetic information as a possible factor in evolutionary changes in life span. Exp. Gerontol. 7, 227.

14 Orgel, L. E. (1963). The maintenance of the accuracy of protein synthe is and its relevance to ageing. Proc. Nat. Acad. Sci. U.S.A. 49, 517.

15 Orgel, L. E. (1973). Ageing of clones of mammalian cells. Nature, 243, 441.

16 Holliday, R. (1975). Testing the protein error theory of aging. Gerontologia, 21, 64.

17 Holliday, R., Huschtscha, L. I., Tarrant, G. M., and Kirkwood, T. B. L., (1977). Testing the committment theory of cellular aging. Science, 198, 366.

18 Kirkwood, T. B. L., (1977). Evolution of ageing. Nature, 270, 301.

19 Kohn, R. R. (1971). Principles of mammalian aging. Prentice-Hall, Inc. Englewood Cliffs, New Jersey.

20 Jackson, D. S. (1973). Some difficulties of the cross-linking theory of ageing of collagen. In Connective Tissue and Ageing Ed. Vogel, H.G. p.191 Excerpta Medica, Amsterdam.

21 Walford, R. L., (1974). Immunologic theory of aging: current status. Fed. Proc. 33, 2020.

22 Harman, D. (1956). Aging: a theory based on free radical and radiation chemistry. J. Geront. 11, 298.

23 Harman, D. (1969). Prolongation of life: role of free radical reactions in aging. J. Amer. Geriat. Soc. 17, 721.

24 Sheldrake, A. R., (1974). The ageing, growth and death of cells. Nature, 250 381.

25 Everitt, A. V., (1973). The hypothalamic-pituitary control of ageing and age-related pathology. Exp. Geront, 8, 265.

26 Lewis, C. M., and Tarrant, G. M., (1972). Error theory and aging in human diploid fibroblasts. Nature, 239, 316.

27 Hayflick, L. (1973). The biology of human aging, Amer. J. Med. Sci. 265, 433.

28 Hayflick, L. (1975). Current theories of biological aging, Fed. Proc. 34, 9.

29 Hayflick, L. (1976). The cell biology of human aging, New Engl.J. Med. 295, 1302.

30 Comfort, A. (1974). The position of aging studies. Mech. Age. Develop. 3, 1.

31 Baird, M. B. and Massie, H. R., (1975). A further note on the Orgel hypothesis and senescence. Gerontologia 21, 240.

32 Gershon, D. and Gershon, H. (1976). An evaluation of the "error catastrophe" theory of ageing in light of recent experimental results. Gerontology, 22, 212.

33 Choe, B-K., and Rose, N. R., (1976). In vitro senescence of mammalian cells. Gerontology, 22, 89.

34 Dreyfus, J-C., Rubinson, H., Schapira, F., Weber, A., Marie, J. and Khan, A. (1977). A possible molecular mechanism of ageing. Gerontology, 23, 211.

35 Martin, G. M., (1977a). Cellular aging - clonal senescence: a review (Part 1). Amer. J. Path. 89, 484.

36 Martin, G. M., (1977b). Cellular aging - postreplicative cells: a review (Part 2). Amer. J. Path. 89, 513.

37 Martin, G. M., Sprague, C. A., and Epstein, C. J., (1970). Replicative life span of cultivated human cells. J. Lab. Invest. 23, 86.

38 Cristofalo, V. J., (1972). Animal cell cultures as a model system for the study of aging . Adv. Geront. Res. 4, 45.

39 Le Guilly, Y., Simon, M., Lenoir, P., and Bourel, M. (1973). Long term culture of human adult liver cells: morphological changes related to in vitro senescence and effect of donors age on growth potential. Gerontologia, 19, 303.

40 Schneider, E. L., Chase, G. A., (1976). Relationship between age of donor and in vitro life span of human diploid fibroblasts. Interdiscipl. Topics Geront. 10, 62.

41 Goldstein, S., Moerman, E. J., Soeloner, J. S.. Gleason, R. E. and Barnett, D.M. (1978). Chronologic and physiologic age affect replicative life-span of fibroblasts from diabetic, prediabetic and normal donors. Science, 199, 781.

42 Puck, T. T., Waldren, C. A. and Jones, C. (1968). Growth stimulation by fetulin. Proc. Nat. Acad. Sci. U.S.A. 59, 192.

43 Buetow, D. E. (1971). Cellular content and cellular proliferation changes in the tissues and organs of the aging mammal. In Cellular and molecular renewal in the mammalian body Ed. Cameron, I.L. and Thrasher, J.O. p.87, Academic Press, New York and London.

44 Reincke, U., Burlington, H., Cronkite, E. P., and Laissue, J. (1975). Hayflick's hypothesis: an approach to in vivo testing, Fed. Proc. 34, 71.

45 Franks, L. M. (1974). Ageing in differentiated cells. Gerontologia, 20, 51.

46 McMillan J. B. and Lev, M. (1964). The aging heart. II The valves, J. Geront. 19, 1.

47 Angrist, A. (1964). Aging heart valves and a unitary pathological hypothesis for aging. J. Geront. 19, 135,

48 Ungar, H. and Ben-Ishay, Z., (1965). Rheumatic and age changes of the heart in Israel. Israel J. Med. Sci. 1; 50.

49 Davies, M. J. and Pomerance, A., (1972). Quantitative study of ageing changes in the human sinoatrial node and internodal tracts. Brit. Heart. J. 34, 150.

50 Harris, R. (1975). Cardiac changes with age. In The Physiology and Pathology of Human Aging. Ed. Golaman,R. and Rockstein, M. p. 109, Academic Press, New York, San Francisco, London.

51 Reiner, L., Mazzoleni, A. Rodriguez, F. L. and Freudenthal, R. R. (1959). The weight of the human heart. I. "normal" cases. Arch. Path. 68. 58.

52 Brody, H. (1955). Organisation of the cerebral cortex. III A study in ageing in human cerebral cortex. J. Comp. Neurol. 102, 511.

53 von Hahn, H. P. (1966). Distribution of DNA and RNA in the brain during the life span of the albino rat. Gerontologia, 12, 18.

54 Franks, L. M., Wilson, P. D. and Whelan, R. D., (1974). The effects of age on total DNA and cell number in the mouse brain. Gerontologia, 20, 21.

55 Vijayashankar, N. and Brody, H. (1972). The neuronal population of the nuclei of the trochlear nerve and the locus caerulus in the human. Anat. Rec. 172, 421.

56 Monagle, B. D. and Brody, H., (1974). The effects of age upon the main nucleus of the inferior olive in the human. J. Comp. Neurol. 155, 61.

57 Brody, H., (1976). An examination of cerebral cortex and brain stem aging. In Neurobiology of Aging, Ed. Terry, R. D. p.177, Raven Press, New York.

58 Andrew, W., Brown, H. M. and Johnson, J. B. (1943). Senile changes in the liver of mouse and man, with special reference to the similarity of the nuclear alterations. Amer. J. Anat. 72, 199.

59 Bachmann, K. -D., (1953). Uber das lipofuscin der Leber. Virchows Archiv. 323, 133.

60 Carr, R. D., Smith, M. J. and Keil, P.G. (1960). The liver in the aging process. Arch. Path. 70, 1.

61 Hollander, C. F., (1970). Model systems in experimental gerontology. Ned. T. Geront. 1, 144.

62 Pieri, C., Nagy, I. Z., Mazzyfferi, G. and Giuli, C. (1975). The aging of rat liver as revealed by electron microscopic morphometry. 1. Basic parameters. Exp. Geront. 10, 291.

63 Schmucker, D. L. (1976). Age related changes in hepatic fine structure: a quantitative analysis. J. Geront. 31, 135.

64 Andrew, W., (1962). An electron microscope study of age changes in the liver of the mouse. Amer. J. Anat. 110, 1.

65 Hasan, M., and Glees, P. (1973). Ultrastructural age changes in hippocampal neurons, synapses and neuroglia. Exp. Geront. 8, 75.

66 Johnson, J. and Miquel, J. (1974). Fine structural changes in the lateral vestibular nucleus of aging rats. Mech. Ageing Dev. 3, 203.

67 Sachs, H. G., Colgan, J. A. and Lazarus, M. L. (1977). Ultrastructure of the aging myocardium: a morphometric approach. Amer. J. Anat. 150, 63.

68 Brock, M. and Hay, R. (1971). Comparative ultrastructure of chick fibroblasts in vitro at early and late stages during their growth span. J. Ultrastruct. Res. 36, 291.

69 Lipetz, J. and Cristofalo, V., (1972). Ultrastructural changes accompanying the aging of human diploid cells in culture. J. Ultrastruct. Res. 39, 43.

70 Tonna, E., (1974). Electron microscopy of aging skeletal ceus. III The periosteum. Lab. Invest., 31, 609.

71 Field, E. and Peat, A., (1971). Intranuclear inclusions in neurons and glia: a study in aging mice. Gerontologia, 17, 129.

72 Mann, D. M. A., Yates, P. O. and Stamp, J. E. (in press). The relationship between lipofuscin pigment and ageing in the human nervous system. J. Neurol. Sci.

73 Adamstone, F. B. and Taylor, A. B. (1972). Nucleolar reorganization in epithelial cells of the jejunum of the rat. J. Morphol. 136, 131.

74 Schmucker, D. L., Mooney, J. S. and Jones, A. L. (1977). Age related changes in the hepatic endoplasmic reticulum: a quantitative analysis. Science, 197, 1005.

75 Moog, F. (1977). The small intestine in old mice: growth, alkaline phosphatase and disaccharidase activities, and deposition of amyloid. Exp. Geront. 12, 223.

76 Tomanek, R. J. and Karlsson, U. L. (1973). Myocardial ultrastructure of young and senescent rats. J. Ultrastruct. Res. 42, 201.

77 Cristofalo, V. J., Parris, N. and Kritchevsky, D. (1967). Enzyme activity during the growth and aging of human cells in vitro. J. Cell. Physiol. 69, 263.

78 Sekhon, S. T. and Maxwell, D. S. (1974). Ultrastructural changes in neurones of the spinal anterior horn of ageing mice with particular reference to the accumulation of lipofuscin pigment. J. Neurocytol. 3, 59.

79 Giuli, C., Pieri, C. and Nagy, I. Zs. (1977). Age-dependent changes of the protein synthetic machinery of liver cell cytoplasm as revealed by electron microscopic morphometry. Aktuel. Geront. 7, 547.

80 Ohnishi, H., Tsukada, S., Hayashi, Y, Ogawa, N., Yajima, G., Masugi, Y., Aihara, K. and Suzuki, K. (1972). Effects of cytochrome C on liver functions of old rats. Nature New Biol. 239, 84.

81 Tauchi, H. and Sato, T. (1968). Age changes in size and number of mitochondria of human hepatic cells. J. Geront. 23, 454.

82 Samorajski, T., Friede, R. L. and Ordy, J. M. (1971). Age differences in the ultrastructure of axons in the pyramidal tract of the mouse. J. Geront. 26,542.

83 Wilson, P. D. and Franks, L. M. (1975). The effect of age on mitochondrial ultrastructure. Gerontologia 21, 81.

84 Herbener, G. H. (1976). A morphometric study of age-dependent changes in mitochondrial populations of mouse liver and heart. J. Geront. 31, 8.

85 Tate, E. L. and Herbener, G. H. (1976). A morphometric study of the density of mitochondrial cristae in heart and liver of aging mice. J. Geront. 31,129.

86 Khent, A., Leibetseder, J. and Burger, H. (1966). Gerontologische Untersuchungen an Rattenherzmitochondien. Gerontologia, 12, 193.

87 Sato, T. and Tauchi, H. (1975). The formation of giant mitochondria in the ageing process of human hepatic cells. Acta Path. Jap. 25, 403.

88 Brunk, U., and Brun, A. (1972). The effect of aging on lysosomal permeability in nerve cells of the central nervous system, and enzyme histochemical study in the rat. Histochemie, 30, 315.

89 Bondareff, W. G. (1957). Genesis of intracellular pigment in the spinal ganglia of senile rats: an electron microscopic study. J. Geront. 12, 364.

90 Malkoff, D. and Strehlet, B. (1963). The ultrastructure of isolated and in situ human cardiac age pigment. J. Cell. Biol. 16, 611.

91 Samorajski, J., Ordy, J. M. and Keefe, J. R. (1965). The fine structure of lipofuscin age pigment in the nervous system of aged mice. J. Cell Biol. 26, 779.

92 Few, A. and Getty, R. (1967). Occurrence of lipofuscin as related to aging in the canine and porcine nervous system. J. Geront. 22, 357.

93 Samorajski, T., Ordy, J. M. and Rady-Reimer, P. (1968). Lipofuscin pigment accumulation in the nervous system of aging mice. Anat. Rec. 160, 555.

94 Reichel, W., Hollander, J., Clarke, J. M. and Strehler, B. L. (1968). Lipofuscin accumulation as a function of age and distribution in the rodent brain. J. Geront. 23, 71.

95 Sekhon, S. S., Andrews, J. M. and Maxwell, D. S. (1969). Accumulation and development of lipofuscin pigment in the aging central nervous system of the mouse. J. Cell Biol. 43, 123a.

96 Fawcett, D. and McNutt, N. (1969). The ultrastructure of the cat myocardium I. ventricular papillary muscle. J. Cell Biol. 42, 1.

97 Brizzee, K. R. and Johnson, F. A. (1970). Depth distribution of lipofuscin in cerebral cortex of albino rat. Acta Neuropath. 16, 205.

98 Nanda, B. S., and Getty, K. (1973). Occurrence of aging pigment (lipofuscin) in the nuclei and cortices of the canine brain. Exp. Geront. 8, 1.

99 Mann, D., and Yates, P. O. (1974). Lipoprotein pigments - their relationship to ageing in the human nervous system. I. The lipofuscin content of nerve cells. Brain, 97, 481.

100 Smarajski, T. and Ordy, J. M. (1967). The histochemistry and ultrastructure of lipid pigment in the adrenal glands of aging mice. J. Geront. 22, 253.

101 Tonna, E. A. (1975). Accumulation of lipofuscin (age pigment) in aging skeletal connective tissues as revealed by electron microscopy. J. Geront. 30, 3.

102 Ives, P. J., Haensley, W. A., Maxwell, P. A. and McArthur, N. H. (1975). A histochemical and ultrastructural study of lipofuscin accumulation in thyroid follicular cells of aging domestic cats. Mech. Age. Dev. 4, 399.

103 Miquel, J., Lundgren, P. R. and Johnson, J. E. (1978). Spectron photometric and electron microscopic studies of lipofuscin accumulation in the testes of aging mice. J. Geront. 33, 5.

104 Whiteford, R., and Getty, R. (1966). Distribution of lipofuscin in the canine and porcine brain as related to ageing. J. Geront. 21, 31.

105 Barden, H. (1970). Relationship of golgi thiamine-pyrophosphatase and lysosomal acid phosphatase to neuromelanin and lipofuscin in cerebral neurones of the aging rhesus monkey. J. Neuropath. Exp. Neurol. 29, 225.

106 Strehler, B. L. (1964). On the histochemistry and ultrastructure of age pigment. Adv. Geront. Res. 1, 343.

107 Toth, S. E. (1968). The origin of lipofuscin age pigment. Exp. Geront. 3, 19.

108 Glees, P. and Gopinath, G. (1973). Age changes in the centrally and peripherally located sensory neurones in rat. Zschr. Zellforsch Mikroskop. Anat. 141, 285.

109 Aune, J. (1976). Ultrastructural changes with age. Interdiscipl. Topics Geront. 10, 44.

110 Haden, H., and Lindstrom, B. (1955). Microspectrographic studies on the yellow pigment in nerve cells. Dis. Faraday Soc. 9, 436.

111 Grinna, L. S. (1977). Changes in cell membrane during aging. Gerontology, 23, 452.

112 Sulkin, N. M. and Sulkin, D. F. (1967). Age differences in response to chronic hypoxia on the fine structure of cardiac muscle and autonomic ganglian cell. J. Geront. 22, 485.

113 Goldfisher, S. and Bernstein, I. (1969). Lipofuscin (aging) pigment granules of the human newborn liver. J. Cell Biol. 42, 253.

114 Goldman, R. (1971). Decline in organ function with aging, In Clinical Geriatrics. Ed. Rossman, I. p.19. Lippincott, Philadelphia, Toronto.

115 Hall, D. A., (1973). Metabolic and structural aspects of aging. In Textbook of Geriatric Medicine and Gerontology Ed.Brocklehurst, J.C., p.17, Churchill Livingstone, Edinburgh and London.

116 Reiner, J. M. (1947). The effect of age on the carbohydrate metabolism of tissue homogenases. J. Geront. 2, 315.

117 Patel, M. S. (1977). Age-dependent changes in the oxidative metabolism in rat brain. J. Geront. 32, 643.

118 Lassen, N. A., Geinberg, I and Lane, M. H. (1960). Bilateral studies of cerebral oxygen uptake in young and aged normal subjects and in patients with organic dementia. J. Clin. Invest. 39, 491.

119 Michenfelder, J. D. and Theye, R. A. (1969). The relationship of age to canine cerebral metabolic rate. J. Surg. Res. 9, 645.

120 Ferendelli, J. A., Sedgwick, W. G. and Suntzeff, V. (1971). Regional energy metabolism and lipofuscin accumulation in mouse brain during aging. J. Neuropath. Exp. Neurol. 30, 638.

121 Fox, J. H., Parmacek, M. S. and Patel-Manolik, K. (1975). Effect of aging on brain respiration and carbohydrate metabolism of syrian hamsters. Gerontologia, 21, 224.

122 Garbus, J. (1955). Respiration of brain homogenates of old and young rats Amer. J. Phsiol. 183, 618.

123 Weinbach, E. C. and Garbus, J. (1956). Age and oxidative phosphorylation in rat liver and brain. Nature, 178, 1226.

124 Barrett, M. C. and Horton, A. (1976). Age related changes in the respiratory control of rat liver mitochondria after brief exposure to hypo-osmotic medium. Biochem. Soc. Trans. 4, 64.

125 Wilson, P. D., Hill. B. T. and Franks, L. M. (1976). The effect of age on mitochondrial enzymes and respiration. Gerontology, 21, 95.

126 van Bezooijen, C. F. A., van Noord, M. J. and Knook, D. L. (1974). The viability of parenchymal liver cells isolated from young and old rats. Mech. Age. Devel. 3, 107.

127 Gold, P. H., Gee, M. V. and Strehler, B. S. (1968). Effect of age on oxidative phosphorylation in the rat. J. Geront. 23, 509.

128 Chen, J. C., Warshaw, J. B. and Sanadi, D. R. (1972). Regulation of mitochondiral respiration in senescence. J. Cell Physiol. 80, 141.

129 Inamdar, A. R., Person, R., Kohnen, P., Duncan, H. and Mackler, B. (1974). Effect of age on oxidative phosphorylation in tissues of hamsters. J. Geront. 29, 638.

130 Brouwer, A. et al. (1977). Respiration activities of hepatocytes isolated from rats of various ages : a brief report. Mech. Age. Develop. 6, 265.

131 Sokoloff, L. (1975). Cerebral circulation and metabolism in the aged. In Aging Ed. Gershon, S. and Rastin, A., Vol. 2. p. 627 Raven Press, New York.

131a Mainwaring, W. I. P. (1969). The effect of age on protein synthesis in mouse liver. Biochem. J. 113, 869.

132 Hrachovec, J. P. (1971). The effect of age on tissue protein synthesis. Age changes in amino acid incorporation by rat liver purified microsomes. Gerontologia, 17, 75.

133 Bustow, D. E. and Ghandi, P. S. (1973). Decreased protein synthesis by microsomes isolated from senescent rat liver. Exp. Geront. 8, 243.

134 Chen, J. C., Ove, P. and Lansing, A. I. (1973). In vitro synthesis of microsomal protein and albymin in aging and old rats. Biochem. Biophys. Acta, 312, 598.

135 Blok, L. N., Krasnitskaya, A. A., Anokhina, G. A. and Nitkin, V. N. (1974). Protein synthesis in a cell free system by microsomes of normal membranes of the liver of rats of different ages. Dokl. Biochem. 217, 340.

136 Beauchene, R. E., Roeder, L. M. and Barrows, C. H. (1970). The interrelationships of age tissue protein synthesis and proteinuria. J. Geront. 25, 359.

137 Du, J. T., Beyer, T. A. and Lang, C. A. (1977). Protein biosynthesis in aging mouse tissues. Exp. Geront. 12, 181.

138 van Bezooijen, C. F. A., Greu, T. and Knook, D. L. (1977). The effect of age on protein synthesis by isolated liver parenchymal cells. Mech. Age. Develop. 6, 293.

139 Ove, P., Obenrader, M. and Lansing, A. (1972). Synthesis and degradation of liver proteins in young and old rats. Biochim. Biophys. Acta 277, 211.

140 Wulff, V. J., Samis, H. V. and Falzone, J.A. (1967). The metabolism of ribonucleic acid in young and old rodents. Adv. Geront. Res. 2, 37.

141 Kanungo, M. S., Koul, O. and Reddy, K. R. (1970). Concomitant sutdies of RNA and protein synthesis in tissues of rats of various ages. Exp. Geront. 5, 261.

142 Szeszak, F., Corradetti, E., and Nagy, I. Z. (1977). Age-dependent alterations of the rate of RNA synthesis in rat brain cell nuclei. Aktuel. Geront. 7, 231.

143 McCreight, C. and Sulkin, N. (1959). Cellular proliferation in the kidneys of young and senile rats following unilateral nephrectomy. J. Geront. 14, 440.

144 Post, J. and Hoffman, J. (1964). Changes in the replication times and patterns of the liver cell during the life of the rat. Exp. Cell. Res. 36,111.

145 Cameron, I. L. and Thrasher, J. D. (1976). Cell renewal and cell loss in the tissues of aging mammals. Interdiscipl. Topics Geront. 10, 108.

146 Litvak, R. and Baserga, R. (1964). An auto-radiographic study of the uptake of 3H-thymidine by kidney cells of mice at different ages. Exp. Cell Res. 33, 540.

147 Thrasher, J. (1967). Age and the cell cycle of the mouse colonic epithelium. Anat. Rec. 157, 621.

148 Thrasher, J. (1971). Age and the cell cycle of the mouse esophageal epithelium. Exp. Geront. 6, 19.

149 Lesher, S., Fry, R. and Kohn, H. (1961). Age and the generation time of the mouse duodenal epithelial cell. Exp. Cell Res. 24, 334.

150 Lesher, S., Fry, R. and Kohn, H. (1961). Aging and the generation cycle of intestinal epithelial cells in the mouse. Gerontologia, 5, 176.

151 Lesher, S. and Sacher, G. (1968). Effects of age on cell proliferation in mouse duodenal crypts. Exp. Geront. 3, 211.

152 Mayer, J., Marwah, A. and Weinmann, J. (1956). Mitotic rate of gingival epithelium in two age groups. J. Invest. Derm. 27, 237.

153 Thrasher, J. and Katzberg, A. (1959). The effect of age on mitosis in the human epidermis, J. Invest. Derm. 33, 35.

154 Slonim, A. and Bedrack, E. (1977). Activity of enzymes associated with the biosynthesis of testosterone by gonads of the old mouse. Exp. Geront.12, 35.

155 Chap, Z. and Bedrak, E. (1977). In vitro testosterone synthesis by testicular tissue of old mouse: the metabolism of 3μ -hydroxy-5-ene steroids. Exp. Geront. 12, 43.

156 Guisti, G., Gonnelli, P., Borrelli, D., Fiorelli, G., Gorm. G., Pazzagli, M. and Serco, M. (1975). Age-related secretion of androstenodione, testosterone and dihyorotestosterone by the human testis. Exp. Geront. 5, 241.

157 Finch, C. E. (1972). Enzyme activities, gene function and ageing in mammals (a review). Exp. Geront. 7, 53.

158 Wilson, P. D. (1973). Enzyme changes in ageing mammals. Gerontologia, 19, 79.

159 Rothstein, M. (1975). Aging and the alteration of enzymes: a review. Mech. Age, Dev. 4, 325.

160 Rothstein, M. (1977). Recent developments in the age related alteration of enzymes: a review. Mech. Age. Dev. 6, 241.

161 Zorzoli, A. (1951). The influence of age on mouse liver acid and alkaline phosphatase. J. Geront. 6, 171.

162 Ross, M. H. (1969). Aging, nutrition and hepatic enzyme activity patterns in the rat. J. Nutrit. 97, Suppl. 1. 565.

163 Wilson, P. D. (.972). Enzyme patterns in young and old mouse livers and lungs. Gerontologia, 18, 36.

164 Surtshin, A. (1957). The influence of age and of renal ischaemia at different levels on renal alkaline phosphatase in the rat. J. Geront. 12, 161.

165 Wilson, P. D. and Franks, L. M. (1971). Enzyme patterns in young and old mouse kidneys. Gerontologia. 17, 16.

166 Bogart, B. I. (1967). The effect of ageing on the histochemistry of the rat submandibular gland. J. Geront. 22, 372.

167 Samorajski, T. and Rolsten, C. (1969). Effect of age on alkaline phosphomonoesterase activity in the adrenals of male mice. Anat. Rec. 163, 473.

168 Suntzeff, V. and Angeletti, P. (1961). Histological and histochemical changes in intestines of mice with aging. J. Geront. 16, 225.

169 Sayeed,M. M. and Blumenthal, H. T. (1968). Age difference in the intestinal phosphomonoesterase activity of mice. Proc. Soc. Exp. Biol. Med. 129, 1.

170 Elens, A. (1969). Age correlated changes in lysosomal enzyme activities: an index of ageing? Exp. Geront. 4, 131.

171 Zorzoli, A. (1955). The influence of age on phosphatase activity in the liver of the mouse. J. Geront. 10, 156.

172 Kurnick, N. B. and Kernen, R. L. (1962). The effect of aging on the deoxyribose nuclease system, body and organ weight and cellular content. J.Geront. 17, 245.

173 Franklin, T. J. (1961). Activity of liver and kidney acid phosphatase at different stages in the life span of the rat. Biochem. J. 79, 34.

174 Ross, M. H. and Ely, J. O. (1954). Aging and enzyme activity. J. Franklin. Inst. 285, 63.

175 Franklin, T. J. (1962). The influence of age on the activity of some acid hydrolases in the rat liver and kidney. Biochem. J. 82, 118.

176 Mainwaring, W. I. P. (1967). The ageing process in the mouse ventral prostate glands: a preliminary biochemical survery. Gerontologia, 13, 177.

177 Ghanadian, R. and Fortherly, K. (1975). Testosterone uptake by prostate tissue from young and old rats. Gerontologia, 21, 211.

178 Höhn, P., Gabbert, H. and Wagner, R. (1978). Differentiasion and aging of the rat intestinal mucosa: morphological, enzyme histochemical and disc electrophoretic aspects of the aging of the small intestinal mucosa. Mech. Age. Develop. 7, 217.

179 Mills, G. T., Paul, J. and Smith, E. E. B. (1953). Studies on u-glucuronidase. III. The influence of age, partial hepatectomy and other factors on the glucuronidase activity of rat liver. Biochem. J. 53, 245.

180 Traurig, H. H. (1976). Lysosomal acid hydrolase activities in the lungs of fetal, neonatal, adult, and senile mice. Gerontology, 22, 419.

181 Barrows, C. H., Falzone, J. H. and Shock, N. W. (1960). Age differences in the succinoxidase activity of homogenates and mitochondria from the livers and kidneys of rats. J. Geront. 15, 130.

182 Leonard, G. L. (1950). Succinic dehydrogenase levels in striated muscle in relation to mice hormone. Endocrinology 47, 260.

183 Barrows, C. H., Yiengst, M. J. and Shock, N. W. (1958). Senescence and metabolism of various tissues of rats, J. Geront. 13, 351.

184 Tonna, E. A. (1959). Post-traumatic variations in phosphatase and respiratory enzyme activities of the periosteum of aging rats. J. Geront. 14, 159.

185 Barrows, C. H., Roeder, L. M. and Flaznne, J. A. (1962). Effect of age on the activities of enzymes and the concentration of nucleic acids in the tissues of female wild rats. J. Geront. 17, 144.

186 Friede, R. L. (1965). Enzyme histochemical studies of senile plaques. J. Neuropath. Exp. Neurol. 24, 277.

187 Limas, C. J. (1971). Aging of the myocardium, Acta Cardiol. 26, 249.

188 Ghiringhelli, E. M. and Gerzeli, G, (1963). Histochemical activities of glandular cells in old rats. J. Geront. 11, 1097.

189 Kanungo, M. S. and Singh, S. N. (1965). Effect of age on the isozymes of lactic dehydrogenase of the heart and the brain of rat. Biochem. Biophys. Res. Commun. 21, 454.

190 Schmukler, M. and Barrows, C. H. (1966). Age differences in lactic and malic dehydrogenases in the rat. J. Geront. 21, 109.

191 Zorzoli, A. and Li, J. B. (1967). Gluconeo-genesis in mouse kidney cortex: effect of age and fasting on glucose production and enzyme activities. J. Geront. 22, 151.

192 Oliveria, R. J. and Pfuderer, P. (1973). Test for missynthesis of lactate dehydrogenase in aging mice by use of a monospecific antibody. Exp. Geront. 8, 193.

193 Lawrie, R. A. (1952). Biochemical differences between red and white muscle. Nature, 170, 122.

194 Singhal, R. L. (1967). Effect of age on the induction of glucose - 6 - phosphatase and fructose - 1, 6 - diphosphatase in rat liver. J. Geront. 22 77.

195 Zorzoli, A. (1962). The influence of age on mouse liver glucose - 6 - phosphatase activity. J. Geront, 17, 359.

196 Singh, S. N. and Kanungo, M. S. (1968). Alterations in lactate dehydrogenase of the brain, heart, skeletal muscle and liver of rats of various ages. J. Biol. Chem. 243, 4526.

197 Wang, R. K. J. and Mays, L. L. (1977). Opposite changes in rat liver glucose - 6 - phosphate dehydrogenase during aging in Sprague-Dawley and Fisher 344 male rats. Exp. Geront. 12, 117.

198 Adelman, R. C. (1976). Age-dependent functional capacities of the mammalian cell: on the maintenance of enzyme adaptation. Interdiscipl. Topics Geront. 9, 2.

199 Kanungo, M. S. (1976). Enzyme patterns and ageing in animals. Interdiscipl. Topics Geront. 10, 100.

200 Bolte, A., Bachmann. K. D., Röhricht E. and Strothmann, G. (1972). Verlängerte Schwangerschaftsdauer und Placentadysfunktion. 1. Häufigkeit und Diagnostik bei den Geburstsjahrgängen. Deutsch. Med. Wschr. 97, 671.

201 Perkins, R. P. (1974). Antenatal assessment of fetal maturity: a review. Obstet. Gynec. Surv. 29, 369.

202 Thomson, A. M., Billewicz, W. Z. and Hytten, F. E. (1968). The assessment of fetal growth. J. Obstet. Gynaec. Brit. Cwlth. 75, 903.

203 Vorherr, H. (1975). Placental insufficiency in relation to postterm pregnancy and fetal postmaturity: evaluation of fetoplacental function: management of the postterm gravida. Amer. J. Obstet. Gynec. 123, 67.

204 Rathbun, L. S. (1943). An analysis of 250 cases of postmaturity. Amer. J. Obstet. Gynec, 46, 278.

205 Gibson, G. B. (1955). Prolonged pregnancy. Brit. Med. J. 2, 715.

206 Wrigley, A. J. (1958). Postmaturity. Lancet i, 1167.

207 Cope, I. (1959). Prolonged pregnancy - its hazards and management. Med. J. Australia 1, 196.

208 Bach, H. G. (1960). Uberreife Syndrum, Verlängerte Schwangerschaft und perinatale Mortalitäs. Gynaecologia 150, 197.

209 McC. Browne, J. C. (1963). Postmaturity. Amer. J. Obstet. Gynec. 85, 573.

210 Evans, T. N., Koeff, S. T. and Morely, G. W. (1963). Fetal effects of prolonged pregnancy. Amer. J. Obstet. Gynec. 85, 701.

211 Lucas, W. E., Ancil, A. O. and Callaghan, D. A. (1965). The problem of postterm pregnancy. Amer. J. Obstet. Gynec. 91, 241.

212 Zwerdling, M. A. (1967). Factors pertaining to prolonged pregnancy and its outcome. Pediatrics 40, 202.

213 Schussling, G. and Radzuweit, H. (1968). Zur Ubertragung in der Schwangerschaft. Zbl. Gynäk. 90, 1705.

214 Sinnathuray, T. A. (1975). A study of uncomplicated prolongation of pregnancy. Aust. N. Z. J. Obstet. Gynaec. 12, 225.

215 Nakano. R. (1972). Post-term pregnancy. Acta Obstet. Gynec. Scand. 51, 217.

216 Clifford, S. H. (1954). Postmaturity - with placental dysfunction: clinical syndrome and pathologic findings. J. Pediatrics 44, 1.

217 Daichman, I. and Gold, E. M. (1954). Postdate labor: effects on mother and fetus. Amer. J. Obstet. Gynec. 68, 1129.

218 Perlin, I. A. (1960). Postmaturity. Amer. J. Obstet. Gynec. 80, 1.

219 Magram, H. M. and Cavanagh, W. V. (1960). The problem of postmaturity. Amer. J. Obstet. Gynec. 79, 216.

220 Mead, P. B. and Marcus, S. L. (1964). Prolonged pregnancy. Amer. J. Obstet. Gynec. 89, 495.

221 Bierman, J. M., Siegel, E., French, F. E. and Simonian, K. (1965). Analysis of the outcome of all pregnancies in a community: Kauai pregnancy study. Amer. J. Obstet. Gynec. 91, 37.

222 Klapholtz, H. and Friedman, E. A. (1977). The incidence of intrapartum fetal distress with advancing gestational age. Amer. J. Obstet. Gynec. 127, 405.

223 Gruenwald, P. and Minh, H. N. (1961). Evaluation of body and organ weights in perinatal pathology. II. Weight of body and placenta of surviving and of autopsied infants. Amer. J. Obstet. Gynec. 82, 312.

224 Rosso, P. (1976). Placenta as an aging organ. Curr. Concepts. Nutr. 4, 23.

225 Winick, M., Coscia, A. and Noble, A. (1967). Cellular growth in human placenta. 1. Normal placental growth. Pediatrics, 39, 248.

226 Winick, M. and Noble, A. (1966). Quantitative changes in ribonucleic acids and protein during normal growth of rat placenta. Nature 212, 34.

227 Jollie, W. P. (1964). Radioautographic observations on variations in desoxyribonucleic acid synthesis in rat placenta with increasing gestational age. Amer. J. Anat. 114. 161.

228 Blecker, O. P., Kloosternam, G. J., Breur, W. and Mieras, D. J. (1977). The volumetric growth of the human placenta: a longitudinal ultrasonic study, Amer. J. Obstet. Gynec. 127, 657.

229 Sands, J. A. and Bobbling, J. In preparation for publication.

230 Geller, H. F. (1957). Uber die sogennanten Hofbauerzellen in der reifen menschlichen Placenta. Arch. Gynäk.188, 481.

231 Becker, V. (1963). Funktionelle Morphologie der Placenta. Arch. Gynäk. 198,3.

232 Fox, H. (1968). Villous immaturity in the term placenta. Obstet. Gynec. 31, 9.

233 Bleyl, U. and Stefek, E. (1965). Zur Morphologie und diagnostischen Bewertung der lockern jungendlichen Zotten in reifen menschlichen Plazenten. Beitr. Path. Anat. Allg. Path. 131, 168.

234 Schuhmann, R. and Wehler, V. (1971). Histologische Unterschiede an Placentazotten innerhalb der maternofetalen Strömungeseinheit: ein Beitrag zur funktioll-en Morphologie. Arch. Gynäk. 240, 425.

235 Geier, G., Schuhmann, R. and Kraus, H. (1975). Regional unterschiedliche Zellproliferation innerhalb der Plazentone reifer menschlicher Plazenten: autoradiographische Untersuchungen, Arch. Gynäk. 248, 31.

236 Aherne, W. and Dunnil, M. S. (1966). Quantitative aspects of placental structure. J. Path. Bact. 91, 123.

237 Aherne, W. (1975). Morphometry. In The Placenta and its Maternal Supply Line, Ed. Gruenwald, P. p .80, Medical and Technical Publishing Co., Lancaster.

238 Bouw, G. M., Stolte, L. A. M., Baak, J. P.A. and Oort, J. (1978). Quantitative morphology of the placenta. II. The growth of the placenta and the problem of postmaturity. Europ. J. Obstet. Gynec. Reprod. Biol. 8, 31.

239 Tedde, G. and Piras, A. T. (1978). Mitotic index of the Langhan's cells in the normal human placenta from the early stages of pregnancy to the term. Acta Anat. 100, 114.

240 Weinberg, P. C., Cameron, I. L., Parmley, T. Jeter, J. R., Pauerstein, C. J. (1976). Gestational age and placental cellular replication. Obstet. Gynec. 36, 692.

241 Gruenwald, P. (1975). The supply line of the fetus: definitions relating to fetal growth. In The Placenta and its Maternal Supply Line Ed. Gruenwald, P. p.1, Medical and Technical Publishing Co., Lancaster.

242 Fox, H. (1976), The histopathology of placental insufficiency. J. Clin. Path. 29 (Suppl. Roy. Coll. Path.), 10, 1.

243 Beischer, N. A., Sivasamboo, R., Vohra, S., Silpisornkosal, S. and Reid, S. (1970). Placental hypertrophy in severe pregnancy anaemia. J. Obstet. Gynaec. Brit. Cwlth. 77, 398.

244 Agboola, A. (1975). Placental changes in patients with a low haematocrit. Brit. J. Obstet. Gynaec. 82, 225.

245 Clavero, J. A. and Botella Llusia, J. (1963). Measurements of the villous surface in normal and pathologic placentas. Amer. J. Obstet. Gynec. 86, 234.

246 Wigglesworth, J. S. (1967). The Langhans layer in late pregnancy: a histological study of normal and abnormal cases. J. Obstet. Gynaec. Brit. Cwlth. 69, 355.

248 Fox, H. (1964). The villous cytotrophoblast as an index of placental ischaemia. J. Obstet. Gynaec. Brit. Cwlth. 71, 885.

249 Kaufmann, P. (1972). Untersuchungen über die Langhans-Zellen in der menschlichen Placenta. Ztschr. Zellforsch. Mikrop. Anat. 128. 283.

250 Fox, H. (1970). Effect of hypoxia on trophoblast in organ culture. Amer. J. Obstet. Gynec. 107, 1058.

251 Buscemi, C. (1957). Riserche istologiche ed istochemiche sulla placenta di gravidanze sesotine. Riv. Obstet, Ginec. 12, 281.

252 Siegel, P. (1963). Die Placenta beim Ubertragenen dystropischen Neugeborenen. Arch. Gynäk. 198, 67.

253 Kubli, F. and Budliger, H. (1963). Beitrag zur Morphologie der insuffizienten Placenta. Frauenheilke Gerburtsch. 23, 37.

254 Fox, H. (1978). Pathology of the Placenta. W. B. Saunders Co. Ltd., London, Philadelphia, Toronto.

255 Tindall, V. R. and Scott, J. S. (1965). Placental calcification: a study of 3025 singleton and multiple pregnancies. J. Obstet. Gynaec. Brit. Cwlth. 72, 356.

256 Wentworth, P. (1965). Macroscopic placental calcification and its clinical significance. J. Obstet. Gynaec. Brit. Cwlth. 72, 215.

257 Fujikuru, T. (1963). Placental calcification and maternal age. Amer. J. Obstet. Gynec. 87, 41.

258 Brandt, G. (1973). Atiologie und Pathogenese der Kalkablagerung in der Placenta. Frauenheilke Gerburtsch 33,119.

259 Eden, T. W. (1897). A study of the human placenta, physiological and pathological. J. Path. Bact. 4, 265.

260 Tenney, B. (1936). Syncytial degeneration in normal and pathologic placentas. Amer. J. Obstet. Gynec. 31, 1024.

261 Vincent, R. A., Huang, P. C. and Parmley, T. H. (1976). Proliferative capacity of cell cultures derived from the human placenta. In Vitro 12, 649.

262 Getzowa, S. and Sadowsky, A. (1950). On the structure of the human placenta with full term and immature fetus, living or dead. J. Obstet. Gynaec. Brit. Emp. 57, 388.

263 Amstutz, E. (1960). Beobachtungen über die Reifung der Chorionzotten in menschlichen Placenta mit besonderer Beruchsichtigung der Epithelplatten. Acta Anat. 42, 12.

264 Burgos, H. M. and Rodriguez, E. M. (1966). Specialized zones in the trophoblast of the human term placenta. Amer. J. Obstet. Gynec. 96, 342.

265 Fox, H. (1967). The incidence and significance of vasculosyncytial membranes in the human placenta. J. Obstet. Gynaec. Brit. Cwlth. 74, 28.

266 Thomsen, K. and Blankenburg, H. (1956). Uber die Entwicklung und Rückbildung der Langhansschen Zellschicht in der menschlichen Placenta. Arch. Gynäk. 187, 638.

267 Traub, A., Jakobovits, A. and Szontagh, F. E. (1964). Ein Beitrag zur Nachweis der Langhanszellen in der Plazenta ausgetragener unkomplizierter Schwangerschaften. Ztschr. Geburtsh. Gynäk. 162, 314.

268 Rodway, H. E. and Marsh, F. (1956). A study of Hofbauer's cells in human placenta. J. Obstet. Gynaec. Brit. Emp. 63, 111.

269 Panigel, M. and Anh, J. N. H. (1964). Ultrastructure des cellules de Hofbauer dans le placenta humain. C. R. Acad. Sci. Paris, 258, 3556.

270 Fox, H. (1967). The incidence and significance of Hofbauer cells in the mature human placenta. J. Path. Bact. 93, 710.

271 Tenny, B. (1935). A study of the collagen of the placenta. Amer. J. Obstet. Gynec. 29, 819.

272 Montgomery, T. L. (1936). Fibrosis of the placenta. Amer. J. Obstet. Gynec. 31, 253.

273 Fox, H. (1968). Fibrosis of placental villi. J. Path. Bact. 95, 573.

274 Fox, H. (1965). The significance of villous syncytial knots in the human placenta. J. Obstet. Gynaec. Brit. Cwlth. 72, 347.

275 Jones, C. P. J. and Fox, H. (1977). Syncytial knots and intervillous bridges in the human placenta: an ultrastructural study. J. Anat. 125, 275.

276 Gerl, D., Eichhorn, H., Eichhorn, K. H. and Granke, H. (1973). Quantitative Messungen synzytialer Zellkernkonzentrationen der menschlichen Plazenta bei normalen und pathologischen Schwangerschaften. Zbl. Gynäk. 95, 263.

277 Hörmann, G. (1953). Ein Beitrag zur funktionellen Morphologie der menschlichen Placenta. Arch. Gynäk. 184, 109.

278 Burstein, R., Frankel, S., Soule, S. D. and Blumenthal, H. T. (1973). Aging of the placenta: autoimmune therapy of senescence. Amer. J. Obstet. Gynec. 116, 271.

279 Liebhart, M. (1971). Some observations on so-called fibrinoid necrosis of placental villi: an electron-microscopic study. Path. Europ. 6, 217.

280 Merrill, J. A. (1963). Common pathological changes in the placenta. Clin. Obstet. Gynec. 6, 96.

281 Wigglesworth, J. S. (1964). Morphological variations in the insufficient placenta. J. Obstet. Gynaec. Brit. Cwlth. 71, 871.

282 Arienzo, F. (1955). Studio anatomo-pathologo delle placente nelle gravidanza protratta. Quad. Anat. Prat. 10, 418.

283 Vanrell-Cluells, J. (1963). Pathologische Veränderungen bei der Übertragenen Placenta. Arch. Gynäk. 198, 71.

284 Mälzer, M., Emmrich, P., Birke, R. and Knaus, T. (1970). Diagnostik und Therapie der sogenannten Ubertragung im Vergleich zu typisch histologischen Placentabefunden. Ztschr. Geburtsh Gynäk. 172, 25.

285 Liebhart, M. and Kuczynska-Sicinska, J. (1971). Microscopic evaluation of the placenta in protracted pregnancy. Ginek. Pol. 42, 883.

286 Justus, B., Justus, J. and Holtoroff, J. (1971). Ubertragene dystrophische Neugeborene und dazugehörige morphologische Plazentabefunde. Ztschr. Geburtsh. Gynäk. 175, 44.

287 Salvatore, C. A. (1971). The placenta in prolonged gestation. Matern. Infanc. 30, 71.

288 Novitsky, I. S., Belomestnova, L. N. and Chernykh, A. P. (1976). The influence of over-term pregnancy on the state of the placenta and the fetus. Akush. Ginec. 1, 29.

289 Wislocki, G. B. and Dempsey, E. W. (1955). Electron microscopy of the human placenta. Anat. Rec. 123, 133.

290 Panigel, M. and Anh, J. N. H. (1914). Ultrastructure des villosités placentaires humaines. Path. Biol. 12, 927.

291 Vacek, Z. (1965). Submicroscopic structure of the human chorion from third month of gestation to term. Folia. Morph. 13, 104.

292 Lister, U. M. (1963). Ultrastructure of the human mature placenta. I. The Maternal surface. J. Obstet. Gynaec. Brit. Cwlth. 70, 373.

293 Jones, C. J. P. (1976). An Ultrastructural and Ultrahistochemical Study of the Human Placenta in Normal and Abnormal Pregnancy. Ph.D. Thesis, University of Manchester.

294 Ludwig, H. (1974). Surface structure of the human placenta. In The Placenta, Biological and Clinical Aspects. Ed. Michissi, K.S. and Hafez, E.S.E., p.40, Charles C. Thomas, Springfield, Illinois.

195 Hashimoto, M., Kosaka, M., Shimoyama, T., Hirasawa, T., Komori, A., Kawasaki, T. and Akashi, K. (1960). Electron microscopic studies on the epithelium of the chorionic villi of the human placenta. (Report 2) J. Jap. Obstet. Gynaec. Soc. 7, 22.

196 Wakitani, T. (1961). Electron microscopic observation on the chorionic villi of the normal human placenta and chorioepithelioma malignum. I. Electron microscopic observation on the chorionic villi of the normal human placenta. J. Jap. Obstet. Gynaec. Soc. 8, 208.

297 Pierce, G. B., Midgley, A. R. and Beals, T. F. (1964). An ultrastructural study of differentiation and maturation of trophoblast of the monkey. Lab. Invest. 13, 451.

298 Inoue, T. (1960). Observations on human placenta chorionic villi under the electron microscope. J. Jap. Obstet. Gynaec. Soc. 7, 173.

299 Strauss, L., Goldenberg, N., Hirota, K. and Okydaira, Y. (1965). Structure of the human placenta with observations on ultrastructure of the terminal chorionic villus. Birth Def. Orig. Art. Series, 1, 13.

300 Tighe, J. R., Garrod, P. R. and Curran, R. C. (1967). The trophoblast of the human chorionic villus. J. Path. Bact. 93, 559.

301 Martin, B. J. and Spicer, S. S. (1973). Ultrastructural features of cellular maturation and aging in human trophoblast. J. Ultrastruct. Res. 43, 133.

302 Tedde, G. and Kujawa, M. (1978) Morphometric study of the syncytiotrophoblast of the normal human placenta from the early stages of the pregnancy to the term. J. Submicr. Cytol. 10, 65.

303 de Palo, G. M. (1967). L'ipersenescenza placentare nella gravidanza oltre il termine con feto ipodistrofico: studio al microscopio elettronico. Riv. Ostet. Ginec. 22, 829.

304 Devizorova, A. S. and Shvirst, E. M. (1970). Ultrastructural characteristics of placental villi in prolonged pregnancy. Akush. Ginek, 46, 49.

305 Jones, C. J. P. and Fox, H. (in press). Ultrastructure of the placenta in prolonged pregnancy. J. Path.

306 Dixon, H. G., Browne, J. C. McC. and Davey, D. A. (1963). Choriodecidual and myometrial blood flow. Lancet, ii 369.

307 Browne, J. C. McC. (1963). Placental insufficiency. Scot. Med. J. 8, 459.

308 Robertson, W. B. and Dixon, H. G. (1969). Utero-placental pathology. In Foetus and Placenta, Ed. Klopper, A. and Diczfalusy, E, p.33, Blackwell Scientific Publications, Oxford and Edinburgh.

309 Yamaguchi, R., Ushioda, E., Nishik-awa, Y. and Shintani, M. (1975). Uteroplacental blood flow in normal and prolonged pregnancies pursued with trager microspheres. Acta Obstet. Gynaec. Jap. 22, 175.

310 Wislocki, G. B. and Dempsey, E. W. (1946). Histochemical age-changes in normal and pathological placental villi (hydatidiform mole, eclampsia). Endocrinology, 38, 90.

311 Thomsen, K. (1955). Histochemische Untersuchungen über die saure phosphatase in der menschlichen Placenta. Arch. Gynäk. 187, 264.

312 Thomsen, K. (1955). Uber die aktivitat der alkalischen Phosphatase in der menschlichen Placenta. Arch. Gynäk. 187, 1.

313 McKay, D. G., Hertig, A. T., Adams, E. C., and Richardson, M. V. (1958). Histochemical observations on the human placenta. Obstet. Gynec. 12, 1.

314 Curzen, P. (1964). Variations in the enzyme histochemistry of the placenta. J. Obstet. Gynaec. Brit. Cwlth. 71, 388.

315 Jones, C. J. P. and Fox, H. (1976). An ultrahistochemical study of the distribution of acid and alkaline phosphatases in placentae for normal and complicated pregnancies. J. Path. 118, 143.

316 Boss, J. H. and Craig, J. M. (1962). Histochemical distribution patterns of oxidative enzymes in the human placenta. Obstet. Gynec. 20, 572.

317 Wielenga, A. C. and Willighagen, R. C. J. (1962). The histochemistry of the syncytiotrophoblast and the stroma in the normal full term placenta. Amer. J. Obstet. Gynec. 84, 1059.

318 Lobel, B. L., Deand, H. W. and Romney, S. (1962). Enzymatic histochemistry of the villous portion of the human placenta from six weeks of gestation to term. Amer. J. Obstet. Gynec. 83, 295.

319 Wachstein, M., Meaguer, J. G. and Ortiz, J. (1963). Enzymatic histochemistry of the term human placenta. Amer. J. Obstet. Gynec. 87, 13.

320 Jones, C. J. P. and Fox, H. (in press). An ultrahistochemical study of the placental content of respiratory enzymes in normal and prolonged pregnancies. Invest. Cell. Path.

321 Wiene, M. (1978). Control of placental 3 μ hydroxy Δ^5 steroid dehydrogenase: partial characteristics of an endogenous inhibitor and an endogenous activator. Mech. Age. Develop. 7, 433.

322 Hellman, L. M., Flexner, L. B., Wilde, W. S., Vosburgh, D. J. and Proctor, N. K. (1948). The permeability of the human placenta to water and the supply of water to the human fetus as determined with deuterium oxide. Amer. J. Obstet. Gynec. 56, 861.

323 Flexner, L. B., Cowie, D. B., Hellman, L. M., Wilde, W. S. and Vosburgh, G. J. (1948). The permeability of the human placenta to sodium in normal and abnormal pregnancies and the supply of sodium to the human fetus as determined with radioactive sodium. Amer. J. Obstet. Gynec. 55, 469.

324 Beling, C. (1977). Estrogens. In Endocrinology of Pregnancy, Ed. Fuchs, F. and Klopper, A., p.76. Harper and Row, Hagerstown, Maryland.

325 Beischer, N. A., Brown, J. B., Smith, M. A. and Townsend, L. (1968). Studies in prolonged pregnancy: clinical results and urinary estriol excretion. Amer. J. Obstet. Gynec. 103, 483.

326 Lindberg, B. S., Nilsson, B. A. and Johansson, E. D. (1974). Plasma progesterone levels in normal and abnormal pregnancy. Acta Obstet. Gynec. Scand. 24, 73.

327 Csapo, A., Knobil, E., Molen, H. v. d. and Wiest, W. (1971). Peripheral plasma progesterone levels during pregnancy and labor. Amer. J. Obstet. Gynec. 110, 630.

328 Turnbull, A. C., Patten, P. T., Flint, A. P. F., Kelrse, M. J. N. C. Jeremy, J. K. and Anderson, A. B. M. (1974). Significant falls in progesterone and rise in oestradiol levels in human peripheral plasma before onset of labour. Lancet, i , 101.

329 Yannone, M. E., McGurdy, J. R. and Goldflen, A. (1968). Plasma progesterone levels in normal pregnancy, labour and puerperium. Amer. J. Obstet. Gynec. 101, 1058.

330 Josimovich, J. B. (1977). Human placental lactogen. In Endocrinology of Pregnancy, Ed. Fuchs F. and Klopper, A. p.191, Harper and Row, Hagerstown, Maryland.

331 Genazzani, A. R., Cocola, F., Neri, P. and Fioretti, P. (1972), Human chorionic somato mammotropin (hCS) plasma levels in normal and pathological pregnancies and their correlation with the placental function. Acta Endocrinol. (Suppl. 167). 71, 1.

332 Chard, T. (1976). Assessment of fetoplacental function by biochemical determinations. J. Clin. Path. Suppl. (Roy. Coll. Path). 10, 18.

333 Wang, H. W. and Hellman, L. M. (1943). Studies in the metabolism of the human placenta. (I). Oxygen consumption in relation to ageing. Bull. Johns Hopkins Hosp. 73, 31.

334 Hellman, L. M., Harris, B. A. and Andrews, M. C. (1950). Studies of the metabolism of the human placenta. (2). Oxygen consumption and anaerobic glycolysis in relation to ageing and severe toxemia. Bull. Johns Hopkins Hosp. 87, 203.

335 Villee, C. A. (1953). The metabolism of the placenta in vitro. J. Biol. Chem. 205, 113.

336 Mackay, R. B. (1958). Studies of the oxygen consumption of fresh placental tissues from normal and abnormal pregnancies. J. Obstet. Gynaec. Brit. Emp. 65, 791.

337 Friedman, E. A. and Sachtleben, M. R. (1960). Placental oxygen consumption in vitro. (I). Baseline studies. Amer. J. Obstet. Gynec. 79, 1058.

338 Friedman, E. A., Little, W. A. and Sachtlenen, M. R. (1962). Placental oxygen consumption in vitro. Amer. J. Obstet. Gynec. 84, 561.

339 Tremblay, P. C., Sybulski, S. and Maughan, C. B. (1965). Role of the placenta in fetal malnutrition. Amer. J. Obstet. Gynec. 91, 597.

340 Paparella, P., Galeotti, T., Bompiani, A. and Terranova, T. (1973). Experimental observations on the energy metabolism of human placenta. J. Obstet. Gynaec. Brit. Cwlth., 80, 627.

341 Beaconsfield, P., Ginsburg, J. and Jeacock, M. K. (1964). Glucose metabolism via the pentose phosphate pathway relative to nucleic acid and protein synthesis in the human placenta. Develop. Med. Child. Neurol. 6, 469.

342 Boime, I., McWilliams, D., Szczeswa, E. and Camel, M. (1976). Synthesis of human placental lactogen messenger RNA as a function of gestation. J. Biol. Chem. 251, 820.

343 Chatterjee, M., Baliga, B. S., Munro, H. M. (1976). Synthesis of human placental lactogen and human chorionic gonadotropin by polyribosomes and messenger RNA from early and full term placentas. J. Biol. Chem. 251, 2945.

344 Lefrowitz, D., Johnson, R. C., Faulk, W. P. and Vincent, R. A. (1978:in press) Undisturbed DNA synthesis (UDS) in mixed cell primarycultures of term human placentae. J. Supramic. Struct. 8.

NEW DEVELOPMENTS IN IMMUNOGERONTOLOGY

Willi Hijmans

1 Schiff, F. & Mendlowicz,L.(1926). Quantitative Untersuchungen über Isoagglutinine mit besonderer Berücksichtigung der Leukaemie.Zeitschr. f. Immunitätsf. 48, 1.

2 Makinodan T., & W. J. Peterson, (1962). Relative antibody-forming capacity of spleen cells as a function of age. Proc. Nat. Acad. Sci. 48, 234.

3 Adler, W.H., Jones, K.H. and Nariuchi, H. (1977) Recent advances in clinical immunology, Churchill Livingstone, Edinburgh, p.77.

4 Makinodan, T. and Yunis, E. (1977) Immunology and Aging, Plenum, New York.

5 Makinodan, T. (1978) Mechanism of senescence of immune response. Fed. Proc. 37, 1239.

6 Hijams, W. and Hollander, C.F. (1977) Immunology and Aging, Plenum, New York, p.23.

7 Day, N.K. and Good, R.A. (1977) Biological Amplification Systems in Immunology, Plenum, New York.

8 Harrison, D.E., Astle, C.M. and Delaittre, J.A. (1978) Loss of proliferative capacity in immunohemopoietic stem cells caused by serial transplantation rather than aging. J. exp. Med. 147, 1526.

9 Vacek, A., Bartonickova, A. and Tkadlecek, L. (1976) Age dependence of the number of the stem cells in haemopoietic tissues of rats. Cell Tissue Kinet. 9, 1.

10 Albright, J.W. and Makinodan, T. (1976) Decline in the growth potential of spleen-colonizing bone marrow stem cells of long-lived aging mice. J. exp. Med. 144, 1204.

11 Hirokawa, K., Albright, J.W. and Makinodan, T. (1976) Restoration of impaired immune functions in aging animals. 1. Effect of syngeneic thymus and bone marrow grafts. Clin. Immunol. Immunopathol. 5, 371.

12 Zharhary, D., Segev, Y. and Gershon, H. (1977) The affinity and spectrum of cross reactivity of antibody production in senescent mice: the IgM response. Mech. Ageing Dev. 6, 385.

13 Abraham, C., Tal, Y. and Gershon, H. (1977) Reduced in vitro response to concanavalin-A and lipopolysaccharide in senescent mice: a function of reduced number of responding cells. Europ.J.Immunol. 7, 301.

14 Kruisbeek, A.M. (1976) Age-related changes in Con-A and LPS-induced lymphocyte transformation. 1. Effect of culture conditions on mitogen responses of blood and spleen lymphocytes from young and aged rats. Mech. Ageing Dev. 5, 125.

15 Kishimoto, S., Takahama, T. and Mizumachi, H. (1976) In vitro immune response to the 2, 4, 6-trinitrophenyl determinant in aged C57BL/6J mice: changes in the humoral immune response to avidity for the TNP determinant and responsiveness to LPS with aging. J. Immunol. 116, 294.

16 Smith, A.M. (1976) The effects of age on the immune response to type 111 pneumococcal polysaccharide (S111) and bacterial lipopolysaccharide (LPS) in BALB/c, SJL/J, and C3H mice. J. Immunol. 116, 469.

17 Callard, R.E., Basten, A. and Waters, L.K. (1977) Immune function in aged mice. 11. B-cell function. Cellular Immunol. 31, 26.

18 Halbrecht, I., Komlos, L. and Strauss, Z. (1977) Lymphocyte reactivity in the aged. J. Am. Ger. Soc. 25, no. 8, 354.

19 Weiner, H.L., Scribner, D.J., Schocket, A.L. and Moorhead, J.W. (1978) Increased proliferative response of human peripheral blood lymphocytes to anti-immunoglobulin antibodies in elderly people. Clin. Immunol. Immunopath. 9, 356.

20 Singhal, S.K., Roder, J.C. and Duwe, A.K. (1978) Suppressor cells in immunosenescence. Fed. Proc. 37, 1245.

21 Roder, J.C., Bell, D.A. and Singhal, S.K. (1977) Regulation of the immune response in autoimmune NZB/NZW F1 mice. 1. The spontaneous generation of splenic suppressor cells. Cellular Immunol. 29, 272.

22 Haaijman, J.J., Schuit, H.R.E. and Hijmans, W. (1977) Immunoglobulin-containing cells in different lymphoid organs of the CBA mouse during its life-span. Immunology 32, 427.

23 Radl, J., Sepers, J.M., Skvaril, F., Morell, A. and Hijmans, W. (1975) Immunoglobulin patterns in humans over 95 years of age. Clin. exp. Immunol. 22, 84.

24 Riesen, W., Keller, H., Skvaril, F., Morell, A. and Barandun, S. (1976) Restriction of immunoglobulin heterogeneity, autoimmunity and serum protein levels in aged people. Clin. Exp. Immunol. 26, 280.

25 Haaijman, J.J., van den Berg, P. and Brinkhof, J. (1977) Immunoglobulin class and subclass levels in the serum of CBA mice throughout life. Immunology 32, 923.

26 Natsuumi-Sakai, S., Motonishi, K. and Migita, S. (1977) Quantitative estimations of five classes of immunoglobulin in inbred mouse strains. Immunology 32, 861.

27 Axelson, U. (1977) An eleven-year follow-up on 64 subjects with M-components. Acta Med. Scand. 201, 173.

28 Englisova, M., Englis, M., Kyral, V., Kourilek, K. and Dvorak, K. (1968) Changes of immunoglobulin synthesis in old people. Exp. Gerontol. 3, 125.

29 Hijmans, W., Radl, J., Bottazzo, F.F. and Doniach, D. Autoantibodies in humans in the age group of 95 years and old. Manuscript in preparation.

30 Radl, J. and Hollander, C.F. (1974) Homogeneous immunoglobulins in sera of mice during aging. J. Immunol. 112, 2271.

31 Makinodan, T., Albright, J.W., Good, P.I., Peter, C.P. and Heidrick, M.L. (1976) Reduced humoral immune activity in long-lived old mice: an approach to elucidating its mechanisms. Immunology 31, 903.

32 Haaijman, J.J. and Hijmans, W. (1978) Influence of age on the immunological activity and capacity of the CBA mouse. Mech. Ageing Dev. 7, 375.

33 Walford, R.L. (1969) The immunologic theory of aging. Munksgaard, Copenhagen.

34 Zanussi, C., Rugard, C., Casal, P., Fabio, G., Perussia, B., Sabbadini-Villa, M.G., Smeralda, R.S. and Duca, G. (1977) Immunological status of aged subjects with reference to serological evidence of autoimmunity. La Ricerca Clin. Lab. 7, 115.

35 Mackay, I.R., Whittingham, S. and Tait, B. (1977) Genetic control of immune responsiveness in man. Vox. Sang 32, 10.

36 Naor, D., Bonavida, B. and Walford, R.L. (1976) Autoimmunity and aging: the age-related response of mice of a long-lived strain to trinitrophenylated syngeneic mouse red blood cells. J. Immunol. 117, 2204.

37 Goidl, E.A., Innes, J.B. and Weksler, M.E. (1976) Immunological studies of aging. 11. Loss of IgG and high avidity plaque-forming cells and increased suppressor cell activity in aging mice. J. exp. Med. 144, 1037.

38 Cazenave, P.-A. (1977) Idiotypic-anti-idiotypic regulation of antibody synthesis in rabbits. Proc. Nat . Acad. Sci. 74, 5122.

39 Urbain, J., Wikler, M., Franssen, J.D. and Collingnon, C. (1977) Idiotypic regulation of the immune system by the induction of antibodies against anti-idiotypic antibodies. Proc. Nat . Acad. Sci. 74, 5126.

40 Kay, M.M.B. (1978) Effect of age on T cell differentiation. Fed. Proc. 37, 1241.

41 Cantor, H., McVay-Boudreau, L., Hugenberger, J., Naidore, K., Shen F.W. and Gershon, R.K. (1978) Immunoregulatory circuits among T cell sets. 11. Physiologic role of feedback inhibition in vivo: absence in NZB mice. J. exp. Med. 147, 1116.

42 Hirokawa, K. (1977) Immunology and Aging, Plenum, New York, p.51.

43 Hirokawa, K. and Makinodan, T. (1975) Thymic involution: Effect on T cell differentiation. J. Immunol. 114, 1659.

44 Pachciarz, J.A. and Teague, P.O. (1976) Age-associated involution of cellular immune function. 1. Accelerated decline of mitogen reactivity of spleen cells in adult thymectomized mice. J. Immunol. 116, 982.

45 Astaldi, A., Astaldi, G.C.B., Schellekens, P.Th.A. and Eijsvoogel, V.P. (1978) Is there a circulating human thymic factor that induces cyclic AMP synthesis? Nature 271, 666.

46 Kruisbeek, A.M., Astaldi, G.C.B., Blankwater, M.-J., Zijlstra, J.J., Levert, L.A. and Astaldi, A. (1978) The in vitro effect of a thymic epithelial culture supernatant on mixed lymphocyte reactivity and intracellular cAMP levels of thymocytes and on antibody production to SRBC by nu/nu spleen cells. Cell. immunol. 35, 134.

47 Niaudet, P. and Bach, M.-A. (1976) Thymic function in NZB mice. 1. Duration of thymic function on New Zealand Black (NZB) mice. Clin. exp. Immunol. 23, 328.

48 Callard, R.E. and Basten, A. (1977) Immune function in aged mice. 1. T-cell responsiveness using Phytohaemagglutinin as a functional probe. Cellular Immunol. 31, 13.

49 Segre, D. and Segre, M. (1976) Humoral immunity in aged mice. 11. Increased suppressor T cell activity in immunologically deficient old mice. J. Immunol. 116, 735.

50 Hallgren, H.M. and Yunis, E.J. (1977) Suppressor lymphocytes in young and aged humans. J. Immunol. 118, 6, 2004.

51 Krogsrud, R.L. and Perkins, E.H. (1977) Age-related changes in T cell function. J. Immunol. 118, 1607.

52 Davey, F.R. and Huntington, S. (1977) Age-related variation in lymphocyte sub-populations. Gerontology 23, 381.

53 Ben-Zwi, A., Galili, U., Russell, A. and Schlesinger, M. (1977) Age-associated changes in subpopulations of human lymphocytes. Clin. Immunol. Immunopath. 7, 139.

54 Preumont, A.M.,van Gansen, P. and Brachet, J. (1978) Cytochemical study of human lymphocytes stimulated by PHA in function of donor age. Mech. Ageing Dev. 7, 25.

55 Antel, J.P., Weinrich, M. and Arnason, B.G.W. (1978) Circulating suppressor cells in man as a function of age. Clin. Immunol. Immunopath. 9, 134.

56 Merhav, S. and Gershon, H. (1977) The mixed lymphocyte response of senescent mice: sensitivity to alloantigen and cell replication time. Cellular Immunol. 34, 354.

57 Hirano, T. and Nordin, A.A. (1975) Age-associated decline in the in vitro development of cytotoxic lymphocytes in NZB mice. J. Immunol. 117, 1093.

58 Weigle, W.O. and Parks, D.E. (1978) Effect of aging on immune and tolerant states. Fed. Proc. 37, 1253.

59 McIntosh, K.R. and Segre, D. (1976) B- and T-cell tolerance induction in young-adult and old mice. Cellular Immunol. 27, 230.

60 Walford, R.L., Meredith, P.J. and Cheney, K.E. (1977) Immunology and Aging, Plenum, New York, p. 183.

61 Jerne, N.K. (1977) Introduction of the 1977 Annual Report of the Basel Institute for Immunology.

62 Scott, D.W., Layton, J.E. and Nossal, G.J.V. (1977) Role of IgD in the immune response and tolerance. J. exp. Med. 146, 1473.

63 Bilder, G.E. and Denckla, W.D. (1977) Restoration of ability to reject xenografts and clear carbon after hypophysectomy of adult rats. Mech. Ageing Dev. 6, 153.

64 Denckla, W.D. (1978) Interactions between age and the neuroendocrine and immune systems. Fed. Proc. 37, 1263.

65 Smith, G.S. and Walford, R.L. (1977) Influence of the main histocompatibility complex on ageing in mice. Nature 270, 727.

66 Greenberg, L.J. and Yunis, E.J. (1978) Histocompatibility determinants, immune responsiveness and aging in man. Fed. Proc. 37, 1258.

LOOKING AHEAD

If you want people to remember something you must tell them, then repeat it, and then say it again.

High expectations are always hard to fulfill. But it did not seem unreasonable when planning this multidisciplinary meeting on the scope for use of the placenta as a research tool, to expect that the specialists invited to participate would do so freely. The wide range of relevant disciplines represented, the informal round-table atmosphere, the total absence of 'third parties' - either audience or reporters - and the time made available for discussion by having the reviews outlined (rather than presented verbatim) should all have contributed to make active interchange of ideas possible. That was the aim agreed by post and confirmed at preliminary meetings with a number of the participants. In their own laboratories and departments, they all talked quite freely, ranging well beyond the bounds of their particular disciplines. At the conference table they did not. Indeed, many did just the reverse of what we had hoped and expected - delving more and more deeply into the minutiae of their specialities.

But why should specialists of repute be so reluctant to venture beyond their own safe ground? Some said that if the meeting had lasted longer we should all have lost our inhibitions. That may be true, but time and money do not permit longer meetings. And, in any case, timidity seems a feeble excuse for established experts not to throw out ideas for debate and possible further investigation. Scientists don't have to be right. But they do have to have open minds, ready to think the unthinkable - and test it. In the event, informed speculation was limited. Thinking horizontally across the board was almost entirely restricted to the clinicians, whose ideas needed expert support they seldom received. Many questions were posed in both reviews and discussion, but few if any were picked up for examination, far less for attempts to answer them. They remain on the page for the discerning reader to cogitate on. Perhaps the organisation of the discussion periods was not tight enough. Maybe we should have planted more provocative ideas. Possibly our expectations were unreasonably high ...

Yet, for all these reservations, the validity of the placenta as an experimental animal was fully unheld. That it provides a useful model for the study of cell replication and immunology, though probably less so for ageing, was generally agreed. Although the discussion on metabolic, hormonal and other biochemical processes failed to bring out any fresh ideas for study, it amply confirmed the value of the placenta as a research tool in these important fields as well.

In editing the proceedings, we have tried to bring out these more positive aspects of each session.

Looking ahead, there is a clear need for more biochemical studies to link the largely isolated islets of knowledge presented by speakers - on metabolic processes and their control, on the role of hormones and prostaglandins in normal development, and on the control of feto-placental growth by DNA. The key to the whole course of intrauterine development from the moment of fertilisation onwards must be held by the DNA of the conceptus. The links between the genetic instructions it contains and all other aspects of development must be biochemical in nature. The human placenta provides unique opportunities for studying them.

From awareness that DNA holds the key to all normal development it is but a step to the idea that mutation(s) in it must be responsible for abnormal development notably neoplasia. The search for such mutations should, I believe, be a major priority of cancer research.

If we accept the work of Watson and Crick, and Jacob and Monod, cancer must affect the DNA in order to be transmissable. So we should be looking for "cancer DNA" and trying to decipher its code. In addition an energy aberration resulting from changes in its atomic arrangement could be the driving force behind malignancy. The proper investigation of these proposals requires the knowledge and techniques of high energy and atomic physicists together with their twin brothers, the mathematicians. An outline proposal for such a study was put forward.

So far as instrumentation is concerned medical science is now roughly in the Newtonian era of physics, and it's time for a change.

In the immunological field, the placenta still has much to teach us, despite the fact that we already possess much more information about its immunology than about cell replication, biochemistry or its other functions. In particular, if further research can clarify the mechanisms by which the placenta prevents rejection of nature's allograft, it should prove possible to manipulate them as practical means of promoting acceptance of grafts and provoking rejection of malignant tissue. And we should not overlook the possibility that DNA may play a directional role in at least some such mechanisms.

Finally, ageing. Maybe the placenta ages, in the true sense, maybe it does not. Our deliberations failed to clarify that question. But they at least suggested the likelihood that here too genetic research - into the role of DNA in the ageing process - would prove rewarding.

Any future meeting in these fields should be able to get off to a better start on the basis of this one, especially if the participants fully appreciate the difference between attending a large meeting which makes comparatively few demands on them, and a small intimate gathering where each person's contribution affects the quality of the whole. New ideas are difficult to get off the ground, particularly as science nowadays boasts more and more technology but seems to apply less and less intellect. Polymaths no longer really exist since our educational system eliminates the possibility somewhere in the middle of the secondary school course, and our culture has made gods of the super-specialists. In fact we have reached a stage where we are frankly suspicious of those rare individuals who know quite a lot about many different things. We talk about multidisciplinary approaches, but I often feel we are only paying lip service to an idea that we do not really want to see implemented. The value of assembling a number of specialists from different disciplines round a table is seriously impaired if they are unwilling to talk to each other, and worse still, if there is no one capable of putting together what they have said so that it can be of use to others.

In these respects the men and women who assembled at Bedford College in October 1978 can be considered true representatives of the society that produced them. And, because of this, many of the problems which confront us today will take much longer than need be to solve - whether they concern cancer, energy supplies or the standard of living. We have to change our habits and start looking at problems as part of a broad spectrum instead of dividing them into narrow compartments - super-specialised isolated phenomena - which compel piecemeal 'solutions' that provide no more than transient relief in one small area - without proper attention either to their longer-term inadequacy or their untoward effects elsewhere.

Our advanced level of technology too often stifles creativity. We need some integration between small-scale science - the personal, academic l'art pour l'art kind - and large scale science, which means involvement with industry (consumer orientated) and politics. We have the potential to achieve so much. If we can return things to a more personal level, we may achieve more as results will depend on the individual and his ideas, rather than on the machine and its backup force.

Most people go to meetings with their own work in mind, looking to see what they can learn from others in the same or closely related fields to enlarge and embellish their own work. As practically all participants have this orientation, little is ever accomplished and science does not advance much at scientific gatherings. We have tried here to translate into practice our idea of a small meeting - one for discussing prospective research - and the somewhat unusual presentation of this book is the result. Ideas take time to percolate and old-established habits are difficult to break. We think we have made a start, and next time such a meeting is convened we hope we can act on the lessons learned here. It has been said that if all scientists were engaged in research there would be no science; equally if all researchers engaged in more thinking while there might be less research more progress would be achieved in terms of alleviating the human condition "created sick, commanded to be sound."

Peter Beaconsfield

London
February 1979

INDEX

Printed in Dunstable, United Kingdom

91338442R00259